VOID

Library of
Davidson College

Studies of Brain Function, Vol. 7

Coordinating Editor
V. Braitenberg, Tübingen

Editors
H. B. Barlow, Cambridge
H. Bullock, La Jolla
E. Florey, Konstanz
O.-J. Grüsser, Berlin-West
A. Peters, Boston

Günther Palm

Neural Assemblies
An Alternative Approach
to Artificial Intelligence

With 147 Figures

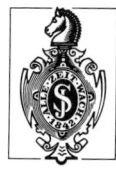

Springer-Verlag
Berlin Heidelberg New York 1982

Dr. Günther Palm
Max-Planck-Institut für Biologische Kybernetik
Spemannstr. 38
7400 Tübingen 1, FRG

ISBN 3-540-11366-5 Springer-Verlag Berlin Heidelberg New York
ISBN 0-387-11366-5 Springer-Verlag New York Heidelberg Berlin

Library of Congress Cataloging in Publication Data. Palm, Günther, 1949– Neural assemblies, an alternative approach to artificial intelligence. (Studies of brain function ; v. 7) Bibliography: p. Includes index. 1. Brain. 2. Artificial intelligence. 3. Neural circuitry. I. Title. II. Series. [DNLM: 1. Cybernetics. 2. Brain–Physiology. 3. Neurophysiology. 4. Intelligence. W1 ST937KF v. 7 / WL 102 P171n] QP376.P34 612'.822 82-3341 AACR2

This work is subject to copyright. All rights are reserved, whether the whole or part of the material is concerned, specifically those of translation, reprinting, re-use of illustrations, broadcasting, reproduction by photocopying machine or similar means, and storage in data banks. Under § 54 of the German Copyright Law where copies are made for other than private use a fee is payable to "Verwertungsgesellschaft Wort", Munich.

© by Springer-Verlag Berlin Heidelberg 1982.
Printed in Germany.

The use of registered names, trademarks, etc. in this publication does not imply, even in the absence of a specific statement, that such names are exempt from the relevant protective laws and regulations and therefore free for general use.

Offsetprinting and binding: Konrad Triltsch, Graphischer Betrieb, Würzburg
2131/3130-543210

Contents, with Outline

Introduction 1

Part I 7

1 The Flow of Information 8
   An introduction to the brain with emphasis on the transmission of information. Digressions 1 and 2 start from here.

2 Thinking as Seen from Within and from Without 15
   Some problems in thinking about thinking are presented; the behavioristic approach to such problems is introduced: What in the observable behavior of somebody else makes us think that he is thinking? This leads to the Turing test for artificial intelligence.

3 How to Build Well-Behaving Machines 19
   "Behavior" is understood as the total stimulus (or situation) → response mapping. For a finite number of different inputs, any such mapping can be constructed. This statement is demonstrated by
   1. coding of any finite set into finite 0,1-sequences
   2. showing that any mapping between finite sets of 0.1-sequences can be built from logical and-, or-, and not-gates.
   3. representing the and-, or-, and not-gate as special threshold neurons of the McCulloch and Pitts type.
   Digression 3 may be of some help here.

4 Organizations, Algorithms, and Flow Diagrams 29
   The chapter contains some general remarks on organizations and cooperativity and introduces the matchbox algorithm.

5 The Improved Matchbox Algorithm 36

The matchbox algorithm is improved by the incorporation of the look-ahead algorithm (e.g., for chess-playing machines) and the associative matrix memory. Appendix 1 starts from here. Chapters 5 and 7 contain the basic constructions needed for the survival algorithm.

6 The Survival Algorithm as a Model of an Animal. 45

The improved matchbox algorithm is interpreted as an algorithm for survival and thus as a model of an animal. If such an algorithm is implemented in terms of neuron-like elements, the result can be checked against experimental data from the neurosciences. Conversely, such data cannot really be understood without a theory (in line with a more general argument as for example in Kuhn 1962).

7 Specifying the Survival Algorithm. 49

Some further specifications of the survival algorithm are given that are necessary in order to implement the algorithm in terms of neurons. A neural realization of the survival algorithm is finally discussed in connection with some basic data on the brain (from Chap. 1) and in order to stimulate interest in further data as supplied in the following chapters. Digression 4 may be entered from here.

Part II 59

8 The Anatomy of the Cortical Connectivity 60

Further data on the connectivity between neurons in the cerebral cortex are presented, leading to some speculations on the flow of neural activity in the cortex.

9 The Visual Input to the Cortex 87

The projection from the retina onto the visual cortex is outlined, to exemplify how sensory input information enters the cortex.

10 Changes in the Cortex with Learning.................. 92

Various experiments correlate differences in the cortex with differences in the environments which had been experienced by experimental animals, and possibly with "learning". Some of these experiments are discussed with the object of obtaining evidence for Hebb's synaptic rule. Digression 4 may be consulted here.

11 From Neural Dynamics to Cell Assemblies 104

Several papers on neural dynamics are discussed in order
 1. *to obtain a more detailed image of the flow of activity in the neural network of the brain (or the cortex)*
 2. *to get a better understanding of the learning- and information processing capabilities of such networks (especially in comparison with the requirements of the survival algorithm of Chaps. 6 and 7).*
The resulting image is fixed in the language of cell assemblies. Appendix 2 and Digression 4 start from here.

12 Introspection and the Rules of Threshold Control 117

The same language of cell assemblies is used to describe some introspections of the author in a more systematic way. This leads to a few strategies for controlling the thresholds of the neurons in a neural network that is used as an associative memory (for example by a survival robot). Appendices 3 and 4 and Digression 5 start from here.

13 Further Speculations............................125

The ideas of cell assemblies and threshold control are carried out further and in a more speculative way. Digression 6 starts from here. Chapters 12 and 13 (together with Digression 5) contain a speculative, algorithmic picture of the information processing in an animal's brain.

14 Men, Monkeys, and Machines 135
It is argued that this picture carries over to humans as well. The acquisition of language, in particular, is regarded as a phenomenon of cultural evolution.

15 Why all These Speculations? 140
The whole book can be understood as an attempt to reduce human behavior to electrophysiological events in the brain and finally to physics, which, of course, does not preclude a heuristic use of teleological arguments (the final purpose being survival and proliferation). Some ethical and epistemological consequences of this attempt are briefly discussed.

References................................147

Digressions 159

1 Electrical Signal Transmission in a Single Neuron 160
2 Basic Information Theory 165
3 Sets and Mappings.............................175
4 Local Synaptic Rules...........................180
5 Flow Diagram for a Survival Algorithm...............186
6 Suggestions for Further Reading...................189

Appendices 191

1 On the Storage Capacity of Associative Memories.......192
2 Neural Modeling 200
3 Cell Assemblies: the Basic Ideas 212
4 Cell Assemblies and Graph Theory 218

Author and Subject Index 241

Introduction

You can't tell how deep a puddle is until you step in it.

When I am asked about my profession, I have two ways of answering. If I want a short discussion, I say that I am a mathematician; if I want a long discussion, I say that I try to understand how the human brain works. A long discussion often leads to further questions:

What does it mean to understand "how the brain works"? Does it help to be trained in mathematics when you try to understand the brain, and what kind of mathematics can help? What makes a mathematician turn into a neuroscientist?

This may lead into a metascientific discussion which I do not like particularly because it is usually too far off the ground.

In this book I take quite a different approach. I just start explaining how I think the brain works. In the course of this explanation my answers to the above questions will become clear to the reader, and he will perhaps learn some facts about the brain and get some insight into the constructions of artificial intelligence.

This book is not a systematic treatment of the anatomy and physiology of the brain, or of artificial intelligence, or of the mathematical tools of theoretical biology; these subjects are only discussed when they turn up in the course of the argument. After a brief introduction (Chap. 1), in Chapter 2 the course of the argument is layed in the direction of artificial intelligence. In Chapters 3 to 7, I discuss the construction of a machine that "behaves well" or shows "intelligent behavior". An algorithm for such a machine is developed; it is called the "survival algorithm"; a possible embodiment of it in terms of neurons is used to stimulate specific questions about real brains. In this way the course of the argument is led through neuroanatomy and neurophysiology (Chaps. 8, 9, 10) to the modeling of neuronal networks as an attempt to get an idea of the flow of activity in the brain (Chap. 11). These considerations are finally combined (Chap. 11 and 12) with the constructive approach in the first part of the book to create a language in which one can talk of thoughts as of states of activity in the brain, or as of events that occur in the operation of a goal-oriented computer (the survival robot). The central term of this language is the term "cell assembly" which was introduced by Hebb (1949). The last three chapters contain extensive speculations based on this language

(Chap. 13) and my personal view on its anthropological and philosophical implications (Chaps. 14, 15).

For those readers who believe that they will never understand mathematics, I should add the consolation that I have tried to keep the mathematical formalism out of the main argument, so that it should be readable and intelligible to anyone who has enough patience and interest in the subject. Chapter 3 is perhaps the most mathematical chapter of the book, and it can be skipped by those who accept the points 3.4 and 3.5. The digressions and appendices which follow the main text are meant to serve as an introduction to those branches of mathematics that I believe to be most useful for this attempt to understand the human brain. In the digressions I have tried to present the mathematics in such a way that it can be understood also by readers with a limited mathematical experience.

The appendices are short self-contained monographs on a few theoretical issues that turn up in the main text.

Let me now answer the last of the introductory questions "What makes a mathematician turn into a neuroscientist?" in a personal way, by just explaining how I came to write this book.

Having finished my Ph.D. thesis at the mathematics department of the University of Tübingen in 1975, I started working at the Max Planck Institut für biologische Kypernetik. I worked on the theory of nonlinear systems, but at the same time I started to read about the brain. I learned several facts on brains and many different opinions or viewpoints on the interpretation of these facts. Quite soon I had to stop reading because I could not decide what to read next. This is not only because the literature on brains is tremendously large, but also because so many different problems opened up.

At the beginning I had learned that the most important things in the brain are the neurons. They transmit and process the information. I also had an idea how neurons work, how, for example, the electrical signal (called "spike") is transmitted along the long output fiber(s) of a neuron. And I had learned that in our brain there are billions of these neurons which are highly interconnected.

But was that enough? What else in the brain might influence the information flow? Do all the neurons work roughly in the same way, i.e., like those few neurons that had been investigated, or could it be that they are more complicated or specialized?

I also looked at Golgi preparations of some mouse brains where one can see the different shapes and arrangements of neurons. It is important to realize that this is possible only because in Golgi preparations just a small percentage of all the neurons is stained, for otherwise you could not distinguish any one neuron, since they are fibrous, highly branched, and

Introduction

so closely and complicatedly interlaced that they fill nearly the whole space.

Such observations again open up more questions than they answer. For example, questions pertaining to the different staining techniques. How does the Golgi technique select the few cells it stains? Does it stain the whole cell? These and many other technical problems even raised some doubts about the basic facts that I had learned up to that point, not to mention the enormous amount of much more detailed experimental results that I had not yet read (and that cannot all be read by any one person anyway).

The whole set of problems seemed to be far too serious for only a few years of reading and thinking about the brain. At first, I had to find out what I really wanted to know. Was my basic knowledge already sufficient to explain this, and if not, where should I go into the details? I started to "think about thinking" again and I read some early works on artificial intelligence, for example the little book by von Neumann (1958).

From a simple argument based on pure logic, I understood that for any well-defined information processing it is possible in principle to produce a device that performs it. And such a device can be built from neurons that all work in essentially the same way as those neurons that had been investigated experimentally (see Chap. 3).

Moreover, if the brain is just a network of interconnected neurons, it is possible in principle to predict the total behavior from the dynamics of single neurons, if one knows how they are interconnected.

So one has to investigate the connectivity between and the dynamics of the single neurons in the brain and one needs some mathematics to convert this kind of knowledge into predictions on the global flow of activity. I started to read papers on "brain modeling", where the dynamics of large (usually randomly) interconnected networks of neurons were analyzed. Here I realized that probably the hardest part was the interpretation of the results (as statements concerning "behavior").

At the same time I thought I should perhaps concentrate on a small part of the brain, and I chose the visual cortex, because there were so many data available on that region of the brain. But this led to several discouraging experiences.

First of all you cannot really understand the visual cortex, unless you have a precise idea of how it is integrated in the working of the brain. Therefore even for the visual cortex it is hard to separate understanding of this part of the brain from understanding of the whole brain. This is what makes "knowledge" on the functioning of isolated parts of the brain so questionable. For example, it can be quite frustrating to contemplate what knowledge might really be expressed in the following figure.

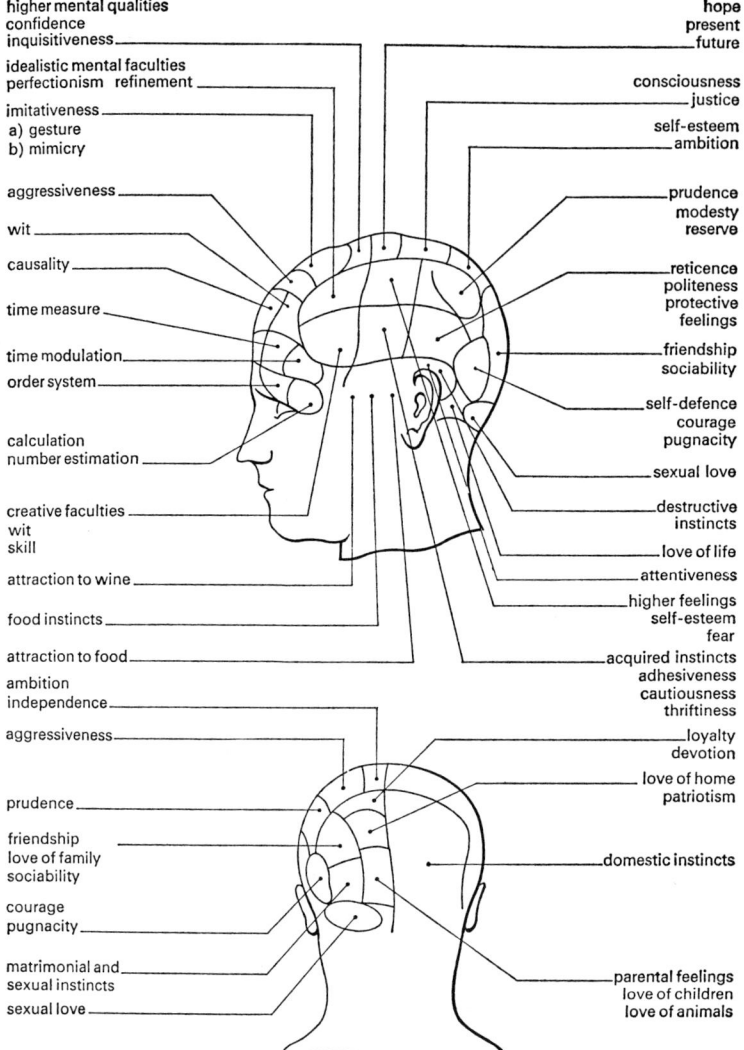

Gall's phrenological chart. (Luria 1973)

Furthermore, if you start getting interested in details you usually find that just the experiment you are interested in has not been performed, or at least those data that you really want to know are not reported (often for technical reasons that are hard to grasp if you do not work experimentally yourself). And you learn that data are not just given (as the word suggests), they are produced, selected, and usually contain a little bit of interpretation. Therefore, it is often not enough to read experimental papers, you have also to talk to the authors and try to find out which theory they have at the back of their minds. Often these ideas are not mentioned in the papers, because they are too hard to express or too easy to falsify. In personal communication, however, I could sometimes manage to discuss these ideas with the authors. In these discussions it often happened that we agreed on a kind of "private language", which was invented in the course of the discussion, and which made it possible to discuss these ideas at all.

It may well be that my mathematical training was helpful for these discussions, although perhaps in a rather unexpected way. When you study mathematics, you learn several mathematical formalisms, like topology, vector spaces, groups, Boolean algebras. But what is more important, you learn quickly to adapt to new formalisms. This means that you learn to handle different notations and you see how an adequate notation can make an understanding much easier and often opens up a whole new field of (mathematical) research. In other words, in mathematics you acquire a high flexibility in the invention and use of new notation. And you learn that the only way of explaining a new idea is often to invent a new language, or at least to define new terms and use new notations.

It may be a lack of this flexibility in the use of language and notation that often makes it impossible to explain the theories an experimenter has at the back of his mind when performing an experiment. Without this unwritten theoretical background even apparently plain descriptive papers often turn out not to be really intelligible.

> Let me use this remark to correct the common image of a mathematician as somebody who manipulates complicated formulas for several pages and finally arrives at some result that is of relevance to nobody except to himself and his few fellow mathematicians. As I said above, in mathematics you learn to handle several formalisms. Such a formalism usually makes it possible to deduce logical consequences from given assumptions (axioms) by doing formal manipulations in a special notation. If you stick to some formalism you can become an expert in the corresponding formal manipulations. This was a common situation historically, since the main field of application of mathematics was physics and most problems in classical physics could be dealt with in the mathematical formalism of differential equations. But today, I think, the situation is different, and the main point in studying mathematics is not to become an expert in handling one formalism, but to learn quickly to adapt to and even to invent new formalisms. A mathematician should worry much more about the "translation" between the actual problem and its representation in the mathematical formalism — although today this is often not yet regarded as part of mathematics.

For a few years I was engaged in several parallel activities: reading of experimental literature on the visual cortex, reading of neuron network theories, and still working on the theory of nonlinear systems. During that time my ideas on the brain were strongly influenced by V. Braitenberg's conception of the cerebral cortex in connection with Hebb's idea of "cell assemblies". In the autumn of 1978, I decided that I should try to fix my own ideas on the brain in terms of a model that shows "intelligent" behavior on the basis of simple neuron-like elements; I even dared to test these ideas by giving a series of lectures at the University of Tübingen. When I prepared these lectures, I found a didactical vehicle that greatly facilitated the explanation (at least from my point of view): this was the matchbox algorithm, a simple algorithm that clearly learns to play (in principle) unbeatable chess (it is explained in Chap. 4 and is, in fact, rather primitive). This book is based on these lectures. I regard it as a starting point for further reading and thinking about the brain.

I am grateful to Valentino Braitenberg who prompted me to begin this book and to my mother who helped me getting it finished. She typed and retyped most of the manuscript. I am obliged to many colleagues at the Max Planck Institut für biologische Kybernetik, especially to Almut Schüz and Christian Wehrhahn who critically read the manuscript and to Ladina Ribi and Claudia Martin-Schubert who prepared the figures.

Part I

1 The Flow of Information

For sheer complexity the cortex probably exceeds any other known structure.   D.H. Hubel and T.N. Wiesel, 1977

1.1 In the brain the information upon which we act comes together. This is visual, acoustical, olfactory, and tactile information about the outside world, as well as information on our own state of motion (proprioception from our muscles and joints) and emotion (e.g., the hormonal concentration in our blood, the condition of our inner organs and glands). On the basis of this information our reaction for this moment is programmed, or sometimes a sequence of reactions is planned for the future.

Thus our brain may be regarded as the middle box in the following simple scheme of the information flow in an organism:

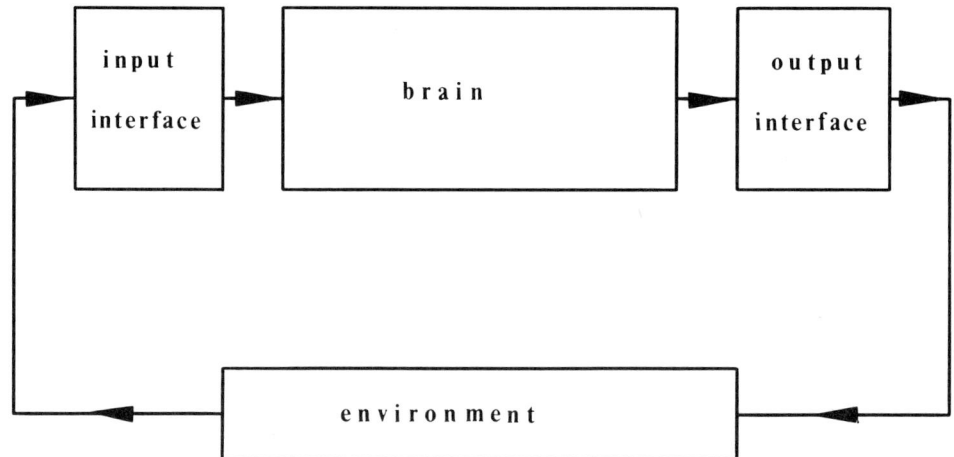

Fig. 1.1

Several precautions should be taken with respect to Fig. 1.1:
a) To carry out movements is itself a fairly complicated task, therefore there are sensory-motor servo mechanisms built into the output interface. Some of them are well known as reflexes, like the pupil reflex or the (knee) tendon reflex.
b) It is important to notice that the middle box − the brain − provides ample possibilities for internal loops in the information flow, which are not mediated through interaction with the outside world.

The Neuron

1.2 Within the nervous system the information is transmitted by the nerve cells or neurons. Let me give a rough description of the shape and functioning of a single neuron (see Fig. 1.2).

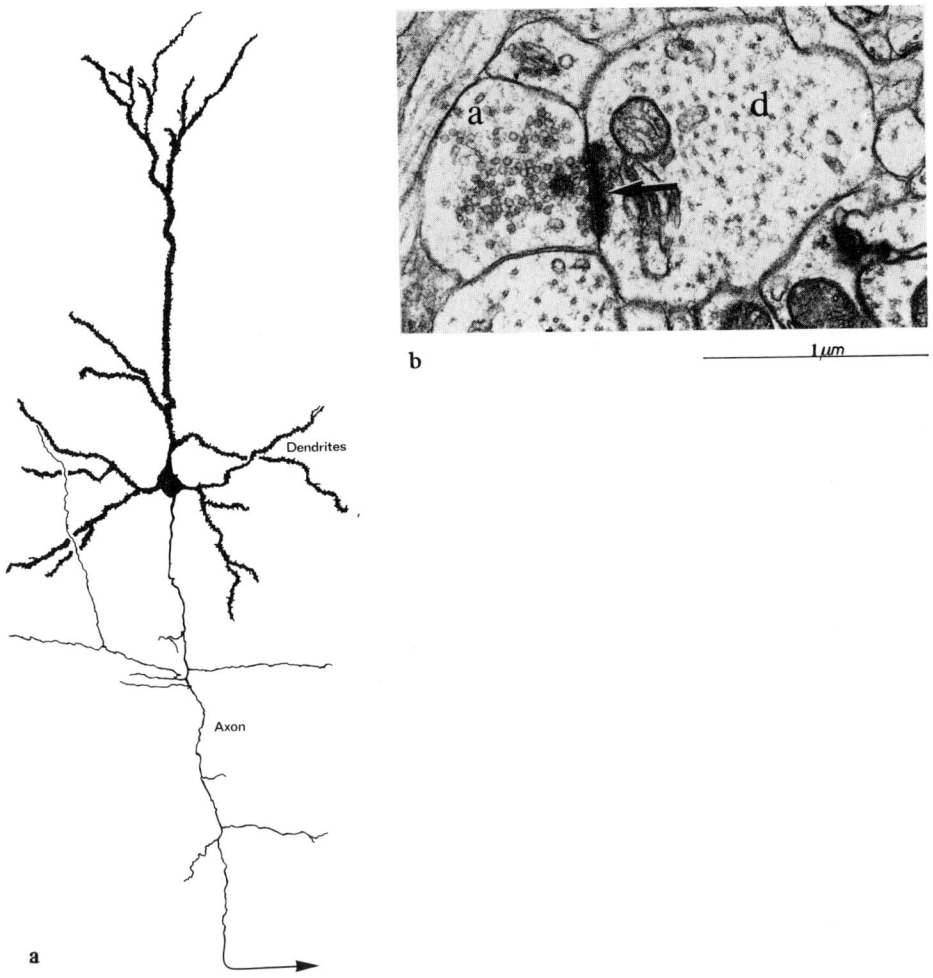

Fig. 1.2. a A neuron (Golgi preparation). (Braitenberg 1978b). **b** A synapse at about 200-fold highr magnification *a* presynaptic axon; *d* postsynaptic dendrite. (Courtesy Dr. A. Schüz)

It has an input tree (dendrites) and an output tree (axon and its collaterals). Incoming signals in the input tree (postsynaptic potentials) are weighted and added en route to the origin of the axon where an output signal is generated, a spike (or a burst of spikes). Its occurrence (or intensity) is therefore a function of a weighted sum of the incoming signals. The output signal runs through all axonal branches, reaching the synapses which connect the axon to dendritic trees of other neurons. Then it passes the synapses and is changed to the new input signal in the adjacent neurons. This new input signal can be positive or negative (excitatory or inhibitory). For more details see Digression 1.

In the human brain there are about 20 billion neurons and on the average one neuron has about 10.000 synapses distributed over its dendritic tree, and of course, the *average* number of synapses on the axon of one neuron must be again about 10.000. Thus a human brain contains in the order of 10^{14} synapses.

1.3 The neurons whose axons provide the input to the brain, in some cases themselves serve to transform their physical input signal to neuronal excitation in their axon (in muscle-stretch receptors, pain receptors, heat or pressure receptors), in other cases they are connected to specialized receptor cells (transforming optical signals in the retina of the eyes, or acoustical ones in the cochlea of the ear, or olfactory ones in the chemoreceptors of the nose or mouth).

At the end of the output (efferent) axons there are special synaptic junctions to the executing organs, e.g., the motor endplates, where neuronal excitation is transformed to contraction of the muscle.

The afferent (or efferent) axons usually enter (or leave) the brain in bundles, called nerves, which consist of up to 10^6 fibers.

1.4 The following diagram (Fig. 1.3) contains a crude subdivision of the brain, distinguishing the more "central" parts from those mainly concerned with preprocessing of the input or postprocessing (organizing) of the output.

1.5 From the numbers given in Table 1.1 we can roughly estimate the information transmitting capacity (more exactly, the "formatal" capacity as defined in Digression 2) of the various channels by multiplying the number of axons in such a channel by the amount of information one neuron can maximally transmit. In fact the estimation of this last number is itself a highly debated subject and the concrete estimates given in the literature (cf. Abeles and Lass 1975, Wall et al. 1956, Holden 1976) vary widely. Just to fix ideas let us say it is 200 bits/s. The information-transmitting capacity only gives an upper bound on the actual information flow passing through these channels under natural conditions, for this depends on the input to the channel (compare the estimates of the actual information flow through a single axon given in Eckhorn et al. 1976).

The Gross Connections

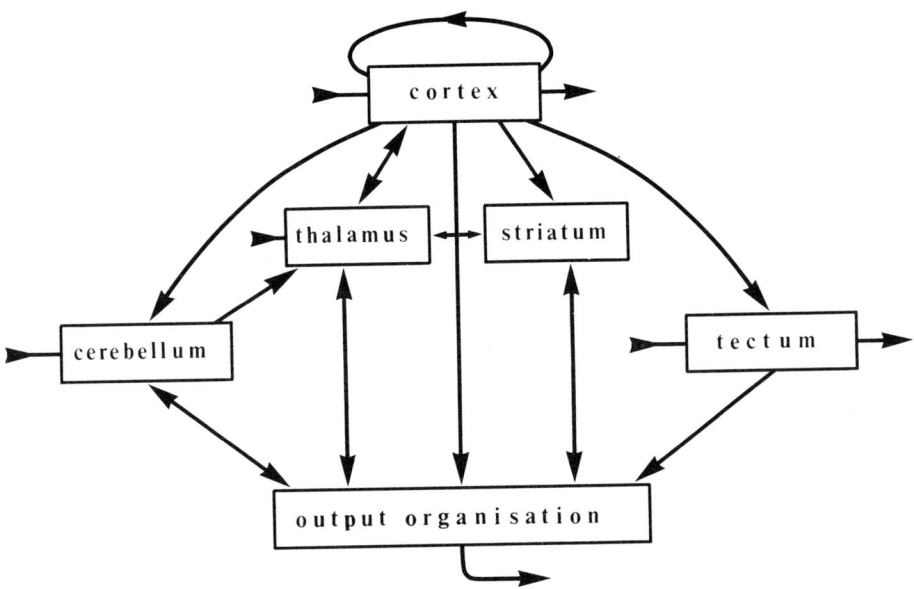

Fig. 1.3. Inputs (from the input interface of Fig. 1.1) are shown as ▶─ ; outputs (to the output interface of Fig. 1.1) are shown as ─▶.

The connections in this figure consist of at least several thousand and at most 10^7 = 10 million fibers, exept from the following connections:
1. The number of cortico-cortical fibers is about 10^{10} (since there are about 10^{10} pyramidal cells that have cortico-cortical axons).
2. The number of fibers between thalamus and striatum (in both directions) is less than 10^8 (this estimation is based on usual fiber densities in fiber tracts and the total surface of the thalamus, which is ≤ 20 cm^2).
3. The number of fibers between thalamus and cortex (in both directions) is less than 10^8 (same argument as in 2).
4. The number of fibers between striatum and cortex (in both directions) is less than $3 \cdot 10^8$ (analogous argument, total surface of striatum is ≤ 100 cm^2).
5. The number of fibers between cerebellum and output organization centers is less than $3 \cdot 10^7$ (from the thickness of the six cerebellar peduncles which is ≤ 6 cm^2).
6. The direct (olfactory) input to the cortex has almost 10^8 fibers, (e.g., Noback and Demarest 1967)

1.6 By psychophysical experiments one could try to determine the information flow through a whole input channel under natural conditions, but here one encounters still another problem.

Let us take the visual input channel as an example. If the capacity of the visual channel is estimated on the basis of spatial and temporal resolution in perceptual experiments, a value can be obtained which comes close to the capacity as estimated from Table 1.1 (which is of the order 10^8 bits/s).

However, if a picture is shortly presented to a person and afterwards he is given time to describe the picture, we see that the information retained about the picture, under optimal conditions, is much less than we

Table 1.1. Estimated order of magnitude of the number of fibers in various connections[a]

Cortex → cortex	10
Input → cortex	7
Thalamus → cortex	≤ 7
Cortex → striatum	≤ 7
Thalamus → striatum	≤ 7
Striatum → thalamus	≤ 7
Cerebellum → output organization	≤ 7
Output organization → cerebellum	≤ 7
Input → cerebellum	6
Cortex → cerebellum	6
Cerebellum → thalamus	6
Input → thalamus	6
Cortex → output	6
All other connections in Fig. 1.3	≤ 6

[a] The order of magnitude of a number is the number of its digits minus 1, e.g., "k is of the order of 10^5" or "the order of magnitude of k is 5" means "k is between 10^5 = 100.000 and 10^6 = 1.000.000" or "k has 6 digits"

would predict from the capacity. Therefore we can say that the bottleneck for the information flow in this experiment is neither in the visual input channel nor in the speech output channel (since the person was given enough time to describe the picture), but in between.

Of course, the visual information has to be recoded before it reaches the speech output channel. Also it has to be stored for a short time in order to be expressed verbally a little later. In addition one can assume that in order to fit into the memory, the information is coded in a different way and is recoded again during the recall. Thus the bottleneck for the "immediate" answer might lie in the speech output channel or in the vision-to-speech coding channel, the bottleneck for the somewhat delayed answers might lie in the coding channel from vision to memory, from memory to speech, or in the memory itself (cf. Fig. 1.4).

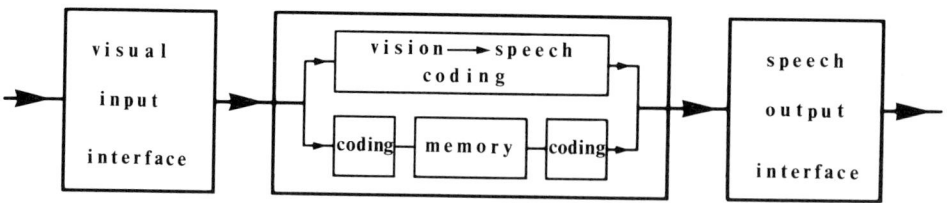

Fig. 1.4

1.7 These problems have been investigated in many psychological experiments, and the result is roughly as follows (for more details see Sanders 1971, Attneave 1959, Massaro 1975, Quastler 1956).

In many different experiments the maximal "throughput" that can be achieved lies around 10–40 bits/s (e.g., experiments on reaction times for the discrimination of various features, see Sanders 1971, Quastler 1956; on reading, piano playing etc., see Attneave 1959, Quastler 1956, Wenzel 1962). It is interesting that this number does not vary too much, even if different sensory modalities are used (see also Wenzel 1962).

Let me give one experiment as an example:

A well-trained pianist is given a "composition" to play at sight. But this composition just consists of notes of equal duration randomly placed inside, say, two octaves. The pianist is told these conditions, and he is able to play the composition at sight, as long as the required speed is sufficiently low. Otherwise he starts to make mistakes. In such a situation one can easily calculate the information flow at the critical speed by multiplying the number of notes per second by the information contained in one note (e.g., $\log_2 25$ for two octaves) and it will be up to 40 bits/s. Of course, the total information impinging on the pianist in this whole situation is much more than 40 bits/s. But most of the things in his surroundings remain constant. The only novel or unpredictable input in this experiment should consist of the random notes themselves.

Thus, in all these experiments it is assumed that the subject can predict the usual evolution of situations, and only the flow of unpredictable (really novel) information through the subject's "mind" is measured.

1.8 Many different experiments (e.g., on "visual masking", Massaro 1975, p. 342ff., or even the fact that in movies we may use 16 frames per second) indicate that for us there is a "shortest time unit" which we may call "moment", below which time differences usually cannot be perceived. The length of this natural human "time unit" is about a tenth of a second.

Thus we can say that only up to 3–10 bits of new (i.e., unpredicted) information can fit into our mind in one "moment" without producing confusion.

1.9 As for the somewhat delayed answers, these rely on the so-called "primary", "immediate" or "short-term" memory, which according to several psychological experiments has a storage capacity of about 30 bits, is very precise, and can be immediately accessed but lasts only for some seconds.

Besides that, we have a long-term memory, which can be divided into two types of memory: "secondary memory", where the storing as well as the recall takes a certain time and "mental" effort, and "tertiary memory" which allows a fast storing and recall without conscious effort, which may be related to the automatic acquisition of all kinds of reflexes and immediate associations. Both long-term memories seem to have a very large storage capacity. For a review of the properties of these three types of memories, see for example Ervin and Anders (1970).

1.10 We have seen that the bottleneck in the information flow through an animal lies between the input and output channels, i.e., in the middle box of Fig. 1.1. Here the different channels have to be connected in a way that the resulting "behavior" is "good" for that animal (it should maximize the chance for survival). Clearly, in the context of Fig. 1.1 the behavior of an animal is determined by its input-output relation, i.e., by the way it reacts to the sensory stimuli, and this in turn is determined by the way these channels are connected.

Therefore, a good coding between these different input and output channels is important, and also previous information should be used for later situations, i.e., information has to be stored there.

This may be a reason why the bottleneck occurs in the middle box, although the number of neurons and connecting fibers in that box is about 10^{10} compared with about 10^7 in all input and output channels summed up.

2 Thinking as Seen from Within and from Without

You can't prove that this statement is true.
Teaser for mathematicians

We have seen that the brain gets all the sensory information necessary to decide what to do. It also possesses the appropriate means for motor control to carry out its decisions. But "who" is making these decisions?

It is clearly necessary that there are devices that transfer sensory activity to the centers for motor control and finally to the muscles, and we have a large number of these devices for transfer of activity: the neurons. But we do not find much else in the brain; just neurons for the fast transfer of electric activity (as described in Chap. 1) and glia cells and blood vessels to supply them with energy. How can this network give rise to what we introspectively experience as thinking, deciding, etc.?

2.1 For example, right now I have a clear picture of my environment in my mind: I feel the chair I am sitting on. I know what kind of chair it is. I feel the pencil in my hand and the paper below it. I have a clear view of many details of the landscape outside the window. I even know exactly where the telephone is on my desk, although I am not looking at it right now. If it started ringing, I could grasp the receiver without looking. I am aware of all this information right now (although I could not really write it all down in one moment). On the other hand I have described experiments showing that not all of that information can really flow through my brain in one "moment".

This paradox is solved, if we remember that my perception of the whole situation I am in at any given moment contains an enormous portion of knowledge about my surroundings. For example, the amount of new information contained in the view outside my window actually is very small right now. Moreover, it seems as if I can only concentrate on a small segment of my total sensory input at any moment. This also decreases the flow of new information I really handle (while concentrating on a special part of my input I assume that other things remain as they were or evolve as they use to evolve, probably without being aware of it).

But what mysterious entity inside my brain is experiencing all this in a single moment? Is there a part of my brain where everything I am "aware of" is represented? And how can all this be represented in one place at the same time? For example, what goes on in my brain when I think about my "awareness" or "thinking", i.e., just about the activity of my brain itself? My brain should then also contain a representation of itself, including its representation of everything I am aware of right now including my thoughts about my brain, etc.

This kind of introspection leads us into problems that are strangely attractive, since they somehow seem to be impossible logically, but on the other hand they seem to be possible physically. I remember that as a child I was very impressed by an advertisement on some product (I think it was margarine), showing a girl presenting that product with exactly the same advertisement on it (see also Fig. 2.1).

I believe many of us have had similar experiences and these are also reflected in many logical or perhaps linguistical paradoxes.

How Can We Deal with These Problems?

2.2 You can indulge in these introspections, that I have only vaguely hinted at. You can think about self-reflection and try to make up your mind as to whether it is possible or not, and whether it may be connected to

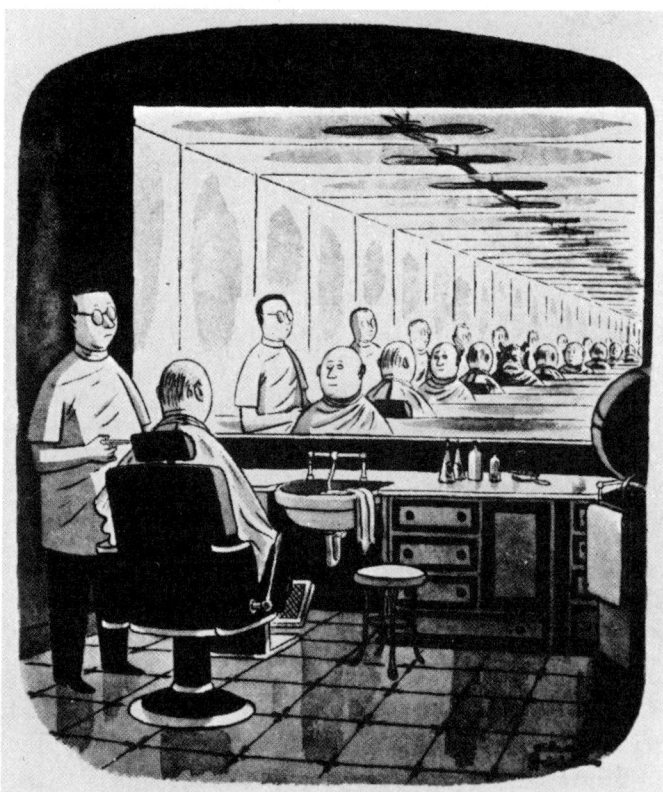

Fig. 2.1. (By Charles Addams)

The Paradox of the Mind

logical paradoxes like the "lyer"; or you can try to classify these paradoxes into classes of similar ones and discuss these. This has been done mainly by philosophers and logicians. I must confess that I personally enjoy thinking about these paradoxes, although I do not have the feeling that it leads to definite communicable results [a famous exception is the theorem of Gödel (1931) and its consequences, which are communicable at least to mathematicians]. There are several books about these paradoxes that have a considerable recreational value (at least for me), for example Smullyan (1978), Hoffstaedter (1979) and the (probably unintentionally recreational) presentation of a blend of feedback, Fichte (1794) and infinite series by Klaczko-Ryndziun (1975).

2.3 You can decide that you cannot decide these problems and therefore had better not worry about things like "awareness" (including "self-awareness").

This leads many people (even scientists working on the brain) to treat input channels and output channels as if they were finally serving a "little man" inside the brain, who is looking at the elegantly preprocessed sensory input and gives commands to the well-designed motor output mechanism. From this point of view it is very satisfying to learn that the visual information from the retina is projected in an orderly, topographic manner (.i.e., preserving "nearness") into the primary visual area, where some features (e.g., small line segments) are detected locally and then projected again in a topographic manner into a secondary visual area, where perhaps somewhat more complicated features are detected and so on. But you had better not follow up this "and so on".

Analogous observations can be made on the output side, where nicely organized feedback loops for motor control are found, which are built on top of each other in a hierarchical manner. In this way most of our quite detailed knowledge on the pre- and postprocessing of information on its way to and from the brain has been obtained. This knowledge is very important, but it is superficial in the following literal sense: it only deals with the outer boxes of Fig. 1.1.

2.4 You can try to circumvent these problems by turning from introspectively studying yourself to studying another human being: Instead of thinking about what makes you think that you are thinking and what is going on in your brain, when you are thinking, you should think about what makes you think that *he* is thinking and what goes on in his brain, when he is.

In this approach the question is the following:

Can we understand how the human brain can produce the behavior that we observe in other humans, for example when we have a talk with them about logical paradoxes or introspection?

What kinds of behavior would be the hardest to "understand" this way?

For these kinds of behavior we would have to invent a mechanism by which the brain could produce them. Of course, the invention of such a mechanism could also be used to build a machine that produces that behavior; and to build such a machine and to observe its behavior would be the easiest way to test that mechanism. Thus we should try to invent machines that we can talk to in natural languages, play chess against, give riddles or problems to solve, etc. This is done by people working in the rather new science called *artificial intelligence*. The obvious test for artificial intelligence in any of these tasks mentioned above is the *Turing test* (Turing 1950): *Can a competent observer connected, say, by telephone to a computer performing the task, tell the computer from a human being?*

2.5 There has been considerable success in the last years in building computers for some of these tasks. The main drawback with regards to the Turing test still is that there is no program for a computer to communicate in a natural language, like English. Some computers (or programs) are growing up now, that you can talk to in a restricted context (Winograd 1974, Minsky 1968, Weizenbaum 1966). There is a computer that can solve some well-defined problems (Newell and Simon 1972, Ernst and Newell 1969), there is one that can prove or disprove theorems from given axioms (Newell et al. 1957, Nilsson 1971), but here again the context is quite restricted. The chess computers probably have gained the greatest popularity, and the better ones indeed can be said to pass the Turing test: it is hard, if not impossible, to tell their playing style from the (highly varying) styles of human players (cf. Frey 1977, Berliner 1978). But this is still a restricted context.

In the following I will describe some mechanisms that can be used to perform these tasks, and that can be realized in the brain by means of the neurons that are there.

3 How to Build Well-Behaving Machines

> *"I could have done it in a much more complicated way"* said the
> Red Queen, immensely proud.   Lewis Carroll

In the following we will discuss how to build such an "intelligent" machine. This machine should work like an organism in an environment, which we again can picture as in Fig. 1.1.

3.1 First the input to the machine is translated into its "internal code". The input could, for example, consist of a visual scene, or of sounds. The visual scene could be scanned by a television camera line by line, as we scan a page when we are reading it; the sound could be detected by a microphone. In any case the original signal is transformed to a sequence of electrical potentials, in a cable: let me call them $p_0, p_1, p_2, \ldots$. In the television example each of these potentials may correspond to the brightness of a single spot in the scanned picture. The exact value of such an electrical potential could be written down as a number; and since these numbers cannot be determined with arbitrary accuracy, it is always sufficient to give them as integer multiples of some small unit potential. Thus the scene or sound could be reconstructed from a sequence of integers $n_0, n_1, n_2, \ldots$, coding the potentials $p_0, p_1, p_2, \ldots$. Moreover, these numbers cannot be arbitrarily large: let us say they are all less than 1000, i.e., every $n_j \in \{0, 1, 2, \ldots, 999\}$, in the language of set theory which is explained in Digression 3. Now the total sequence of numbers can be coded into just one number:
For example the sequence 13,750,62,7,365
is coded into 0 1 3 7 5 0 0 6 2 0 0 7 3 6 5.
Thus, if one "sound" can be coded by 8 such numbers, it can also be coded by one number n with $8 \cdot 3 = 24$ digits, i.e.,
$n \in \{0, 1, \ldots, 999999999999999999999999\}$.
This means that there are at most
999999999999999999999999 + 1 = 1000000000000000000000000
different situations.

In this way we can code any situation into a number: usually there is only a finite number N of different situations, and we could just enumerate these situations $s_1, s_2, \ldots, s_N$ and code each situation s_j by its number j. The numbers can then be coded into sequences of digits 0,1,2,3,4,5,6,7,8,9 (as we usually do it), but also into sequences of just 0 and 1, for example in the following way:

$$0 \mapsto 0000$$
$$1 \mapsto 0001$$
$$2 \mapsto 0010$$
$$3 \mapsto 0011$$
$$4 \mapsto 0100$$
$$5 \mapsto 0101$$
$$6 \mapsto 0110$$
$$7 \mapsto 0111$$
$$8 \mapsto 1000$$
$$9 \mapsto 1001$$

This procedure would code for example the number 013750062007365 into 0000000100110111010100000000011000100000000001110011o-1100101. In a similar way the output of our machine will be performed by motors that could be controlled again by electrical potentials, which again can be coded by numbers, or by sequences of 0s and 1s.

3.2 Now we can concentrate on the construction of the middle box in Fig. 1.1, which has to produce the right type of behavior by transforming its input 0,1-sequence just into the correct output 0,1-sequence. Of course, this transformation should work correctly for a large set of input sequences — maybe even for all possible 0,1-sequences as inputs.

How Can We Build up a Mechanism Performing Such a Transformation?

Firstly, we can reduce the problem to output "sequences" consisting of just one digit. Indeed, if every single digit in the output sequence contains exactly the predescribed value -0 or 1- for every possible input sequence, we correctly obtain the whole predescribed output sequence.

Now we need a machine m, that assigns the output 1 to one predescribed class of input sequences and the output 0 to the remaining input sequences.

We would probably give the prescription for such a machine m by writing down explicitly the input sequences $s_1, s_2, s_3, \ldots, s_n$ which should yield the output 1 and requiring the output to be 0 otherwise. Thus the output should be 1, if (and only if) the input is s_1 *or* s_2 *or* s_3 *or* ... *or* s_n.

Then we can describe the inputs digit by digit:
Say $s_1 = 011001$, then the input is s_1, exactly if there is a

0 in the 1st place *and* a
1 in the 2nd place *and* a
1 in the 3rd place *and* a

The Logical Construction

0 in the 4th place *and* a
0 in the 5th place *and* a
1 in the 6th place.

Thus the condition for the output to be 1 can be written as a disjunction (*or*) of conjunctions (*and*) of conditions on single digits of the input sequence.

Now we can write 1 for "true" and 0 for "false" and then we can figure out these "truth values" for any complicated condition on many digits of the input sequence. We can even construct a machine for this task. To this end, we construct little conjunction (*and*) machines working on the truth values 0 and 1, and also disjunction (*or*) machines; and we need machines that produce the prescribed "truth value" (1 or 0) for a condition on a single digit of the input sequence.

Such a machine is indeed easy to build: The condition "the jth digit should be 1" is true exactly if the jth digit is 1, i.e., the jth digit d_j itself can be used as truth value for this proposition. The condition "the jth digit should be 0" is true exactly if the jth digit is 0: $d_j = 0$, i.e., $1-d_j = 1$. Thus $(1-d_j)$ can be used as truth value for this proposition.

Here we needed a little machine performing the mapping $x \mapsto 1-x$ for the values 0 and 1, i.e., $\begin{matrix}0 \mapsto 1 \\ 1 \mapsto 0\end{matrix}$. It is called the logical *not* machine; the logical symbol for it is $\sim$. It is defined as $\sim : \begin{cases} 0 \mapsto 1 \\ 1 \mapsto 0 \end{cases}$

or in form of a little table:

x	$\sim$ x
0	1
1	0

We can describe the logical *and*- and *or*-machines in the same way: The following mapping defines the *and*-machine, its logical symbol is "$\wedge$"; it has two inputs which can be 0 or 1, and one output.

$\wedge$: $0,0 \mapsto 0$ i.e.

x	y	x$\wedge$y
0	0	0
0	1	0
1	0	0
1	1	1

i.e. $0 \wedge 0 = 0$
$0 \wedge 1 = 0$
$1 \wedge 1 = 0$
$1 \wedge 1 = 1$

$0,1 \mapsto 0$
$1,0 \mapsto 0$
$1,1 \mapsto 1$

Note that $x \wedge y = x \cdot y$ for $x,y \in \{0,1\}$.

The following mapping defines the *or*-machine, its logical symbol is "$\vee$":

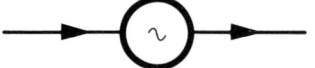

Fig. 3.1. a The *not*-machine; b the *and*-machine; c the *or*-machine

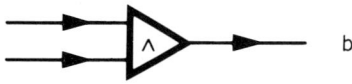

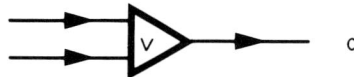

$$
\begin{array}{llll}
v: & 0,0 \to 0 & \text{i.e.} & \begin{array}{c|c|c} x & y & x v y \\ \hline 0 & 0 & 0 \\ 0 & 1 & 1 \\ 1 & 0 & 1 \\ 1 & 1 & 1 \end{array} & \text{i.e.} & \begin{array}{l} 0 v 0 = 0 \\ 0 v 1 = 1 \\ 1 v 0 = 1 \\ 1 v 1 = 1 \end{array} \\
& 0,1 \to 1 & & & & \\
& 1,0 \to 1 & & & & \\
& 1,1 \to 1 & & & &
\end{array}
$$

Note that $x v y = x + y$, for $x, y \in \{0,1\}$, with the only exception that $1 + 1 = 2$ (see Fig. 3.1).

Now we can build our machine m by connecting *not*-, *and*-, and *or*-machines in the appropriate way. First the single digits of the input sequence are passed through *not*-machines if necessary, to produce the correct truth value for the conditions on these digits. Then they are joined through *and*-machines, until only one output digit is left; this output indicates the truth of the condition "the input sequence was s_1". This is also done for every other input sequence $s_2, \ldots, s_n$, and finally all these outputs are joined by *or*-machines (see Fig. 3.2).

For any well-defined input-output behavior we can construct a machine that performs it.

Moreover, this machine can be constructed — up to input and output coding into 0,1-sequences — by a network of *not*-, *or*-, and *and*-machines.

3.3 Now one could ask whether it is also possible to use other basic machines to construct any input-output relation. This can indeed be done, and we can show that a set M of basic machines can produce everything, by just showing that the *not*-, *or*- and *and*-machines can be produced by combining machines of the set M.

For the moment let me call a set M of machines *complete*, if every input-output behavior can be produced by appropriate combinations of

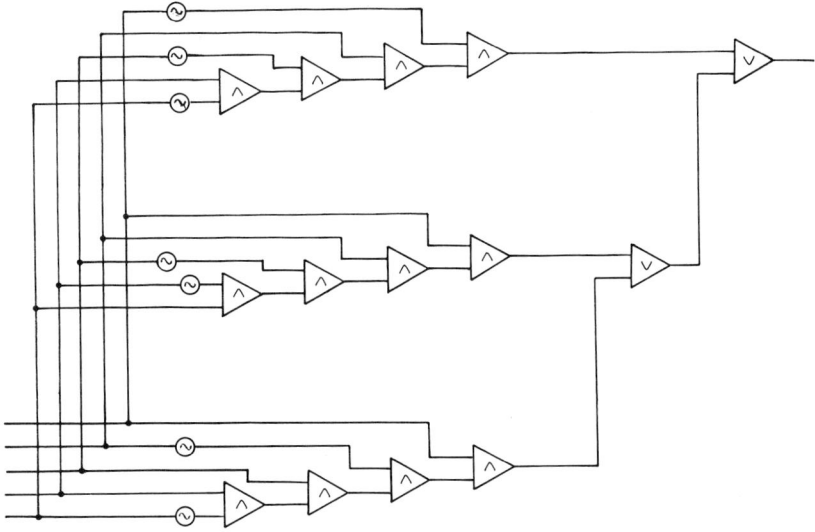

Fig. 3.2

machines from M (given a fixed input-output coding into some fixed alphabet, like {0,1} in our case).

Using this new term, we can restate what we have shown above.

Proposition 1: M = {*not, or, and*} is complete.
Next we show the following.

Proposition 2: M = {*nand*} is complete.
nand means "not and", and the *nand*-machine is defined as follows:

x,y	x *nand* y
0,0	1
0,1	1
1,0	1
1,1	0

That is, the *nand*-machine can be described by Fig. 3.3, and "x *nand* y" means "*not* (x *and* y)".

To understand that the *nand*-machine is universal, we have to construct the *not-, and-,* and *or*-machines from *nand*-machines:

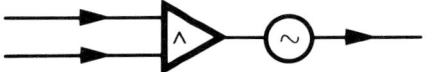

Fig. 3.3. The *nand*-machine

a) $\sim x = x$ *nand* x, since 0 *nand* 0 = 1 = ~ 0
    and 1 *nand* 1 = 0 = ~ 1
b) x *and* y = $\sim$ (x *nand* y) = (x *nand* y) *nand* (x *nand* y)
c) x *or* y = ($\sim$x) *nand* ($\sim$y) = (x *nand* x) *nand* (y *nand* y)

The first equality holds since

	x	y	$\sim$x	$\sim$y	($\sim$x) *nand* ($\sim$y)
Case 1	0	0	1	1	0
Case 2	0	1	1	0	1
Case 3	1	0	0	1	1
Case 4	1	1	0	0	1

and the last column is in every case identical with the column defining x *or* y.

Proposition 3: M = {nor} is complete.
Nor means "not or", and the machine is defined as follows:

x	y	x *nor* y
0	0	1
0	1	0
0	0	0
1	1	0

The reader should try to verify the above proposition himself.

Proposition 4: Threshold neurons are complete.

A *threshold neuron* is a machine that was introduced by McCulloch and Pitts (1943) as a "logical" device that roughly models the input-output behavior of a single neuron. The synaptic inputs x_i to the neuron are weighted (i.e., multiplied by numbers w_i, that reflect the different conductivity properties of the synapses, as well as the different distances of the synapses to the beginning of the axon) and added.

If this sum is greater than the threshold Θ of the neuron, the output will be 1, otherwise 0.

In other words a threshold neuron is specified by the numbers w_i (i = 1, ... ,n) and Θ, and is given by the mapping

$$m: (x_1, \ldots, x_n) \mapsto \begin{cases} 0 \text{ if } \Sigma w_i x_i < \Theta \\ 1 \text{ if } \Sigma w_i x_i \geq \Theta. \end{cases}$$

Now we can convince ourselves that the set M of all threshold neurons is universal (see also Muroga 1971).

Completeness of Elementary Machines

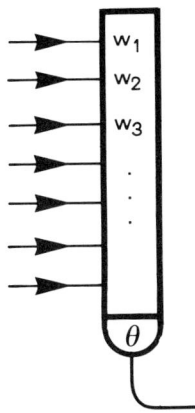

Fig. 3.4. A threshold neuron. $w_1, w_2, \ldots$ weights, Θ threshold

First argument: *not, or* and *and* can be constructed by them:

$m_\sim$ is specified by $w_1 = -1, \Theta = -\frac{1}{2}$;

then $m_\sim(0) = 1$ thus $m_\sim = \sim$.
$m_\sim(1) = 0$

$m_\wedge$ is specified by $w_1 = 1, w_2 = 1, \Theta = 1\frac{1}{2}$;

then $m_\wedge(0,0) = 0$,   thus $m_\wedge = \wedge$.
$m_\wedge(0,1) = 0$
$m_\wedge(1,0) = 0$
$m_\wedge(1,1) = 1$

$m_\vee$ is specified by $w_1 = 1, w_2 = 1, \Theta = \frac{1}{2}$;

then $m_\vee(0,0) = 0$,   thus $m_\vee = \vee$.
$m_\vee(0,1) = 1$
$m_\vee(1,0) = 1$
$m_\vee(1,1) = 1$

Second argument: *nand* can be constructed by them:
m_{nand} is specified by $w_1 = -1, w_2 = -1, \Theta = -1\frac{1}{2}$;
The reader should check himself, whether $m_{nand} = nand$.

Third argument: *nor* can be constructed by them:
How?

By the way, it is clear that there are many more possible threshold neurons than just $m_\sim$, $m_\vee$ and $m_\wedge$. Therefore many input-output relations can be wired in a much simpler way with threshold neurons than with *or-*, *not-*, and *and*-machines. For example Fig. 3.2 can be wired as in Fig. 3.5.

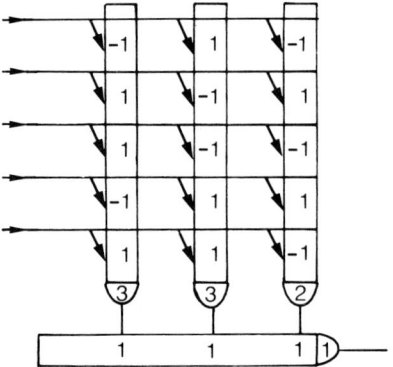

Fig. 3.5. Here the weights w_i are $+1$ or -1, corresponding to the possible insertion of not-gates in Fig. 3.2. The threshold of the vertical elements is set equal to the number of $+1$'s in their weights to perform the *and* operation. The weights and the threshold of the horizontal element are set to 1 to perform the *or* operation

This arrangement is the same as in the so-called perceptron (cf. Minsky and Papert 1969).

3.4 Let me summarize the arduous constructive work of this chapter. A behavior can be defined as a mapping associating outputs (actions) to inputs (situations). The input- and output-signals can be coded into 0,1-sequences. In this way the problem of constructing a machine that displays a predescribed behavior is reduced to the problem of constructing a machine that performs a predescribed mapping between 0,1-sequences. Such a machine can indeed be constructed from "logical machines" that correspond to the logical operations of "not", "and", and "or". It can also be constructed from "threshold neurons", which are neuron-like machines.

Thus for any predescribed behavior we can build a machine performing it, and we even can build it from very simple neuron-like elements.

For didactical reasons I have used simple logical arguments to make this statement clear, but the "discontinuous" or "decision-like" behavior of the logical operations (and the threshold neurons as well) is in no way essential for the demonstration. This can already be seen from the facts that the logical *and* operates on 0s and 1s in the same way as multiplication, and that the logical *or* operates nearly in the same way as addition.

Furthermore we can also replace a threshold neuron with threshold Θ by a similar device which does not "jump" at Θ, but is 0 until $\Theta-\epsilon$, moves continuously up to 1 between $\Theta-\epsilon$ and Θ, and remains at 1 for values bigger than Θ. A third argument is given in Palm (1979), where I have shown that so-called "sandwich"-elements are universal. The universality of any class of simple elements can also be interpreted as a negative result: the knowledge that a system is built from (many of) these elements leads to no predictions or restrictions on its information-processing capabilities.

Further investigations on the functioning of single neurons will not lead to "global" predictions on the behavior of large neural networks (of course, one can predict and even simulate the all-over behavior of a *given* network with known connections from exact knowledge on the functioning of its parts).

3.5 We have seen that for any predescribed behavior we can build a machine performing it, and we even can build it using neuron-like elements.

This statement, however, is only true "in principle", and this very much so: if we would record one hour's conversation between two people, code it into 0-1-sequences and then try to build a machine performing exactly the input-output behavior of one of the two, we would get 0-1-sequences of an enormous length and accordingly we would need an even more enormous amount of "neurons" if we proceed as in Fig. 3.5. Also an exact wiring of all these "neurons" would be required and this wiring would take many more hours than the original conversation. An exact blueprint for the wiring would probably take thousands of pages.

But in any case it is good to know that in principle we can build a machine for any predescribed behavior. In this way we can fully concentrate on the problem of reducing the complexity of the described machine. We are faced with a square engineering problem: how to build such a machine in an economic way.

I have just hinted at the two main points we can try to save on:
1. *On elementary machines* (i.e., neurons).
2. *On blueprint* (i.e., genetic pre-organization).

The second point leads us to the next chapter. The question is: how much information is really needed to build up a highly organized structure?

We will see that this question is hard, if not impossible to answer, since there are many cases known, even from physics, where a structure emerges apparently without any goal-oriented instruction. This phenomenon is called "self-organization", and we would of course like to employ such a kind of mechanism in building up our machine, since it seems to be a way of saving blueprint. Therefore organization and "self-organization" are discussed in the next chapter.

The construction of a well-behaving machine will be taken up again after this discussion in Chapter 5 (and 7).

4 Organizations, Algorithms, and Flow Diagrams

> *Roghly, by a complex system I mean one made up of a large number of parts that interact in a nonsimple way. In such systems, the whole is more than the sum of the parts, not in an ultimate, metaphysical sense, but in the important pragmatical sense that, given the properties of the parts and the laws of their interaction, it is not a trivial matter to infer the properties of the whole.*
>
> H.A. Simon, 1969

In the last chapter we considered the task of building a complicated network that is designed to perform a certain kind of behavior. In this chapter we shall concentrate on the question of how to save blueprint in the description of this task.

This leads to the more general problem of finding the "simplest" instruction (to give to a machine or a person or even several machines or persons) for a complicated task.

4.1 Heuristically, we use the following approach to find a simple instruction or a simple way of proceeding, when faced with a complicated task:

We organize the task into simpler tasks (which we then may organize again into still simpler subtasks).

Such an organization can be written down in a *diagram:* (as in Fig. 4.1)

In human cooperation we use this way of organizing tasks all the time: e.g., in organizing the production of TV sets or cars, in structuring big companies, etc.

4.2 It is usually easy to find a quite simple organization of a given task, but it is very hard to make sure that there is not a much simpler organization of that task.

There are tasks that can be organized in a surprisingly simple way such that the result of the task looks (and perhaps is) much more complicated and intricate than the description of the algorithm performing the task.

As an example for this consider the taks of constructing a machine that plays unbeatable chess and the following algorithm that leads to exactly such a machine (compare Gardner 1969).

The Matchbox Algorithm

4.3 The procedure is the following:

You need a chess set and a huge pile of empty matchboxes. Chose an opponent and start playing.

If it is your move, do the following:

1. Look through your stock of "prepared" matchboxes for a box that shows the position on the board.
2. If you don't find it, take an empty matchbox and "prepare" it:
   a) Print the position at hand on the matchbox.
   b) Knowing the rules of the game, find out all possible moves, write them on sheets of paper and put these into the matchbox.
   c) If no move is possible, check whether your king is attacked; if this is not the case, put in a sheet with "draw" written on it, otherwise leave the matchbox empty.
   Now you have a "prepared" matchbox with the position on the board printed on it.
3. Read the top sheet in the box and perform that move.
   In case you find "draw", say that it is a draw and stop playing.
   Keep this matchbox at hand until your next move.
4. If the box is empty, give up and take out the top sheet of the last box you used.

Roughly speaking the strategy consists of listing all possible moves and discarding all moves that lead to a loss (see Fig. 4.2).

4.4 These are only "local" rules and they are easy to follow. However, in the course of many games the machine operating according to this procedure will assemble millions of matchboxes and it will eventually play better chess than any of our grandmasters of today.

Since the strategy of the procedure is very simple, this fact is conceivable with a bit of thought, although it would be unrealistic to try to implement this procedure on a computer and see it work.

Moreover, this procedure clearly works with any two-person game, irrespective of the special rules of the game. For the general theory of games, including "games against nature", see the illuminating book of Luce and Raiffa (1957).

In the following I shall use this "algorithm" as a prototype for the organization of the task of building a well-behaving robot. I can do this because the task of playing good chess can be generalized to the task of optimizing situation-response behavior, and because the algorithm itself has so many nice features.

It is a good example of a simple algorithm that creates a complex structure (namely the heap of prepared matchboxes). It needs only a few

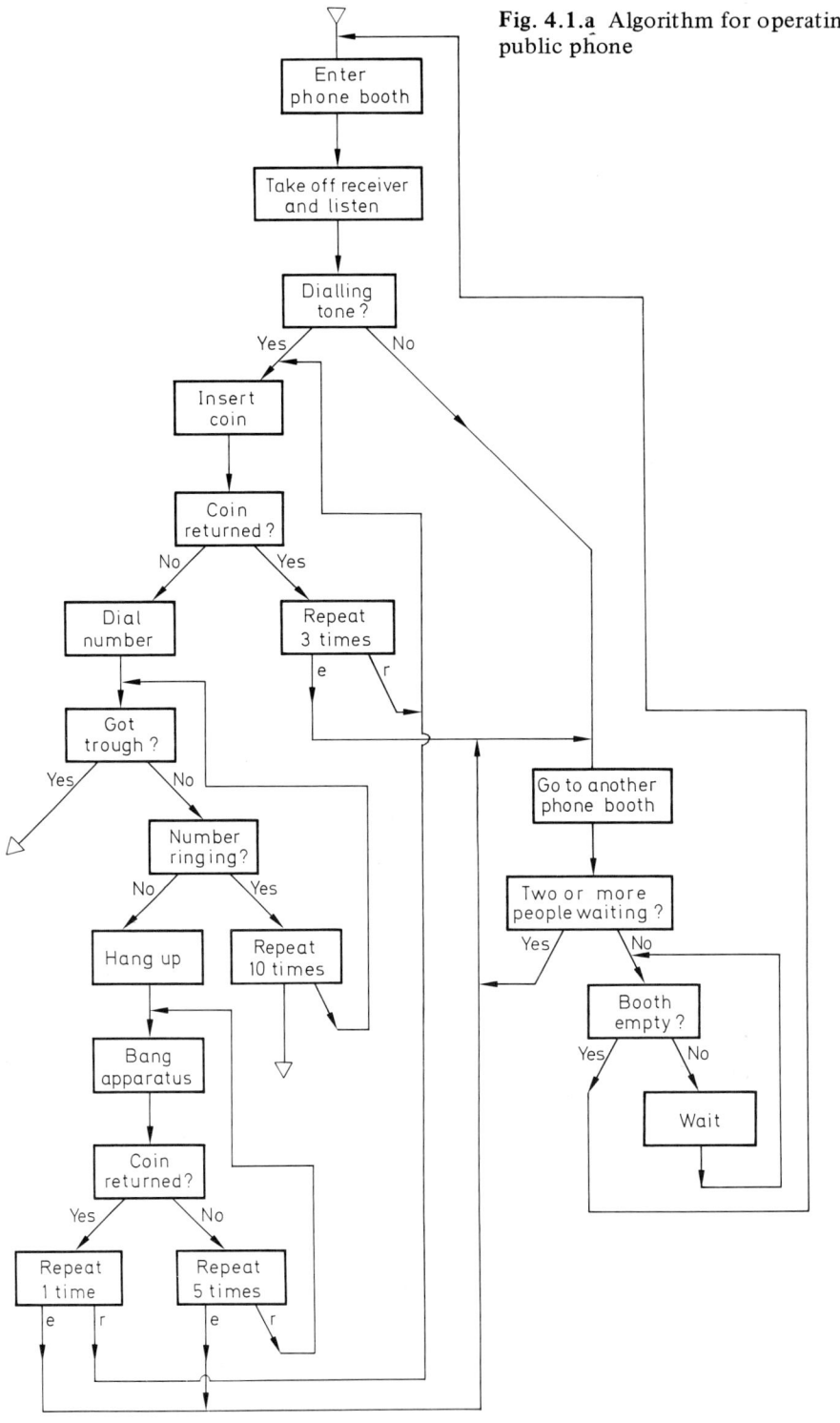

Fig. 4.1.a Algorithm for operating public phone

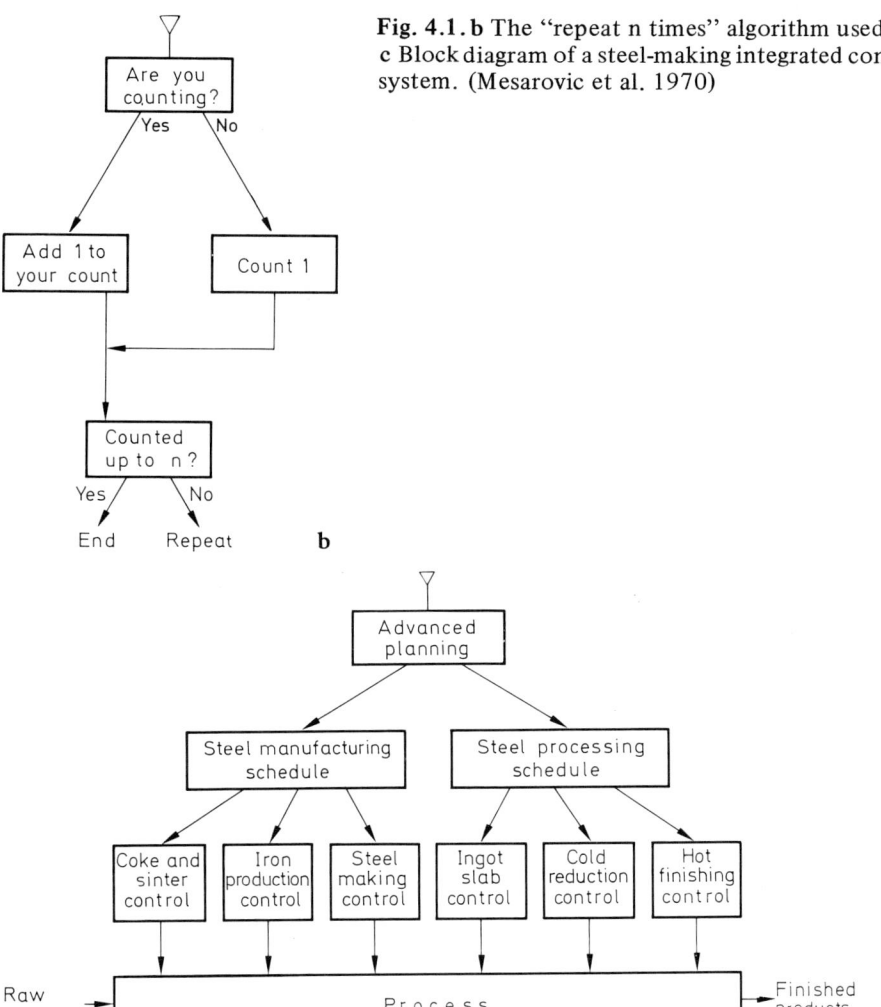

Fig. 4.1. b The "repeat n times" algorithm used in **a**. **c** Block diagram of a steel-making integrated control system. (Mesarovic et al. 1970)

subtasks that are much simpler than the original task and that are repeated very often. Furthermore it is more serial than parallel and we would perhaps refrain from calling its work cooperative or even self-organization.

4.5 In the context of computing, such an organization of a complicated task into simpler tasks is called on *algorithm*.

In a flow diagram two boxes (representing tasks) are connected by an arrow if some result of the first task is under some conditions passed to the second task (at least as a trigger signal). There are many different kinds of organizations, or diagrams representing them; some special cases are illustrated in Fig. 4.3.

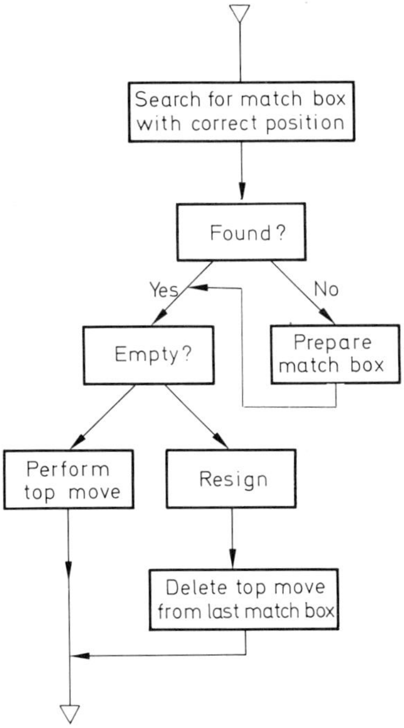

Fig. 4.2. The matchbox algorithm

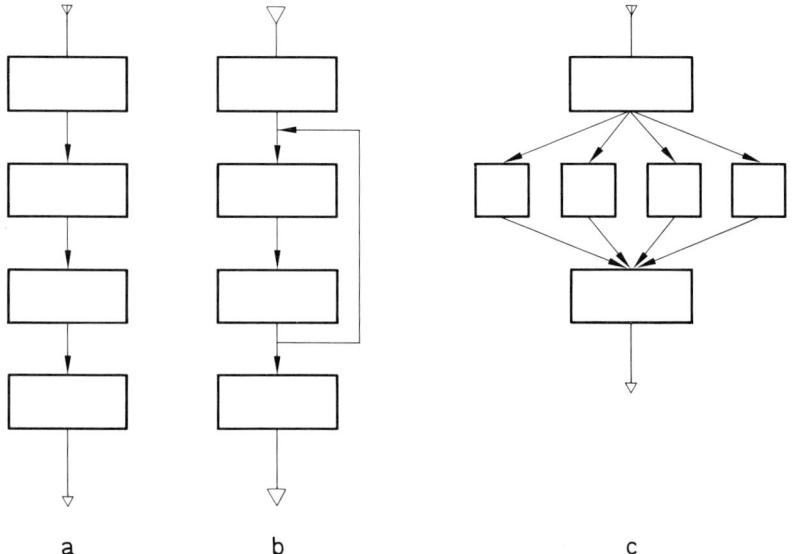

Fig. 4.3. a Serial organization; **b** recurrent organization; **c** parallel organization

Types of Organizations

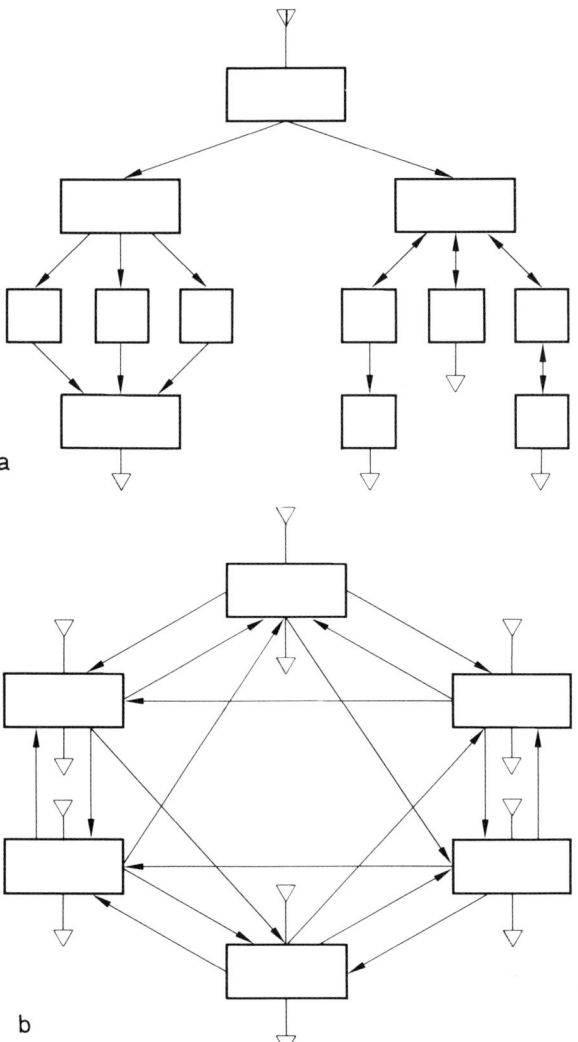

Fig. 4.4. a Hierarchical; **b** cooperative

In Fig. 4.3c several arrows converge on one box. This implies that the corresponding subtask cannot be too simple itself: it has to contain at least some instruction concerning the possible convergence of information along these arrows.

Note that in the recurrent flow diagrams of Fig. 4.1a and b no convergence of arrows on one subtask occurs. Combining recurrent connections and parallel organization one can obtain all sorts of diagrams (see Fig. 4.4).

Of course, these are only extreme cases and usually we find mixtures of them, and perhaps there are even entirely different types that we cannot classify yet.

The problem of classifying diagrams is another aspect of the problems treated in Appendix 4.

Roughly we may say that an organization is *hierarchical,* if it is described by a diagram that can be reasonably divided into different levels (mainly according to the "distance" of the different boxes to the input and/or output), where the flow of information occurs mainly between the boxes at different levels and not inside any one level, and that an organization somehow is "more" *cooperative,* if it is "less" hierarchical. Of course, the word "cooperative" as well as the word "organization" also implies that all the different boxes in the flow diagram are interconnected along some way. I will come back to the problem of characterizing cooperative organizations in (4.7) and in Appendix 4. The invention and investigation of cooperative organizations (and algorithms) is a rather new field of research (see for example Dijkstra 1968, Dal Cin 1976, Chap. 3.3 and 1978); one example of a cooperative organization is the "stereo algorithm", which I have analyzed together with T. Poggio and D. Marr (Marr et al. 1978).

4.6 In this context the notions of "cooperative phenomena" and "self-organization" come to mind, and I want to finish this section by pointing out an important difference between cooperative phenomena and cooperative algorithms.

The term "cooperative phenomena" stems from physics and a typical example is the hexagonal pattern (Fig. 4.5) that emerges when water is heated from below, and the regions of upstream of warmer water and downstream of colder water are made visible.

Generally, the formation of a global pattern may be termed a *cooperative phenomenon,* if it arises by the interaction of a large number of similar "components". Moreover, the laws governing the interaction of these "components" should be "local", i.e., any given component should interact only with few other components; the laws should be the same for all components, and they should not contain the "symmetries" of the global pattern that evolves through the interactions.

4.7 On the other hand we may say that a cooperative algorithm is the organization of a complex task (e.g., formation of a complex pattern) into very few types of simpler tasks, each of which occurs very often in the diagram and is always connected in a typical way to other tasks (of the same type and also of other types).

In this respect one may say that a cooperative phenomenon is the physical realization of a cooperative algorithm at work, where the components are the physical realizations of the simple tasks.

Cooperative Phenomena

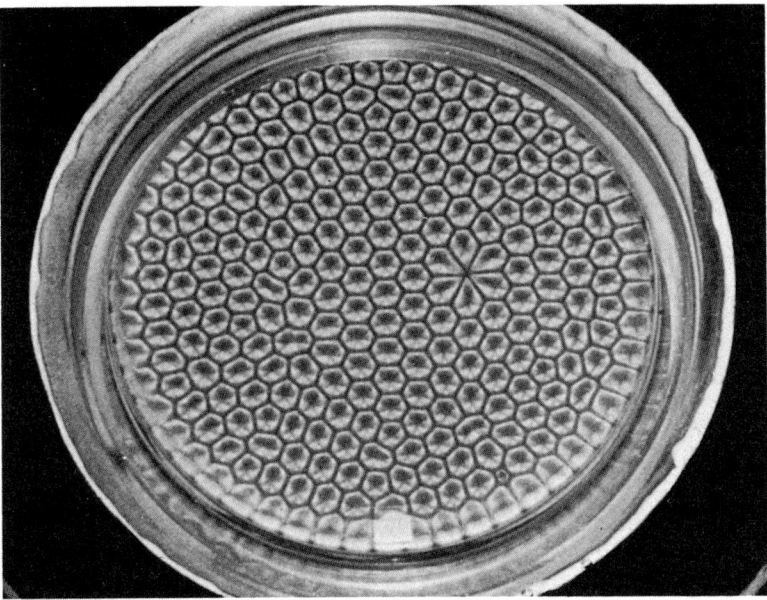

Fig. 4.5. Convection cells in silicone oil under an air surface. Visualization with aluminum powder. *Dark lines* indicate vertical motion; *bright areas* indicate predominantly horizontal motion

But there still is an important difference:

A cooperative algorithm has been *designed* to its task, therefore it is usually clear to which end it works. On the contrary, a cooperative phenomenon represents a hard problem to the physicist, because it is usually extremely difficult to predict the type of global pattern that will finally arise from the local interactions. This is implicit in the word "self-organization", and it is emphasized by the requirement that the laws governing the local interactions should *not* contain the symmetries of the arising global patterns.

5 The Improved Matchbox Algorithm

Dem Ingenieur ist nichts zu schwör. Daniel Düsentrieb

In this chapter we shall take up the "square engineering problem" posed at the end of Chapter 3. Namely, how to build a "well-behaving" machine in an economic way. Our first concern will be how to save "blueprint" in the description of this machine. In Chapter 7 we shall finally arrive at the question: of how many building blocks (i.e., neurons) are needed for such a machine.

In the last chapter we introduced the matchbox algorithm as an example of a cooperative algorithm, whose final performance can be predicted heuristically without any knowledge about the exact way leading to it. Indeed, in the long run the algorithm will never lose the game. The algorithm achieves this by slowly learning to perform a good move in every possible situation of the game. Obviously this comes close to what we would like to build into an organism:

We would like to save blueprint for building up a complicated behavior by using a comparatively simple cooperative algorithm to produce a machine performing that behavior. The matchbox algorithm is a simple cooperative algorithm that — given a valuation for situations — will learn to produce that kind of reaction in every situation, that finally leads to a "good" situation. Thus we only have to give the valuation, but this does not seem to be such a great problem, since we can argue that evolution has selected for those valuations, that define situations to be "good", if they are good for the survival and reproduction of the organism (or his genes).

Is a matchbox algorithm with an evaluation for situations developed by evolution, a realistic model for a learning animal — or perhaps even for a man?

There are some reasons why the behavior of such an algorithm would not qualify compared to learning animals or humans:

1. As I already pointed out, in the course of time the algorithm will pile up an enormous number of prepared matchboxes. In every situation it would have to search through this pile to find out whether that particular situation has occurred before. How can this be done fast enough if a fast reaction is necessary? Or can the searching be avoided altogether?
2. The learning of the matchbox algorithm is very slow, i.e., it takes too many losses until the algorithm starts to perform better.

How to Avoid Searching

3. Animals and humans can anticipate bad events in the near future and try to avoid them.
4. If a bad event has happened, the individual can perhaps trace further back for its "fault" that probably "caused" that event; in the analogous situation the matchbox algorithm can only change the very last decision before the loss.
5. An animal can transfer a solution it has arrived at in one situation to other "similar" situations.

In this chapter we try to find strategies that deal with these problems in such a way that we can incorporate them into a machine — in this case we shall try to incorporate these strategies into the matchbox algorithm.

5.1 *How to avoid searching* (1st problem). The problem is to store a large number of associations between situations and moves suggested for these situations. This can be done by accumulating a huge pile of "prepared matchboxes" as in our first description of the matchbox algorithm. But the appropriate type of memory for this problem would be a *mapping memory* (cf. Appendix 1): it yields a machine that works on its input, in this case the situation, and in a very short time yields the predescribed output, in this case the move or the list of moves.

How can such a mapping memory be built?

Let us say, we have to store a mapping associating to a number of situations the appropriate moves.

$$f: s_1 \mapsto m_1, s_2 \mapsto m_2, s_3 \mapsto m_3, \ldots, s_n \mapsto m_n$$

We may assume that the input information characterizing the situation is coded into a 0,1-sequence and the output information defining the move as well. Let us start with just one situation:

$$s_1 \mapsto m_1$$

The task is the following:
Given a situation s_1 and a move or lists of moves m_1 we have to construct a machine that works on the input s_1 and rapidly produces the output m_1.

Here is a possible machine for this: see Fig. 5.1.

The horizontal and vertical lines can be imagined as wires, the "connecting elements" c_{ij} between the i-th horizontal and j-th vertical wire work like this: at the beginning they give no connection, once there is a current (or voltage) in both lines the element can connect between, it does so. After that the connection remains constant.

To produce our mapping memory machine we just have to "apply" the patterns s_1 and m_1 to the matrix, i.e., set voltage to the horizontal

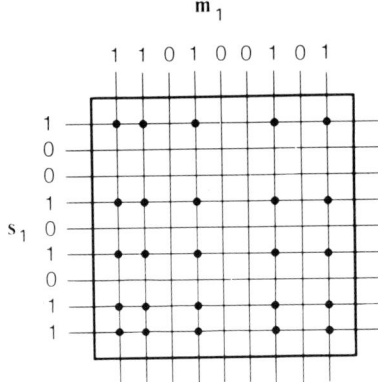

Fig. 5.1. Associative matrix memory. The *dots* represent the connections formed by storage of the pair (s_1, m_1)

lines that correspond to the 1s in s_1 and to the vertical lines that correspond to the 1s in m_1. After that the machine will immediately respond with m_1 on the vertical lines to the input s_1 on the horizontal lines. For a more detailed treatment of associative memories, see Appendix 1.

But what do we do with more than one pair of patterns to associate?

One way of solving this problem is to use a matrix for every pair. If we make sure that the inputs s_i are all coded into 0,1-sequences containing the same number of 1s — call it k —, and that the voltage or current or, more generally, the "strength of excitation" in the vertical output cables of the matrix reflects the number of horizontal input cables they are connected to, we can use the design shown in Fig. 5.2.

Clearly this mechanism would still work very fast. The main objection to this scheme is that we need too many elements to build up all these matrices.

Now one could try to save matrices by using the same matrix for more than one (s_i, m_j)-pair. This will still work out well for a few pairs per matrix, since we can get rid of interfering connections by using only those output lines that have a strength of excitation corresponding to k inputs. But if the number of (s, m)-pairs stored in such a matrix gets too high, the interferences between different pairs of patterns can get serious enough to produce errors, i.e., the machine can only tell that the predescribed output m was one of several equally possible ones, say, $m_1, \ldots, m_n$. In this case it is still possible to estimate the severity of such errors by calculating the average information per (s, m)-pair stored in such a matrix about the correct output m.

The results are rather encouraging: in an association matrix built from x storage elements (switches between horizontal and vertical wires), about 2/3 x bits can be stored (for large x) (cf. Palm 1980).

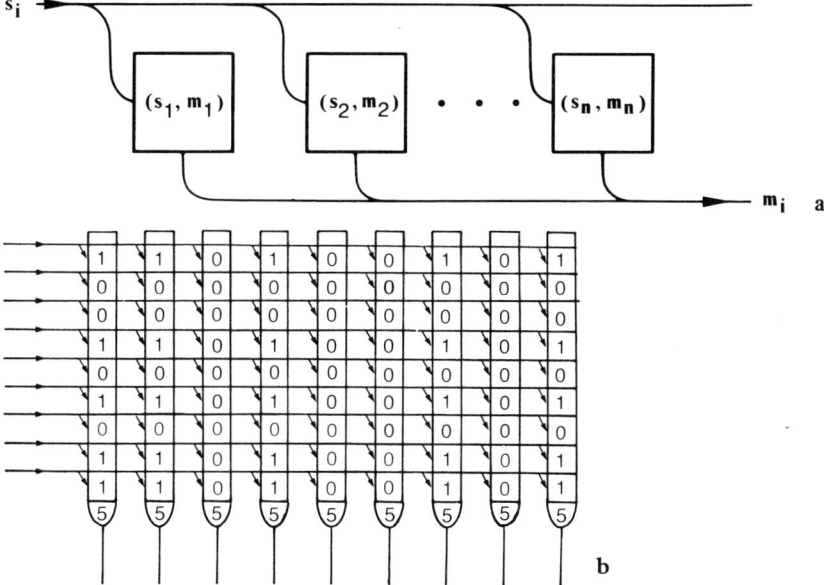

Fig. 5.2. a Each matrix can be realized as in **b. b** The matrix for (s_1, m_1) corresponding to Fig. 5.1. The "vertical wires" of Fig. 5.1 are realized as threshold neurons (Fig. 3.4) with threshold k (= 5). The weights correspond to the dots of Fig. 5.1

5.2 *How to speed up learning* (2nd problem). The algorithm can be improved by the strategies described in (3) (4) and (5), and I think this will be enough.

5.3 *How to anticipate* (3rd problem). For game-playing machines there is an obvious way of looking ahead a number of moves. It is called the *Minimax-Algorithm* and it is used for example in the little chess-playing machines sold today.

Let us say the machine has to look ahead three full-moves (a full-move consists of one move of the machine and one move of the opponent, which are therefore sometimes called half-moves). Then it can proceed as follows:

Pick any possible move, perform it, pick any possible move for the opponent in the resulting situation, perform it, do this again for two more times. This yields one possible situation three moves ahead. Evaluate this situation (using a predescribed evaluation, such as adding the values of the machine's pieces and subtracting the values of the opponent's pieces in simple chess machines) (see Fig. 5.3).

Then pick another possible move in the previous situation and evaluate again the resulting situation (see Fig. 5.4).

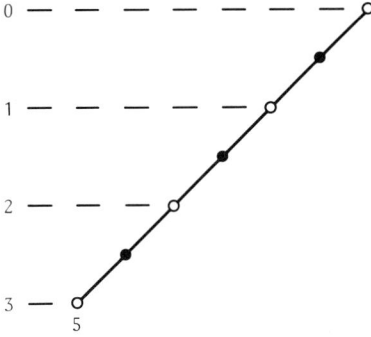

Fig. 5.3. Evaluation of a certain position, 3 moves ahead (depth 3), yields the value +5. *White dots* indicate positions where it is the machine's move, *black dots* indicate positions where it is the opponent's move

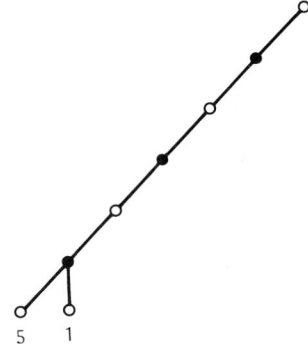

Fig. 5.4

If the last move you have just changed is the opponent's move, remember the lower of the two values. This is reasonable, since the opponent will prefer to carry out the move yielding the lower value for the machine.

If the last move you have just changed is your own move, remember the higher of the two values.

In this way try out all possibilities and assign the resulting value to the previous situation (Fig. 5.5).

Then the same is done for the previous situation again, i.e., we now start to vary and evaluate the possible moves in the situation two full-moves ahead (Fig. 5.6).

In our example now the maximum value has to be taken (see Fig. 5.7).

In this way every possibility is checked until we obtain an evaluation for the situation at hand (depth 0) together with a sequence of best moves realizing it.

This simple procedure again has a number of drawbacks. First of all it is very time-consuming to check all the possibilities up to a certain depth. One can, however, speed it up considerably by the method of "pruning" (cf. Samuel 1967). For example in Fig. 5.8 it is clear that the value of the situation at arrow a does not exceed 0, thus in comparison with the situation of arrow b we will have to remember the higher of the two values, i.e., 1.

Thus it is not necessary to try all the other possibilities in that situation (arrow a). The move leading to b is anyway better than the move leading to a. The same type of arguing also applies higher up in the search tree, i.e., at lower depth (see Fig. 5.9).

How to Anticipate

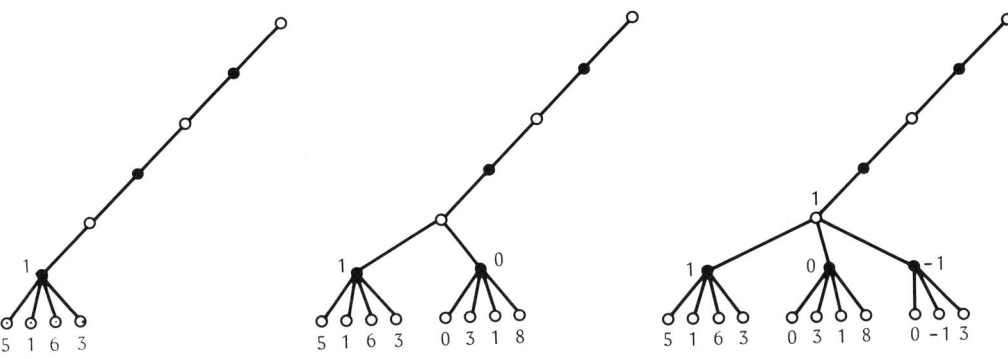

Fig. 5.5. All moves of the opponent have been tried and evaluated (values *5, 1, 6, 3*) and the resulting value (the minimum) has been assigned to the previous situation (5 half-moves ahead)

Fig. 5.6

Fig. 5.7. In the situation two full-moves ahead (depth 2), three moves are possible for the machine, with the values 1, 0, −1. The maximum 1 has been assigned to this situation

Here the computer need not try other possibilities for his move in situation a, since the one tried already shows that the value of situation a is at least 1. Thus the opponent might as well (or better) perform the move leading to position b with value 1.

In a particular case the pruned tree might finally look like Fig. 5.10.

Obviously the pruning cuts down the search tree further, if we manage to try the best moves in every situation first.

Thus it would be helpful to develop intuitive ideas as to which moves are probably good in a given situation. In the matchbox analogy we would make our way through the search tree using the matchboxes for generating the moves in the order of the sheets of paper inside. In this case a proper ordering of these sheets of paper could speed up the search considerably.

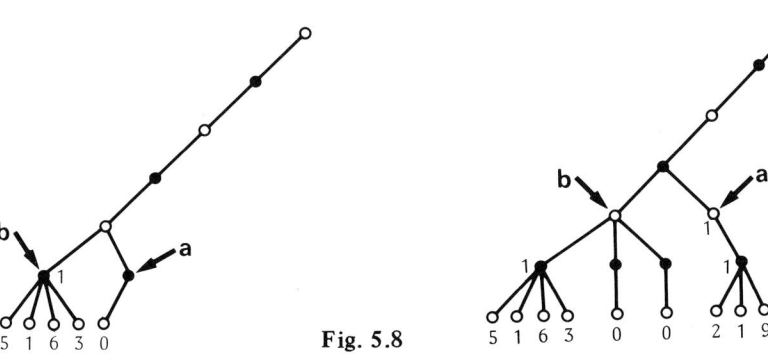

Fig. 5.8

Fig. 5.9

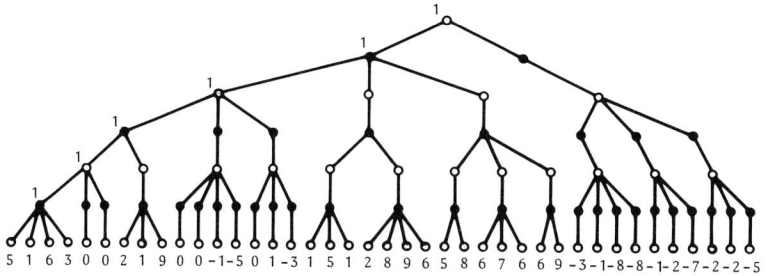
Fig. 5.10

Moreover, this making use of the same matchboxes during search and play would considerably speed up the learning of the matchbox algorithm, since now we can also take out of the boxes the moves leading to hopeless situations (i.e., empty boxes) that occur during the search and not in the actual game. This, by the way, already partially solves the fourth problem.

5.4 *How to trace back* (4th problem). One may be tempted to argue that in view of the prediction algorithm, backtracing is not important anymore, since the evaluation of a predicted future situation can be associated to the situation at hand and to the move leading to it, already during prediction. We do not have to wait for this situation to occur. But even so, eventually, unfavorable situations do occure (or become inexcapable) and then it may be reasonable to trace back for the reason for it. Apart from the above, a more detailed discussion of this problem is postponed to Section 13.10.

5.5 *How to use similarities and analogies* (5th problem). After our discussion of the minimax searching and especially the pruning algorithm the use of analogies seems to be even more important, since now the look-ahead-algorithm can be viewed in quite a different way:

1. We have a criterion for the "goodness" of situations (evaluation).
2. We have a criterion by which we can order the possible moves in a given situation — the comparatively better moves first. I will call this "urgentness" of moves.

This criterion can in particular be used to generate the most probable (or most urgent) move in any situation. Then we let the present situation evolve in the most probable way for a number of moves and evaluate the resulting situation.

This value can be corrected by checking less probable off-roads, the general tendency being to try more alternative moves on the part of the opponent if the value is higher, and to try more alternative moves on the

How to Anticipate 43

computer's part if the value is lower. The better the criteria for "goodness" and "urgentness", the less is the required deepness of search and the need for rechecking the "most probable" prediction.

Thus one should try to use analogies especially to develop good criteria for "goodness" of situations and "urgentness" of moves.

If we use an associative matrix memory (Fig. 5.1) to associate to a situation not only a list of possible moves, but also values for their respective urgentness and a value for the goodness of the whole situation, we can perhaps do this.

I have mentioned that a correlation matrix can sometimes produce "errors" in the sense that it sometimes may not distinguish between two situations, and thus may mix up the codings for the corresponding moves. This occurs only if many (s,m)-pairs are stored in the same matrix, and most easily between two situations, that are very "similar" in the sense that their codings into 0,1-sequences differ only in a few places.

If we could invent an input-output coding such that similar input 0,1-sequences correspond to situations similar in the sense that they have a similar value and a similar list of urgent moves – or, more generally, that they lead to a similar output 0,1-sequence, then the failure of the matrix to distinguish between some inputs could be regarded as prediction by analogy.

Therefore, an intelligent input-output coding is very important, and probably crucial for a reasonable performance of a learning machine based an a correlation matrix.

But of course such an intelligent input-output coding requires some insight into the nature of the game, which can be quite difficult to obtain.

5.6 By inventing additional algorithms for the problems listed at the beginning of this chapter, we have obtained quite a different picture of the matchbox algorithm. It can now predict the future from familiar situations and transfer bad experiences to analogous situations in an associative way. This is achieved by an additional look-ahead algorithm and the use of correlation matrices instead of matchboxes.

The additional notions of "pruning" and "urgentness" provide further advantages. For example, in chess-playing machines, that use the minimax algorithm for a fixed depth, people have discovered the problem of the "horizon effect": If the computer cannot avoid a big drop in the evaluation function during the next few moves, but can delay it beyond the fixed depth of analysis, for example by admitting smaller drops at first, it will do so.

In other words: the computer will try to delay a loss beyond its fixed "horizon", although often this strategy results in an even bigger loss a few moves later.

By the concept of "urgency" this fallacy can be avoided. We could imagine the urgency-value to be given by a number; then we could require that after a certain depth the prediction may only be stopped, if in the next whole-move the (two) most urgent moves for both opponents have a sufficiently low urgency. In this case the computer could never, for example, delay the capturing of his queen beyond the horizon.

Moreover, the notions of "pruning" and "urgentness" have turned the picture of the look-ahead algorithm from a complete search, trial-and-error minimax algorithm more to an algorithm of modified "most probable" prediction. This is even more reasonable, if one is not dealing with a chess-playing machine but with an animal.

For an animal the part of the opponent is played by nature, and it may be more reasonable to use a most-probable prediction (compared to a worst-case prediction as in the proper minimax algorithm) on the part of nature. In this case one would only have to check less "urgent" alternatives on one's own part, not on the opponent's part.

In summary, we have incorporated basically two new ideas into the matchbox algorithm of Chapter 4: the use of associative matrix memories and the minimax look-ahead algorithm. This has resulted in an algorithm quite different from the naive original matchbox algorithm. This improved matchbox algorithm will now be taken as a model for the organization of a learning animal, and will be called the *survival algorithm* in this context. In the next chapter this crucial step is discussed.

6 The Survival Algorithm as a Model of an Animal

> *I am never content until I have constructed a mechanical model of the subject I am studying. If I succed in making one, I understand; otherwise I do not.*
>
> Lord Kelvin

Can the improved matchbox algorithm (constructed in the last chapter) be taken seriously as a model for a learning animal? The algorithm has been introduced as a simple example for a cooperative type of mechanism, where the final goal it will attain is intuitively clear, although the detailed way to that goal is impossible to predict.

Then it has been improved to learn faster and to avoid immediate fallacies. In the final presentation of the algorithm in the last chapter it could indeed be imagined to "behave" very much like a simple learning animal.

We have already noted that the problem solved by the matchbox algorithm, namely to find fairly good moves in every situation it gets into during actual play, is quite analogous to the problem solved by animals. In this case the criteria for "good" moves are defined genetically, since during evolution genes have developed that program their organism to survive and proliferate them as efficiently as possible. How such a statement can be explained on purely physical grounds is very well illustrated by the book of Dawkins (1976).

From now on we shall use the improved matchbox algorithm in this behavioral context. In this context I shall address it as the *survival algorithm*.

That this kind of algorithm as applied to the game of checkers really can show a quite intelligent behavior was illustrated by Samuel (1959), who actually built a similar machine. This machine was able to beat its constructor after some learning.

In the following we shall try to find criteria for comparing the improved matchbox algorithm in more detail with the working of the human brain — or perhaps at first with the brain of a higher mammal like a cat, a monkey, or a camel.

To do this, we will have to specify many of the details of that algorithm, although it often may be clear that alternative specifications are nearly equally possible. For example, we have to get a more detailed image of the processing of input and output, of the way the associative prediction and evaluation of situations is actually carried out, how the learning — i.e., throwing bad moves out of the corresponding matchboxes — is actually implemented as a change in the prediction and/or evaluation.

Then we have to specify how all these mechanisms are built into the brain — to a certain degree of accuracy we should be able to say what is done where. The next chapter is devoted to these specifications.

Only after that will we be able to compare the algorithm with the huge body of knowledge about our brain that has accumulated

1. by introspection,
2. by measurements on the total input-output behavior of animals and people,
3. by measurements of the electrical activity of single neurons and of the mass-activity on the brain surface,
4. by inspecting the anatomical arrangement and shape of neurons,
5. by analyzing the chemical composition of parts of the brain,
6. by clinical observations, which usually correlate some abnormal kind of behavior with some irregularities in the "hardware", for example, parts of the brain may be missing or look differently, or have an unusual chemical composition; more generally, clinical experiences suggest correlations between changes in 4,5 and changes in 1,2,3,
7. by investigating changes in 1,2,3,4 following artifical manipulations of animals' brains (deprivation, lesions, chemical injections).

It is plainly impossible to get an overview of all the information that has accumulated in hundreds of journals over many decades. I think it will even be impossible for me to mention everything I have learned concerning the brain in a few years. Therefore I will follow a different strategy:

I will use the necessary specifications of the survival algorithm — taken as a model for the brain — as a guideline for the presentation of facts about the brain (in Chaps. 8, 9, and 10). This does not mean that I am going to search through the literature for facts that "fit the model"; on the contrary, perhaps even a fair and unbiased overview of the results in any one of the fields (1–7) listed above cannot be done without the light of some kind of theory.

6.1 For introspection (1) this is obvious: here it seems nearly impossible to separate facts and theories.

6.2 As far as behavioral or psychophysical experiments (2) are concerned: here at first it may seem possible just to make a lot of observations without any modeling. It quickly turns out, however, that there is such a huge number of possibilities to make experiments, that one has to concentrate

Electrophysiology 47

on certain questions, which are usually derived from models —although these models often are quite superficial phenomenological ones.

Thus theories are very important in this field; this is witnessed by nearly every book on experimental psychology. The fact that theories are important for the choice and also the reception of experiments is equally true for the other fields yet to be mentioned.

6.3 Concerning electrophysiology (3): As for the electrical activity of single neurons, the need for a theory has probably already become clear in this field of research.

Here experimenters typically stick to clear-cut input and output areas of the brain, where the activity of a single neuron can be correlated with events in the outside world. For example, in a sensory area one can try to find that sensory stimulus, to which the neuron responds "best" (this usually means with highest spike frequency). Here one abstraction can be made offhand:

The neuron is regarded as a "detector" for that stimulus (cf. Lettvin et al. 1959).

One could then build detectors for more complicated stimuli from detectors for simpler stimuli — until one finally gets the well-known (but, of course, fictive) "grandmother detectors". But how many different detectors or neurons for how many different objects do we need? How rarely will those specialized neurons be active? What do we do with these neurons, i.e., how do we connect them to the output neurons whose activity is for example correlated to a particular limb movement?

These questions merely indicate that the "theory" of a neuron as a detector of something is not enough (see also John 1972). Electrophysiology, especially if carried out outside the primary input and output areas, needs a theory!

As for the electrical activity on the surface of the brain (EEG, evoked potentials), these measurements can be used in two ways:

a) As a superposition of single neuron activities they can be used as an additional source of information about the electrical activity of all the single neurons contributing to surface potentials. In this case theories are needed in the same way as in single neuron studies; moreover, there is a need for a physical theory that can to some degree of accuracy predict how the activity of single neurons is really combined to form a surface activity.

b) They can be used in a correlative way in cases of dysfunction, i.e., in (6) and (7).

6.4 Concerning anatomy (4): Of course, it is possible just to describe the shape of "regions" and neurons within the brain. But if one interprets information on the shape and arrangement of neurons, as information on the connectivity of the actual neuronal network in the brain, one immediately starts to look for implications of the shape of neurons concerning their function; and this requires some theory.

6.5 Chemical analysis (5) is mainly used in connection with clinical observations (6) and artificial manipulations (7).

As for (6) and (7): Experiences of correlation between abnormalities in behavior and anatomical or biochemical abnormalities have been assembled for many years for clinical use without any obvious immediate need for theory-building. But since the refined techniques of measuring and experimenting in psychology have gone hand-in-hand with some theory-building, theories clearly play a role in analyzing these correlations. Moreover, even the correct documentation of these correlations requires some theoretical thinking, besides a profound knowledge of all the fields of research involved, (1)–(5).

6.6 This has become particularly obvious in the study of cortical lesions (see for example Lashley 1931, 1950, Sperry 1947, Luria 1973, Doty 1973) where – apart from primary sensory and motor regions – it usually turned out to be impossible to define the function that is performed in any brain region in a simple way. The reason for this seems to be that we cannot find the right terms in which to define "function", as long as we do not ask how such a function may be performed. For example the terms used in the figure in the Introduction have turned out not to be the right terms.

Already the early experiments of Lashley suggested that a particular content of an animal's memory cannot be located in a particular part of the brain, i.e., the contents of memory are somehow stored in a distributed way, all over the brain. Thus – apart from primary areas – brain lesions seem to have no clear-cut effect on the performance of learned tasks: the memory just seems to get worse diffusely, in proportion only to the cortex volume that has been removed. This feature, by the way, especially seems to call for an explanation in terms of associative memory. It also shows the immense flexibility of the mammalian brain in recovering from lesions.

7 Specifying the Survival Algorithm

> *Like objects, placed in like circumstances, will always produce like effects.*
> D. Hume, 1739

In this chapter I shall provide some possible specifications of details of the survival algorithm, in order to see whether these specifications fit with known data on real brains.

7.1 *Input-output coding.* As mentioned in Chapter 5, coding should be done in such a way that similar situations, as well as similar actions, are coded similarly. Here the meaning of similarity for the coded 0-1 sequences is obvious, whereas the meaning of similarity for acts and situations requires knowledge about the "world outside" or the "rules of the game": In any case the following statements should be true for the notion of similarity:

1. Similar acts lead in similar situations to similar situations.
2. Similar situations, if evaluated, get a similar value.

To build up the appropriate pre- and postprocessing, i.e., the appropriate similarities, in the coded 0-1 sequences is a very complicated problem. The long process of evolution has led to reasonable solutions of this problem, for example in the preprocessing of sensory inputs to the cerebral cortex.

This task can be analyzed in its own right. The analysis must involve
a) accumulating relevant knowledge about our world,
b) inventing algorithms for perception of objects and performance of simple actions that make use of this knowledge,
c) seeing what kind of algorithms are realized in the wiring of animals.

Of course, this kind of analysis is very important, and it is actually carried out in many laboratories today, by scientists working in the fields of artificial intelligence, psychophysics, electrophysiology, and also anatomy.

It is, however, not the main object of this book to expand extensively on these more peripheral problems. The interested reader should rather consult for example Winston (1975, 1977) or Marr (1981) for the artificial intelligence approach to input coding.

Some facts concerning (c) will be briefly presented in Chapter 9.

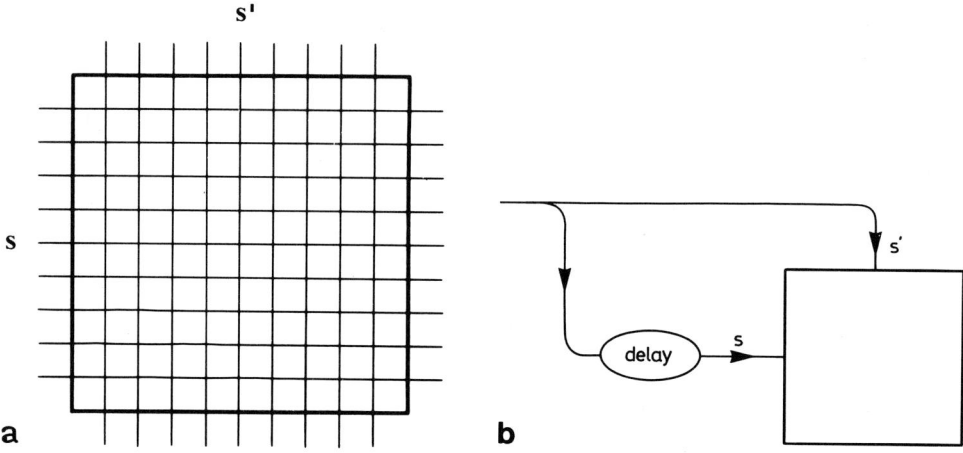

Fig. 7.1a,b. A situation s is associated with the next situation s' by the mechanism of Fig. 5.1

7.2 *Associative prediction.* Basically, we need a mapping m assigning to any situation s the "next" situation s'.

m: s → s'   or   m: $s_1 → s_2, s_2 → s_3, s_3 → s_4, \ldots$

and so on through life.

This can be done by the correlation matrix as in Fig. 7.1.

If we have stored in this way a long sequence of situations, we can re-run the whole sequence, if we provide additional feedback connections (see Fig. 7.2).

Now the storing as well as the read out can be done in a very simple way (Figs. 7.3, 7.4).

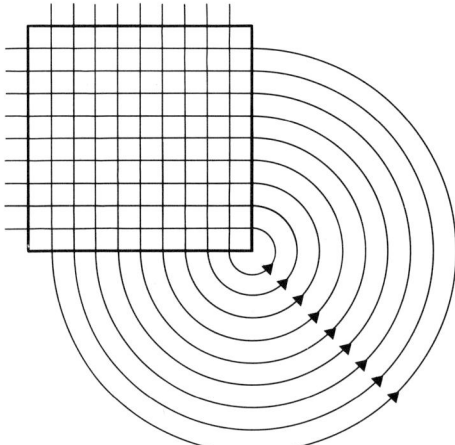

Fig. 7.2. The associative matrix of Fig. 7.1a with additional feedback connections

Associative Generation of Moves

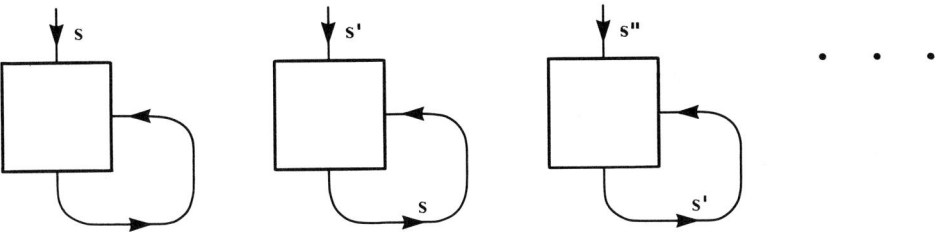

Fig. 7.3. Storing: at time t = 0 the situation *s* comes in; at time t = 1 the "next" situation *s'* comes in and is associated with s; at time t = 2 the "next" situation *s"* comes in and is associated with s', and so on

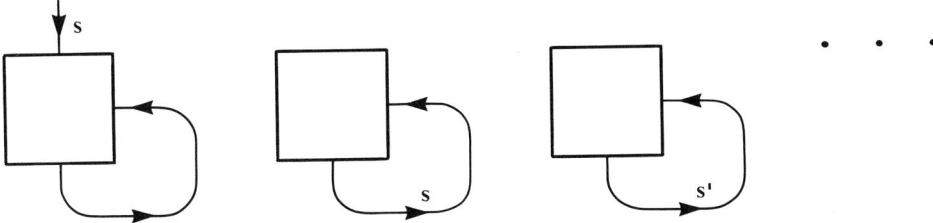

Fig. 7.4. Recall: through the connections formed during storing, the pattern *s* calls forth *s'*. s' calls forth s", and so on

In principle, the recall will only work correctly if in each situation the same move is always made. Remember that a "situation" is meant to represent everything on the basis of which the evolution for the future is determined. Thus in any short temporal sequence of situations there will usually be a large part of the corresponding patterns that remains constant and that can be said to represent the "context" in which that particular sequence takes place.

7.3 *Associative generation of moves and evaluation.* Here we need a mapping assigning to the input situation or *circumstances,* cs, the appropriate list of moves or *actions,* a, and their expected *values,* v:

m: cs ↦ (a,v).

Using a correlation matrix this can be done in the usual way (see Fig. 7.5).

It can, however, also be done differently, namely by associating the whole situation s = (cs,a,v) with itself (Fig. 7.6).

The readout in this case is done by *pattern completion* (as in Fig. 7.7).

If only the part cs (or any other sufficiently large part) of s = (cs,a,v) is fed into the matrix, the whole pattern s will emerge.

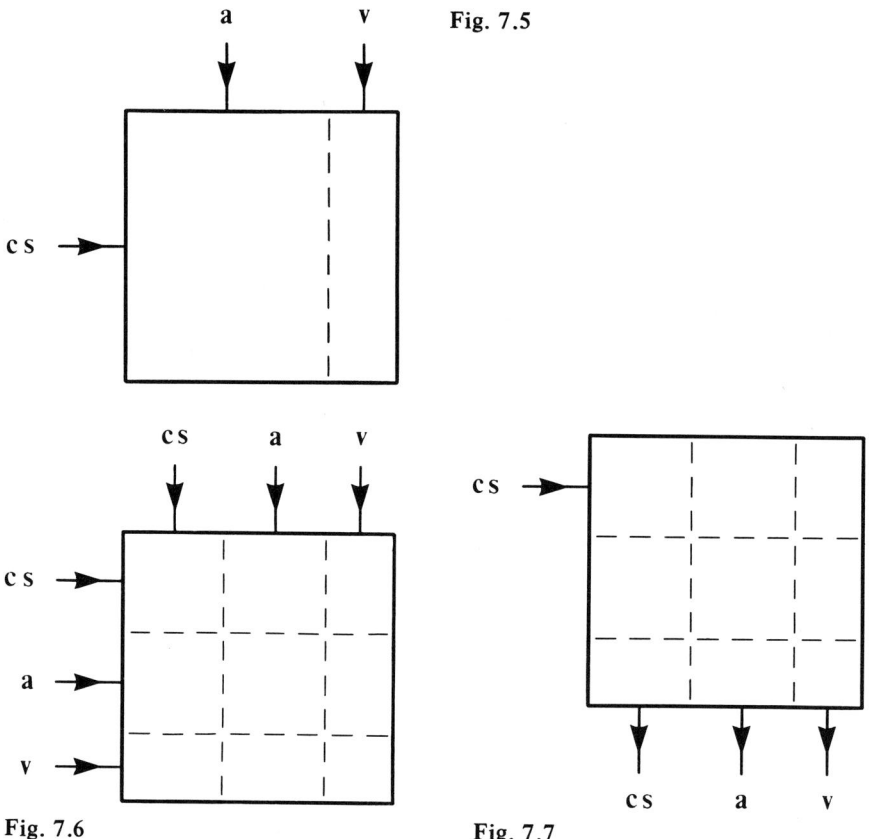

Fig. 7.5

Fig. 7.6   **Fig. 7.7**

Fig. 7.6. The pattern (cs,a,v) is associated with itself

Fig. 7.7. In this case cs is applied as an input to the horizontal lines of the matrix and the resulting output on the vertical lines is the whole pattern (cs,a,v)

For the pattern completion to work properly it should, of course, be required that no stored pattern be the completion of another stored pattern. Obviously this is another requirement on the preprocessing or input coding (see Sect. 7.1), which could simply be realized by having the same number of 1s in every proper input pattern (compare Chap. 5.1).

The duplication of the pattern s = (cs,a,v) which is required in Fig. 7.6 can be avoided by using the same feedback connections as in Section 7.2 (Fig. 7.8).

Here we only have to present the input (cs,a,v) at one side of the matrix, but just for a slightly longer time.

The recall procedure is shown in Fig. 7.9.

Changes in Prediction or Evaluation 53

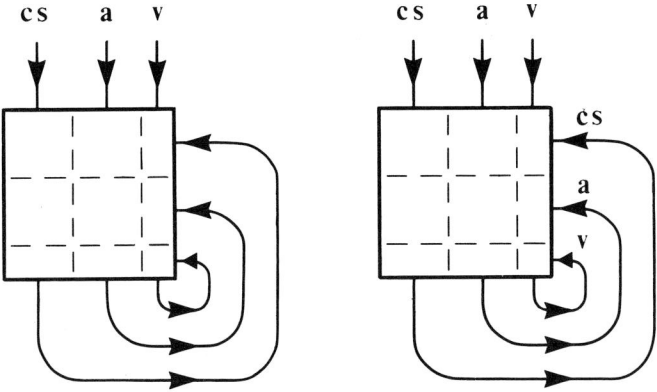

Fig. 7.8. (*cs,a,v*) is applied as an input to the vertical lines and — via the feedback connections — comes back into the matrix along the horizontal lines. If the input (cs,a,v) to the vertical lines is held fixed until this moment, an association of (cs,a,v) with itself can be performed

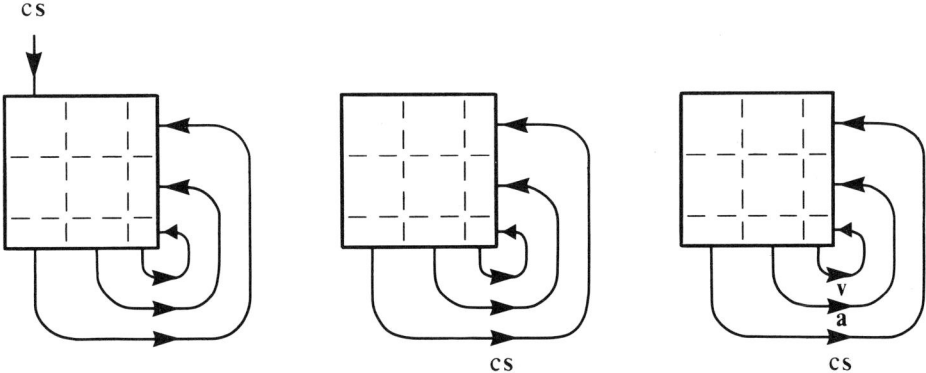

Fig. 7.9. *cs* is applied to the vertical lines, comes back in along the horizontal lines and yields the full output pattern (*cs,a,v*) by the previously formed association of (cs,a,v) with itself

7.4 *Changes in prediction or evaluation.* These are performed by using just the "storage" procedure of Sections 7.2 and 7.3. This will, of course, not immediately replace the new information by the old one, but yield a mixture of both at first. If the storing of the new association cs → (a,v) or (cs,a,v) is repeated for some time, it will completely overwrite the old association.

To this end it would be necessary to have a mechanism that can "hold" a situation or pattern for a variable extended time in order to present it for a variable time to the matrix in the learning phase (cf. Fig. 7.8).

Since Sections 7.2 and 7.3 can be done with essentially the same arrangement of a feedback matrix, it seems possible that they can be done in one and the same matrix. This indeed seems to be possible, although there are reasons to use different matrices for the processes of prediction and evaluation. I will come back to this problem in Chapters 11 and 13.

7.5 Finally I want to discuss the possibility of realizing all these mechanisms by using neurons as building blocks. This will turn up several experimental questions that may help in guiding the reader's interest through the next chapters.

The matchbox algorithm itself is logically very simple. The same is true for the look-ahead algorithm, although this algorithm needs a short-time storing of evaluations obtained at intermediate steps, of possibilities that have already been checked, etc. (see also Digression 5). This storing can probably be done by a mechanism for "holding" some information for a variable, but rather short time. Remember that such a mechanism was also needed for the mechanism of Fig. 7.8.

We have shown (in Chap. 3) that any kind of predescribed input-output behavior can be performed by an appropriate network of threshold neurons. Thus the simple logic of the two algorithms can easily be performed by a neuron network, which will probably take comparatively few neurons. The bulk of the neurons will probably have to be used for the various storing tasks:

1. We need one — or several — network(s), that can "hold" a pattern. One way of achieving this, is to use the mechanism of Figs. 7.8 and 7.9 for pattern completion, i.e., a correlation matrix with feedback.
2. We need the associative evaluation, which can again be done by the mechanism of Figs. 7.8 and 7.9, i.e., by a correlation matrix with feedback.
3. We need the associative prediction, which can also be done by a feedback correlation matrix, as explained in Section 7.2.

Thus, apart from a small logical network and the appropriate input-output coding, we can do with a number of correlation matrices.

How can such a matrix be realized by neurons?

The basic idea of Fig. 7.10 is that the neurons are employed in the same way as the formal neurons in Fig. 5.2, with the important additional requirement that the excitatory synapses (which provide the "weights" in Fig. 5.2) change their effectivity (or strength) in a systematic way: coincident activity in the presynaptic axon and the postsynaptic dendrite must improve the effectivity of the synapse.

If we try to use Fig. 7.10 as a realization for Fig. 7.1, we have to be able to give two input patterns to the matrix in the learning phase, i.e, we need an additional input controlling the dendrites in Fig. 7.10: see Fig. 7.11.

In this scheme the synapses between the vertical axons and the vertical dendrites need not change in strength, and each of these axons would con-

Neural Realization

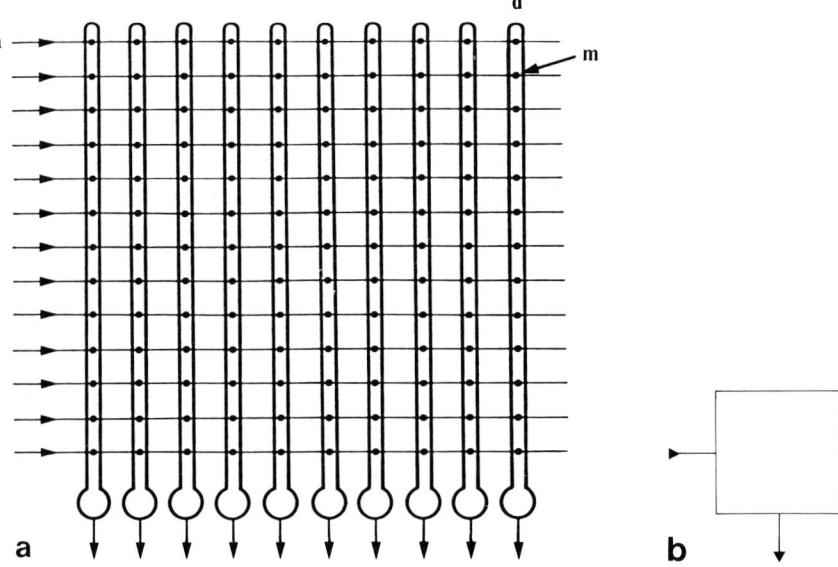

Fig. 7.10. a A schematic neuronal realization. *a* axon; *d* dendrite; *m* modifiable synapse. **b** shorthand for **a**

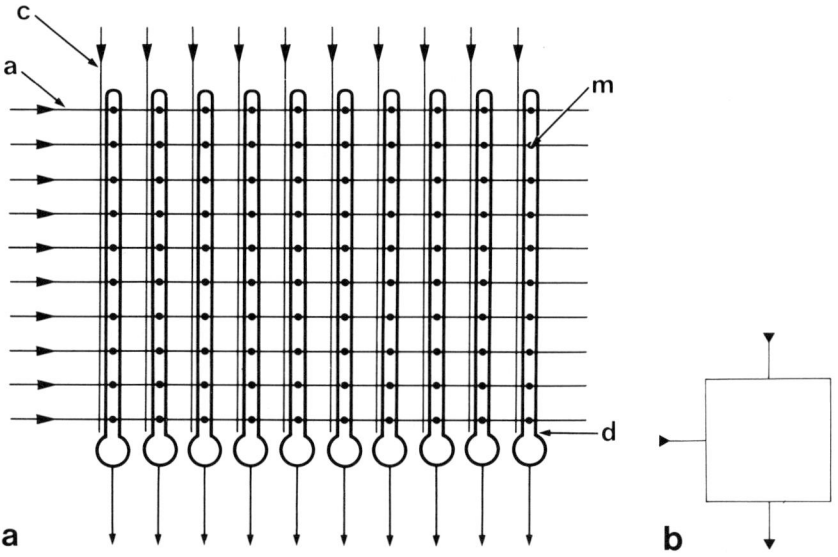

Fig. 7.11. a A schematic neuronal realization of Figs. 5.1 or 7.1. *a,c* axons; *d* dendrite; *m* modifiable synapse. **b** shorthand for **a**

trol a dendrite in a 1-to-1 fashion. This would imply a rather peculiar arrangement of axons and dendrites: the axons would have to run along the dendrites. Such an arrangement is only very rarely found in the brain, with one important exception: the climbing fibers of the cerebellum (Cajal 1911).

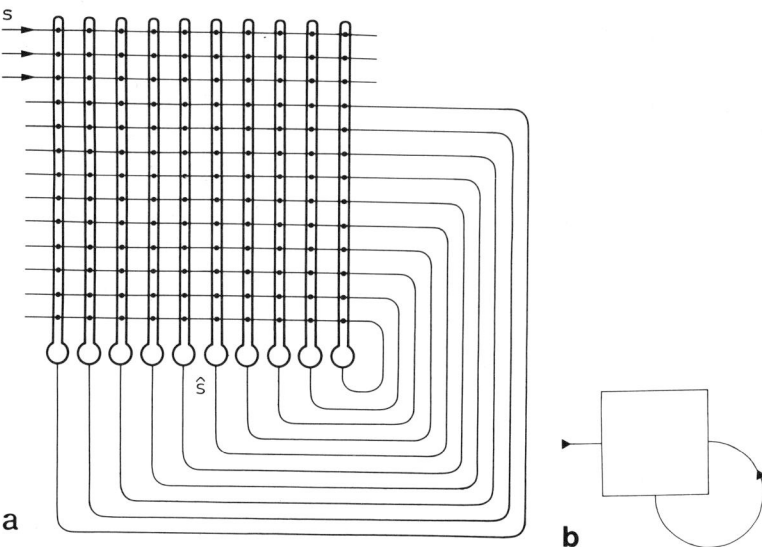

Fig. 7.12. a See text. **b** shorthand for **a**

The cerebellum occupies in men only a small volume of the brain and is mainly involved in output control.

Therefore we should look for another anatomically inconspicuous scheme for providing the vertical input in Fig. 7.11 and similarly in Figs. 7.3, 7.4, 7.8 and 7.9.

If we remember that in our schemes the input s is always assumed to be already preprocessed, i.e., that it is only a representation of the original input, we may as well have it processed through another mapping, yielding a different representation $\hat{s}$, as in Fig. 7.12.

One can now easily try out this scheme for the storing and readout paradigms of Figs. 7.8 and 7.9; I suggest this as an exercise to the reader.

The learning rule of the correlation matrix, applied to Figs. 7.11 and 7.12, requires that the strength of the synapses (i.e., connections) between the horizontal axons and the vertical dendrites increases due to common activity in the two. This rule for the modification of synaptic effectivity (or connectivity), was first formulated by Hebb (1949), and I shall call it *Hebb's rule*.

Since 1949 there have been many debates about this rule and similar *synaptic rules*. But it turned out to be very hard to verify or falsify the validity of such a rule, for example in the mammalian cortex (or in the cerebellum, but see Ito 1981). In Digression 4 I classify the simplest local synaptic rules. Concerning possible biophysical or biochemical mechanisms for synaptic modification, see for example Stent (1973), or Nathanson and Greengard (1977).

7.6 There is still quite a strong anatomically testable assumption in Fig. 7.12: taken strictly, it requires that a connection can be formed, if necessary, between any axon and any dendrite of the cells forming the matrix. Thus, if the matrix is formed of N neurons, there should be N^2 possible connections. From Palm (1980) we may take the result that in a well-filled matrix the number of actual connections should be around $\frac{1}{2} N^2$ (see also Appendix 1). Even if we take, say, $\frac{1}{10} N^2$ as a low estimate, we would be led to the conclusion that there are around 10^5 such matrices in our brain, each containing around 10^5 neurons, for only this high number of matrices could account for "only" $10^{14} = \frac{1}{10} (10^5)^2 \cdot 10^5$ synapses for $10^{10} = 10^5 \cdot 10^5$ neurons. On the other hand it is intuitively clear that the matchbox algorithm will need only a few such matrices, say 3 or 10 or so.

Moreover, if we have many such correlation matrices in the brain, we also need neuronal channels for the flow of information between these matrices. Such a channel has to consist of quite a large number of axons if it is to carry a reliable picture of the state of the matrix M to the matrix M'. The number of these connecting channels has to be at least as large as the number of matrices (it could well be three or five times as large, but it should not be much larger). Thus the total number of synapses needed for these channels will not be completely negligible.

Therefore one should ask to what degree the requirement of N^2 possible connections for N elements in the matrix can be relaxed? Clearly, it cannot be relaxed too far, since, after all, the point of forming such a correlation matrix is that it should be possible to detect any correlation. Thus the whole set of neurons forming such a matrix has to be "highly interconnected", but it is a severe mathematical problem what this should really mean. Some aspects of this problem are discussed in Appendix 4. For a random distribution of less than N^2 variable connections in an N x N matrix, I have obtained the following result (see Palm 1981a, and Appendix 1). If k switches are distributed at random in an N x N matrix (where $K < N^2$), and if this arrangement is used as an associative memory (cf. Chap. 5.1), then at least $\frac{1}{20}$ k bits can be stored (for large k). This is still an encouraging result (although it is worse than the result cited in Chap. 5.1), because it provides a simple strategy by which 10^{14} variable synapses can be used to store at least $5 \cdot 10^{12}$ bits. On the other hand, from Chap. 1.7 we may infer that we can maximally take up 40 bits of new information per second, i.e., about 10^{11} bits in 100 years.

These last problems that have occurred in our attempt to implement the improved matchbox algorithm in terms of neuronal networks will hopefully motivate the reader to learn some more detailed facts about real brains in the next section.

Part II

8 The Anatomy of the Cortical Connectivity

The cortex is an information mixing machine.   V. Braitenberg

8.1 You can get a first idea about the global organization of the human brain by inspecting it carefully (Fig. 8.1):

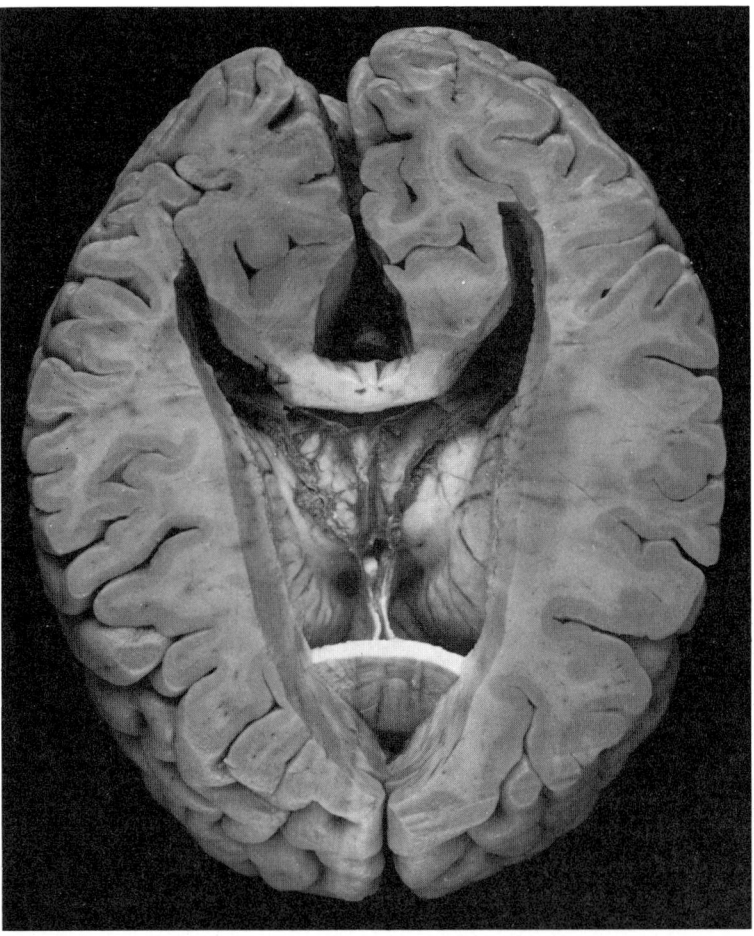

Fig. 8.1. Lower half of a human brain, cut horizontally (Gluhbegovic and Williams 198

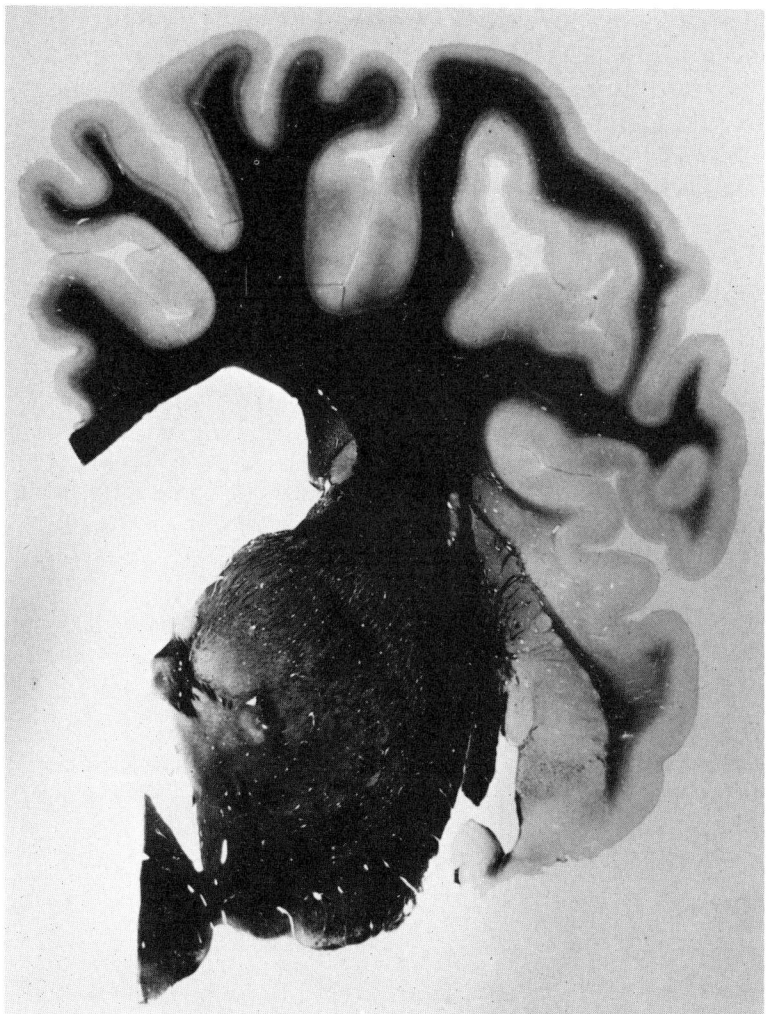

Fig. 8.2. Section through a cerebral hemisphere of an adult cow, stained for myelin. The darkest parts of the picture represent dense masses of myelinated fibers. (Courtesy V. Braitenberg)

With the naked eye you can distinguish lighter and darker regions: *White matter* and *grey matter*. The grey matter consists of a network of dendrites, axons, and cell bodies of nerve cells. The white matter consists of myelinated fibers which connect different regions of the brain with each other and with sense organs and muscles. This distinction between grey and white matter (shown as grey and black in the myelin-stained brain section – Fig. 8.2) provides a natural organization of the brain into processing units of grey matter and their connections through white matter.

The cerebral cortex forms the surface of the brain and I am told by comparative anatomists that it is also the "newest" part of the brain. In the following we shall distinguish between cortical and subcortical regions of the brain: the main connections between the cortex and subcortical structures have been sketched in Fig. 1.3.

The two cortices (right and left) are the two largest continuous portions of grey matter. Together they make up about half of the brain's volume.

Due to the abundance of cortico-cortical fibers (cf. Table 1.1) the cortex seems to work mainly on its own output. Therefore, it seems to be the only part of the brain that defies description as a mere relay station. Most loops of connections inside the brain occur in the cortex.

8.2 The speculations of the last paragraph suggest that one looks exactly for a large, highly connected part of the brain as the possible location for the postulated correlative memories. Therefore we will now have a closer look at the cerebral cortex.

If we imagine the cortex of both hemispheres flattened out, we obtain the following schematic picture (Fig. 8.3):

Table 8.1 gives estimates of the "strength" of the connections drawn in Fig. 8.3.

Each of the two pancakes has a surface of about 800 cm², which corresponds to a radius of 16 cm, a volume of about 200 cm³, and a highly varying thickness around 2–3 mm.

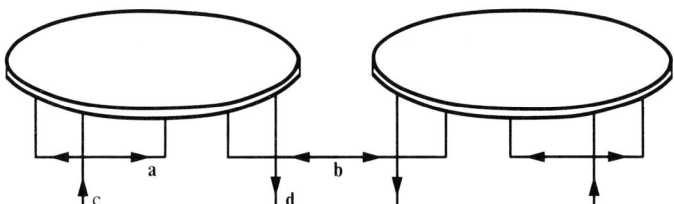

Fig. 8.3. Cf. Table 8.1

Table 8.1. Estimated number of fibers in the connections of Fig. 8.3

a		$5 \cdot 10^9$
b		$2 \cdot 10^8$
c	Olfactory input	10^7
	sensory input	10^6
	all input	10^8
d	Motor output	10^6
	all output	10^8

Layers 63

Inside each pancake, in spite of some local variation, the organization is surprisingly uniform: the cells are arranged in horizontal layers (see Fig. 8.4).

There are two main types of cells:

1. Pyramidal cells (Fig. 8.5): They always have spines on their dendrites and their dendritic tree can be split into apical dendrites (which usually reach up into the first layer), and basal dendrites. Their axon gives off collaterals into the grey matter, but one branch always leaves the grey matter and enters the white matter. There is a considerable variation in the size of pyramidal cells, as indicated in Fig. 8.5b.

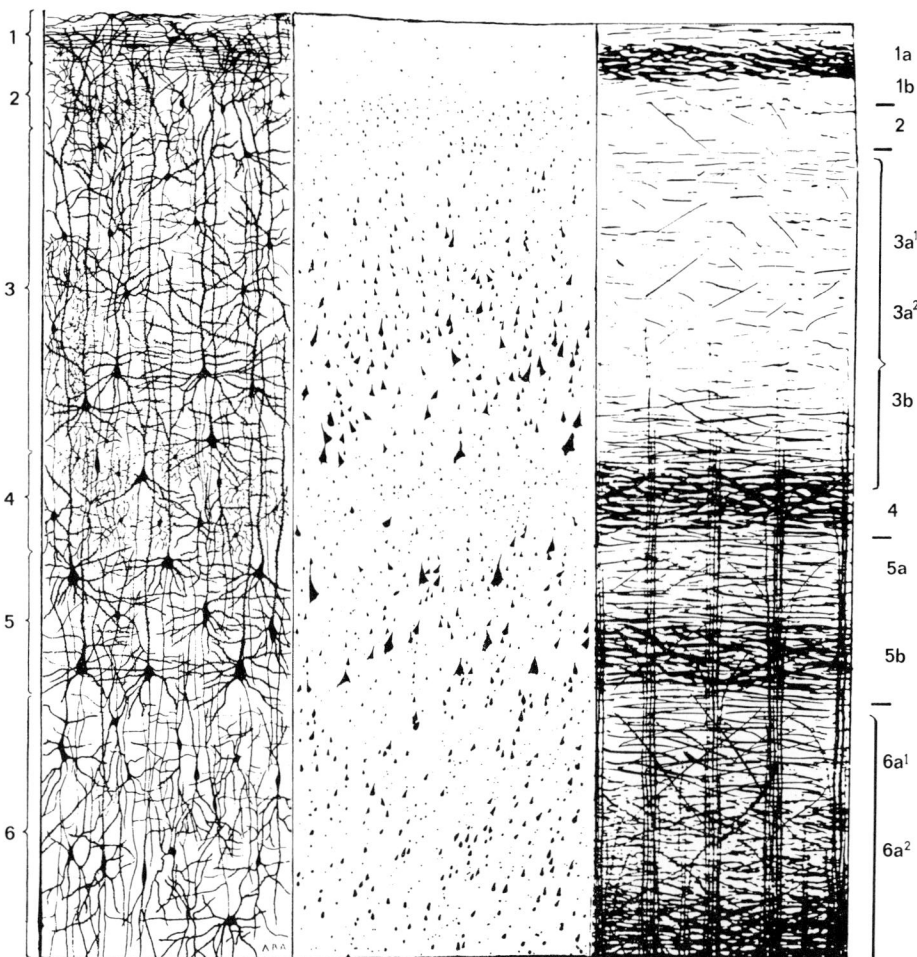

Fig. 8.4. a Distribution of cells and myelinated filters in different layers of the cortex (I–VI) (Carpenter 1976)

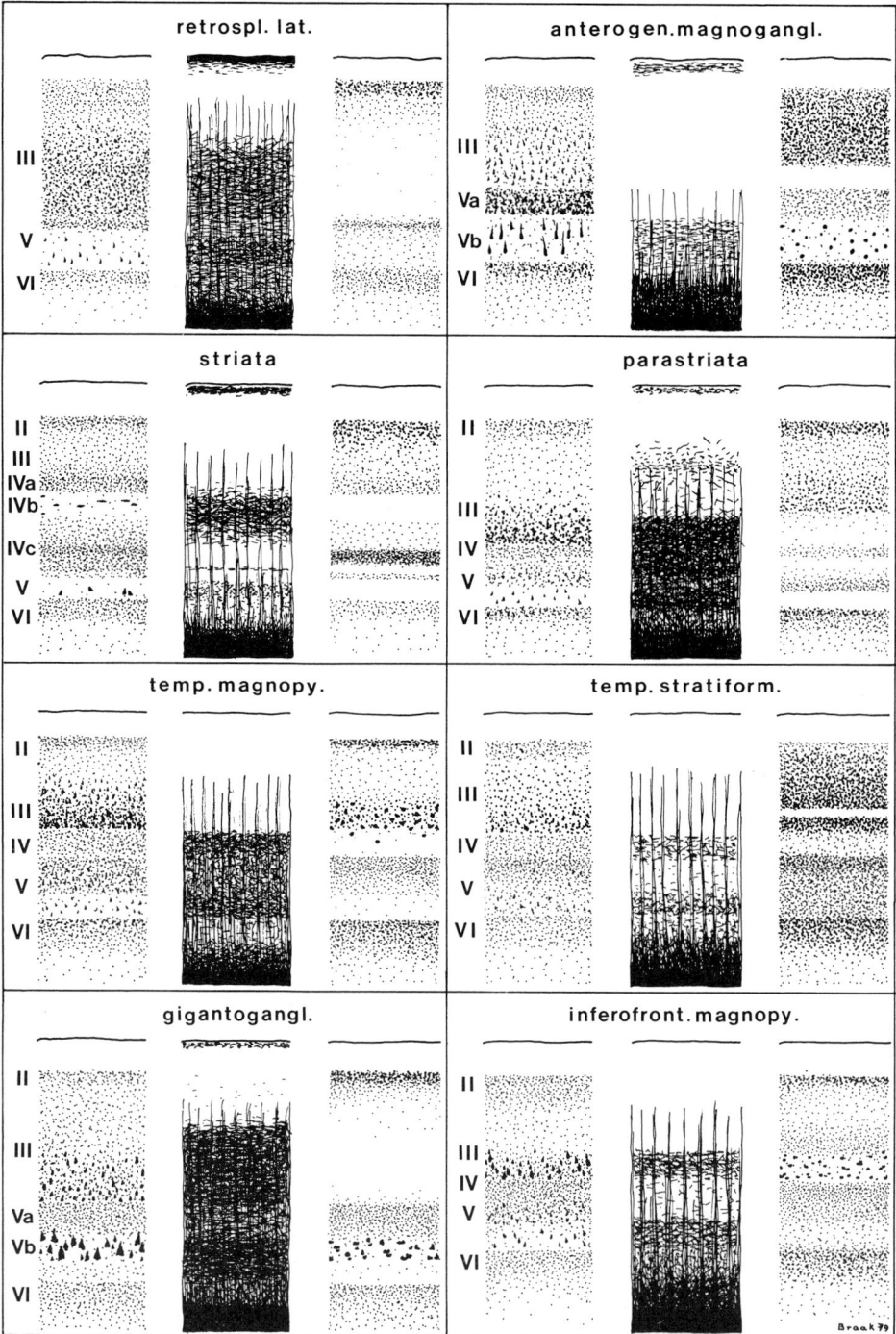

Fig. 8.4b Variations of the histological picture (Nissl, myelin, and pigment preparation) in different areas of the cortex (Braak 1980)

Cell Types

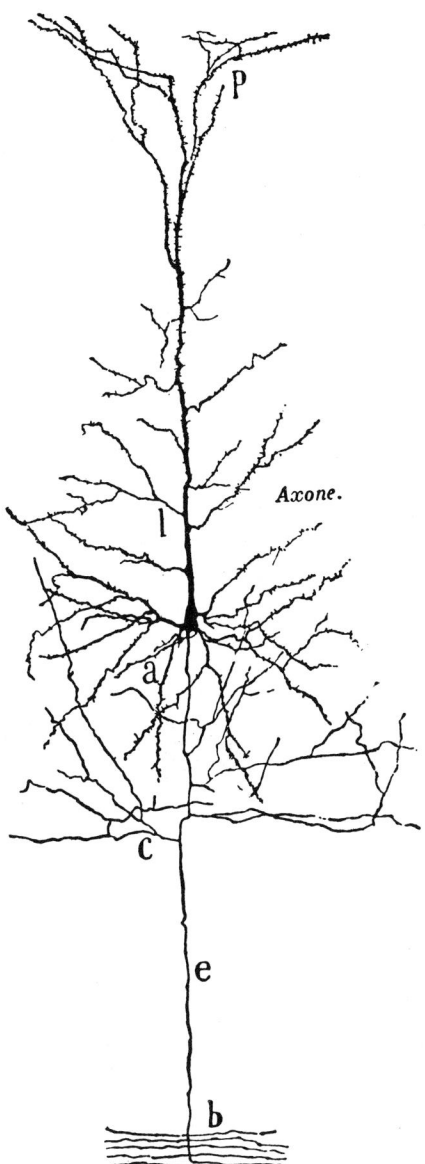

Fig. 8.5. a A pyramidal cell of the cerebral cortex. (Cajal 1911). The axoncollaterals are not shown in full length (cf. **b**). **b** Two pyramidal cells injected with horseradish peroxydase (Gilbert and Wiesel 1979). (The figures on the *left* define the layers)

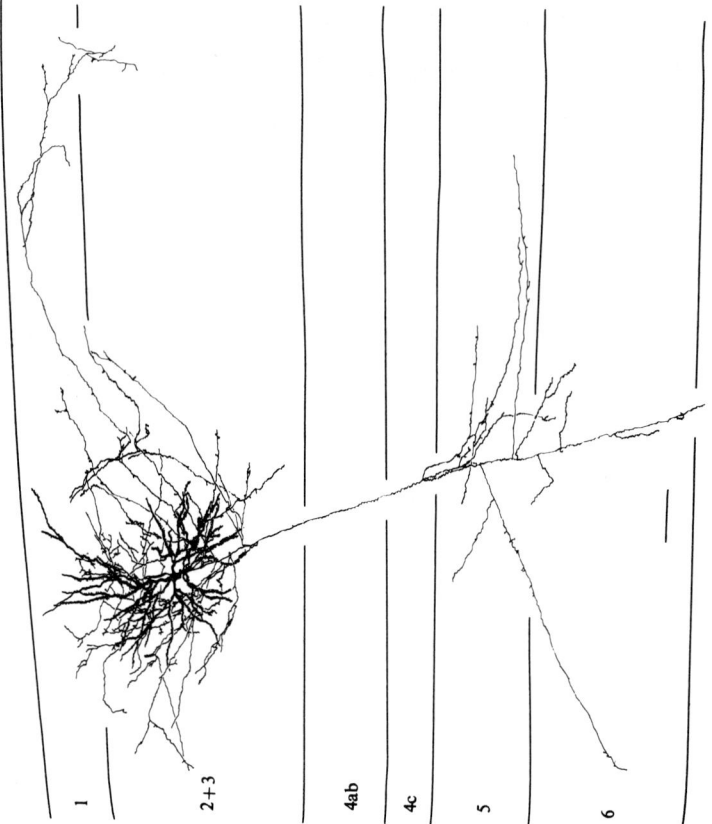
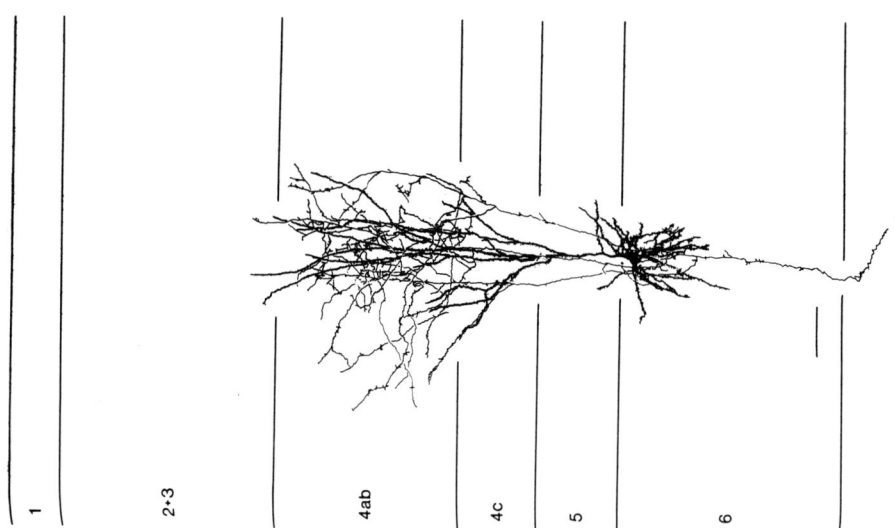

Fig. 8.5.b Legend see p. 65

Cell Types

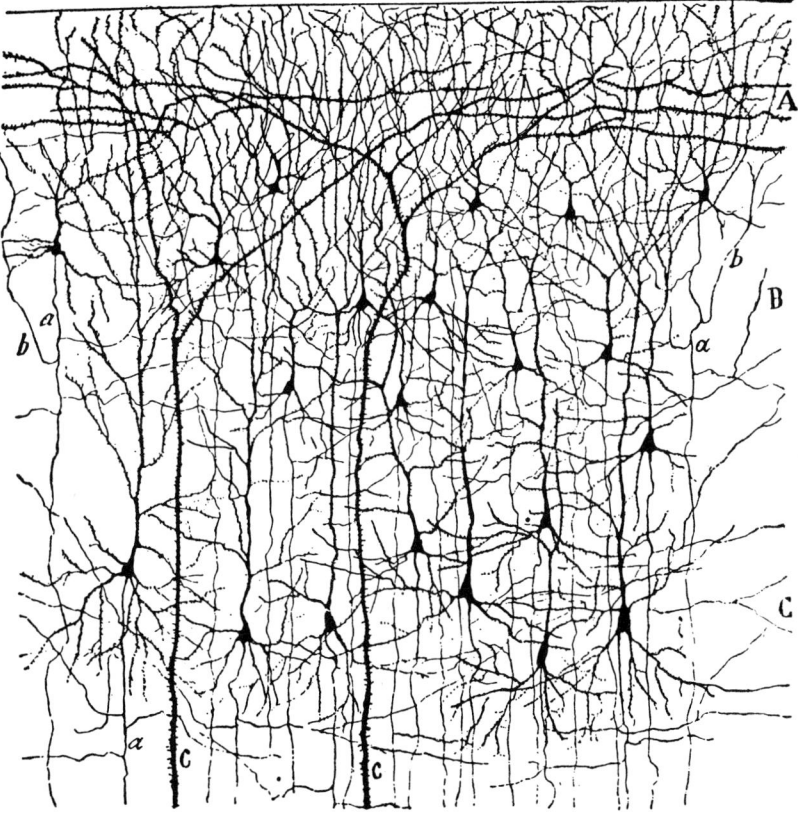

Fig. 8.5c. Many pyramidal cells of the upper layers of the cortex (Cajal 1911)

2. Local cells: These cells are characterized by the fact that both their dendritic and axonal arborizations ramify in the neighborhood of the cell body. Several subtypes of local cells can be distinguished since their dendritic and axonal arborizations can have various shapes (Fig. 8.6), but I will mention only two common subtypes here.

a) Stellate cells, which have a roughly spherical arborization (Fig. 8.7a)
b) Martinotti cells, whose dendrites spread in the lower layers and whose axon goes up to the first layer (Fig. 8.7b).

Their relative frequencies are hard to estimate; they also vary a little from animal to animal and from region to region (of cortex), and of course every author uses a slightly different classification.

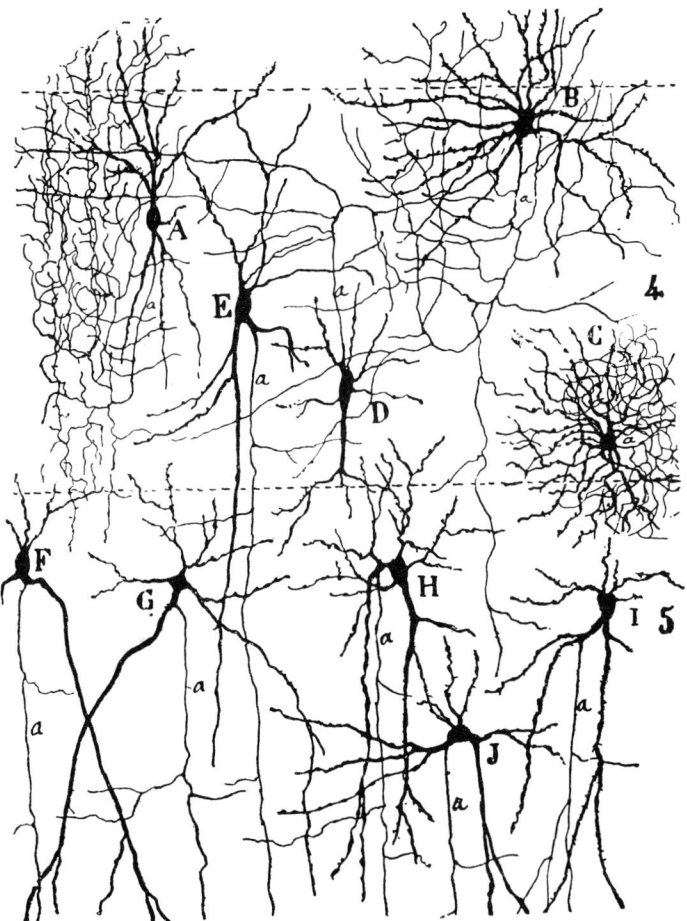

Fig. 8.6. Various shapes of neurons in the cortex (Cajal 1911)

Cell Types

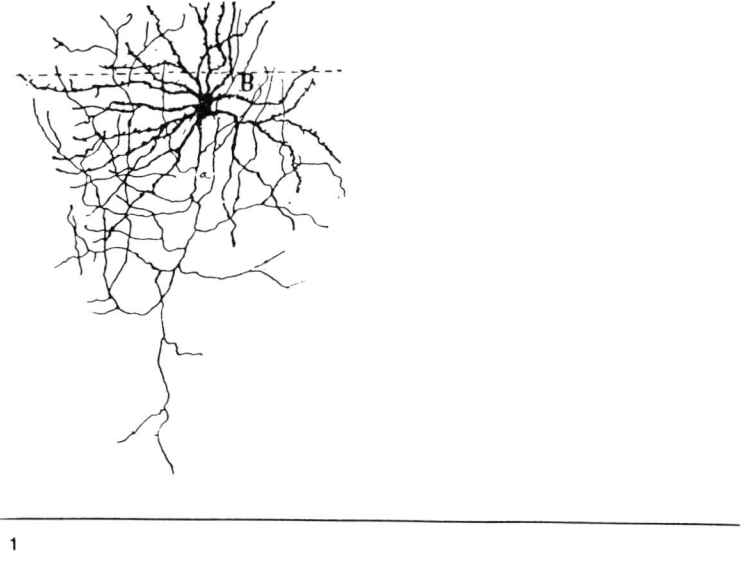

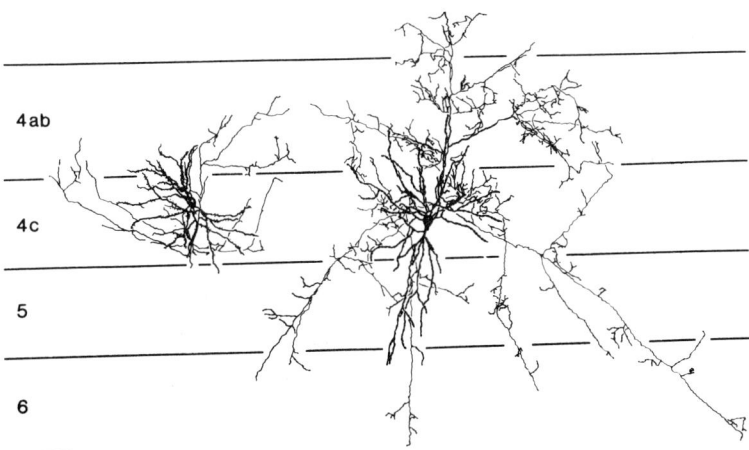

Fig. 8.7a. Stellate cells (Cajal 1911 and Gilbert and Wiesel 1979)

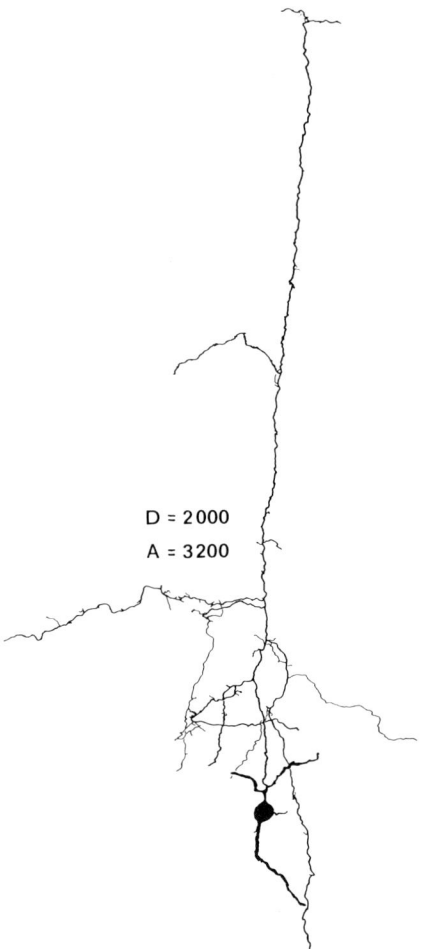

Fig. 8.7b. A Martinotti cell (Braitenberg 1978b)

Rough figures are given in Table 8.2, taken from Mitra 1955 and Winfield et al. 1980. Obviously, most cells can be grouped as pyramidal cells or stellate cells.

Combining these numbers, the Nissl pictures of Fig. 8.4, and perhaps the beautiful drawings of Cajal (like Fig. 8.8) one can – with a little fantasy – get an impression of the shape and arrangement of the neurons in the cortex. The basic image indeed has not changed substantially since 1911 (see for example the more recent drawings by Parnavelas et al. 1977, Peters and Fairen 1978, Peters and Feldman 1977, Lund et al. 1979, and Valverde 1978).

Cell Types

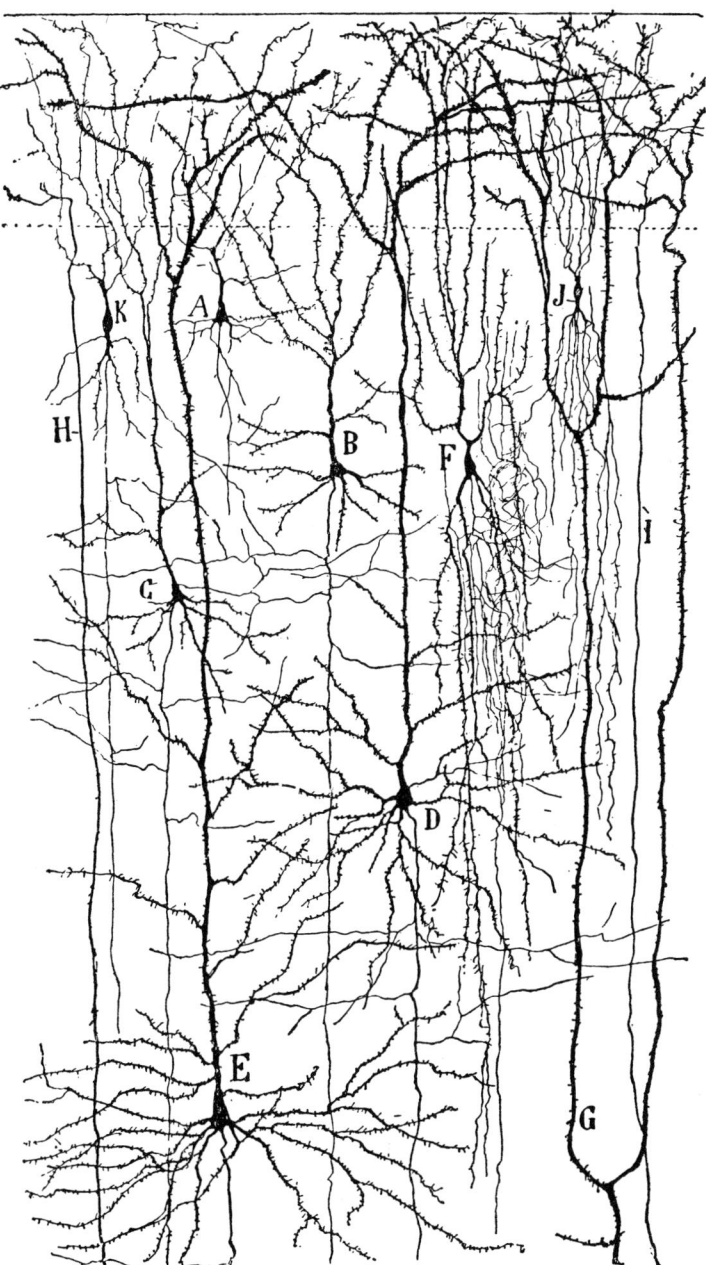

Fig. 8.8a. Shows some pyramidal cells (*B,C,D,E*) and some local cells (*F,J*) in the upper half of the cortex. *G* is part of the dendrite of a pyramidal cell. The axons of *A* and *K* are probably incompletely stained and go down to the white matter. In this case *A* and *K* are grouped as pyramidal cells. *H* and *I* are hard to classify from this picture (Cajal 1911)

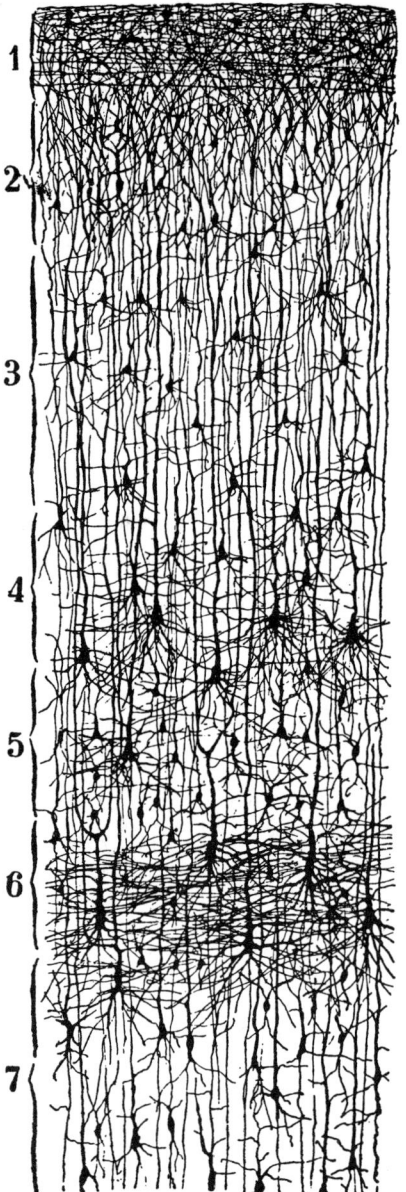

Fig. 8.8b. Even in this picture only a few percent of all the cells have been stained (Cajal 1911)

Cell Types

Table 8.2a. Relative proportions of the cell types in certain cortical areas of different mammals (Mitra 1955)

Animal and area		Cell types expressed as percentages of the total number of classified neurons		
		Pyramidal	Stellate	Fusiform
Monkey visual	4a	54	44	2
	4b	51	47	2
Cat visual	190a	62	34	5
	190b	63	34	3
	190c	57	37	6
	236	63	33	5
	307	61	37	2
	244 (6 weeks)	66	31	3
Rabbit visual	2366a (adult)	66	32	2
	2366b (adult)	69	28	3
	2357a (adult)	65	32	3
	2357b (adult)	64	32	4
	2436 (adult)	69	29	2
	2487 (adult)	65	30	6
	2303 (17 days)	74	23	3
	2557 (10 days)	85	13	2
Cat somatosensory	307a	64	35	1
	307b	62	36	2
Monkey motor	4a	75	21	4
	4b	73	23	4
Cat motor	273a	84	10	6
	273b	86	8	6
	265a	86	8	5
	265b	84	12	5
Human prefrontal		72	26	2
Rabbit visual (adult)		66.0	31.0	3.0
Cat visual (adult)		60.0	35.0	5.0
Monkey visual (adult)		52.0	45.0	3.0
Cat somatosensory (adult)		63.0	35.0	2.0
Monkey motor (adult)		74.0	22.0	4.0
Monkey parastriate (adult)		66.0	29.0	5.0
Cat motor (adult)		85.0	9.0	6.0
Human prefrontal (adult)		72.0	26.0	2.0
Kitten visual (6 weeks)		66.0	31.0	3.0
Rabbit visual (17 days)		74.0	23.0	3.0
Rabbit visual (10 days)		85.0	13.0	2.0

Table 8.2b. The proportion of different cell types in the motor and visual cortices of the cat, rat and monkey (Winfield et al. 1980)

Animal		Pyramidal	Non-pyramidal		Total sample
			Large stellate	Small stellate	
Cat 526	Motor	64 (67%)	3 (3%)	29 (30%)	96
	Visual	66 (66%)	5 (5%)	30 (29%)	101
Cat 543	Motor	67 (67%)	5 (5%)	28 (28%)	100
	Visual	67 (67%)	5 (5%)	28 (28%)	100
Rat 1	Motor	73 (65%)	7 (6%)	32 (29%)	112
	Visual	85 (72%)	4 (3%)	29 (25%)	118
Rat 2	Motor	68 (64%)	8 (8%)	30 (28%)	106
	Visual	80 (69%)	9 (8%)	27 (23%)	116
Rat 3	Motor	67 (67%)	6 (6%)	27 (27%)	100
	Visual	62 (62%)	5 (5%)	33 (33%)	100
Monkey 126	Visual	62 (62%	5 (5%)	33 (33%)	100

8.3 From Fig. 8.4 it is already clear that this arrangement varies a little from one cortical region to another. These variations have led to a so-called cyto-architectonic distinction between different cortical areas (see Fig. 8.9).

These distinctions can be compared with the rather vague ideas on the function of different regions of the human cortex that have been obtained from studying patients with brain lesions (see Fig. 8.10).

Such a correspondence is, of course, hard to establish, especially when the "function" itself is characterized in rather vague terms (see also Chap. 6.5).

A comparatively recent method (of blood flow analysis, see Lassen and Ingvar 1978) may provide more insight into these problems (e.g., Fig. 8.11).

Those cytoarchitectonic regions, which can be best identified in terms of their function as well, are the sensory input and motor output areas of the cortex.

Each sensory input region of the cortex receives input through a dense (apparently excitatory, e.g., Mitzdorf and Singer 1978, Peters and Feldman 1976) projection from a specific thalamic nucleus. Other cytoarchitectonic areas can be related to a more general input-output fiber system of the cortex:

Areas

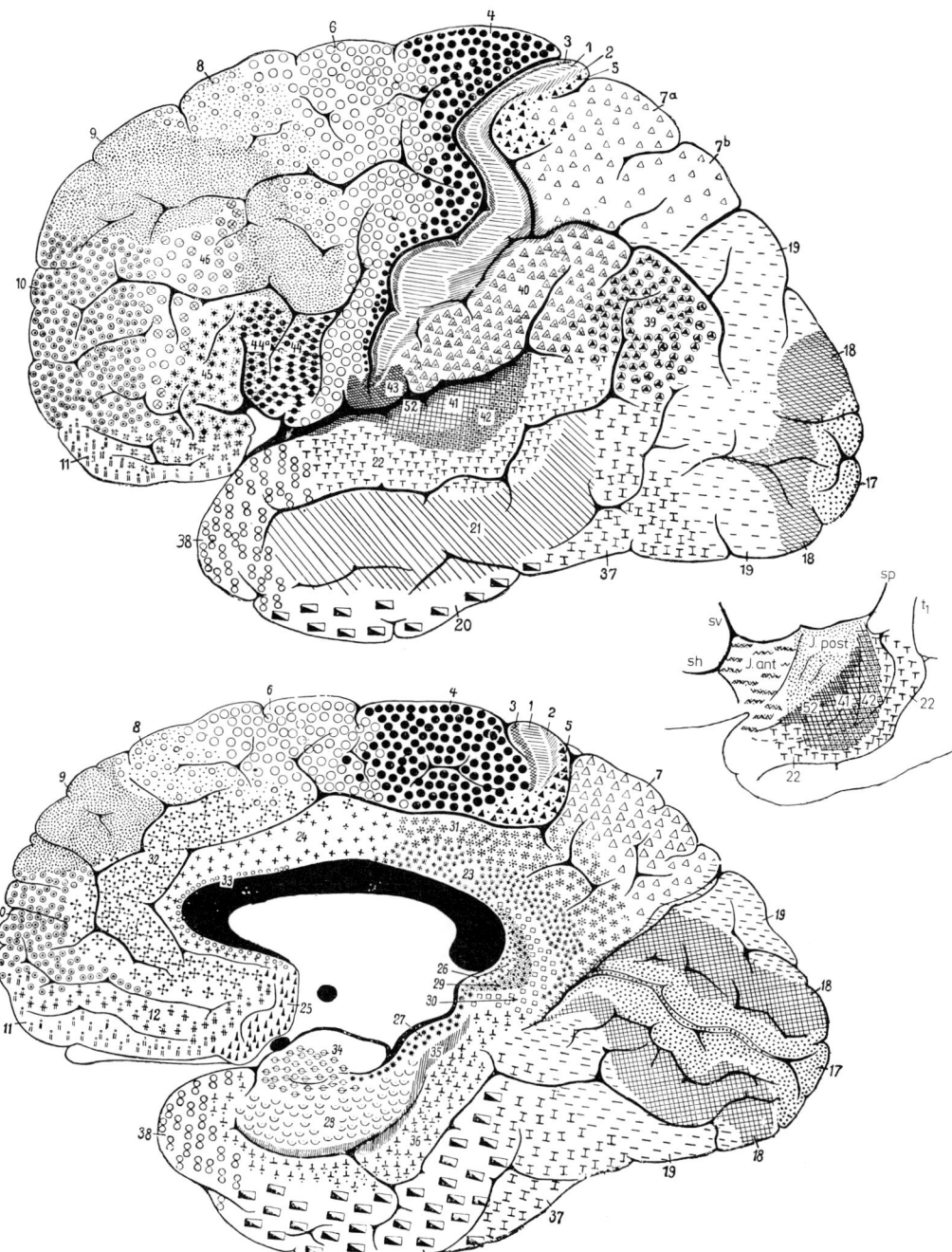

Fig. 8.9. Brodmann's famous chart of cortical areas (Brodmann 1909)

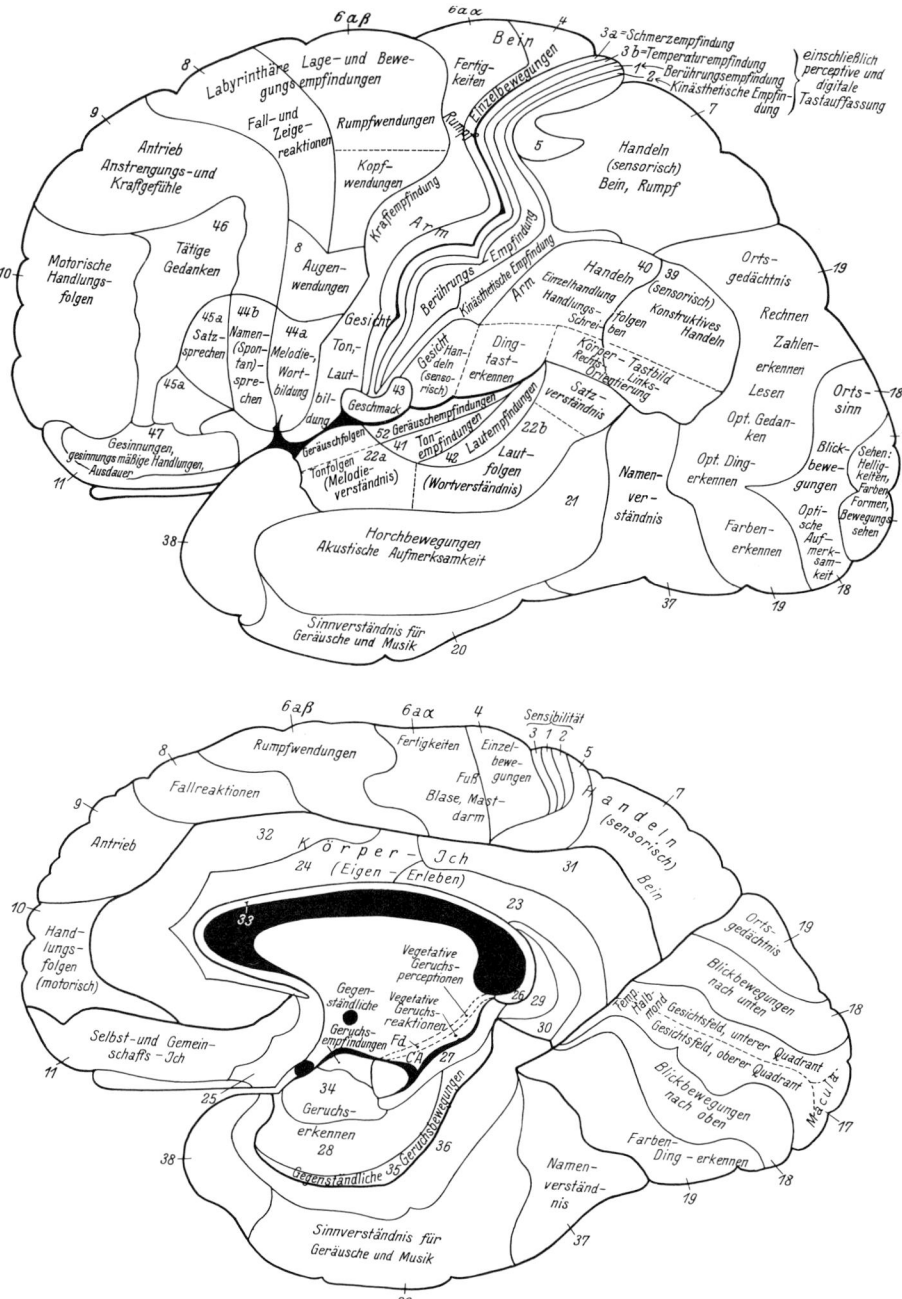

Fig. 8.10. Kleist's chart of cortical localization (Kleist 1934)

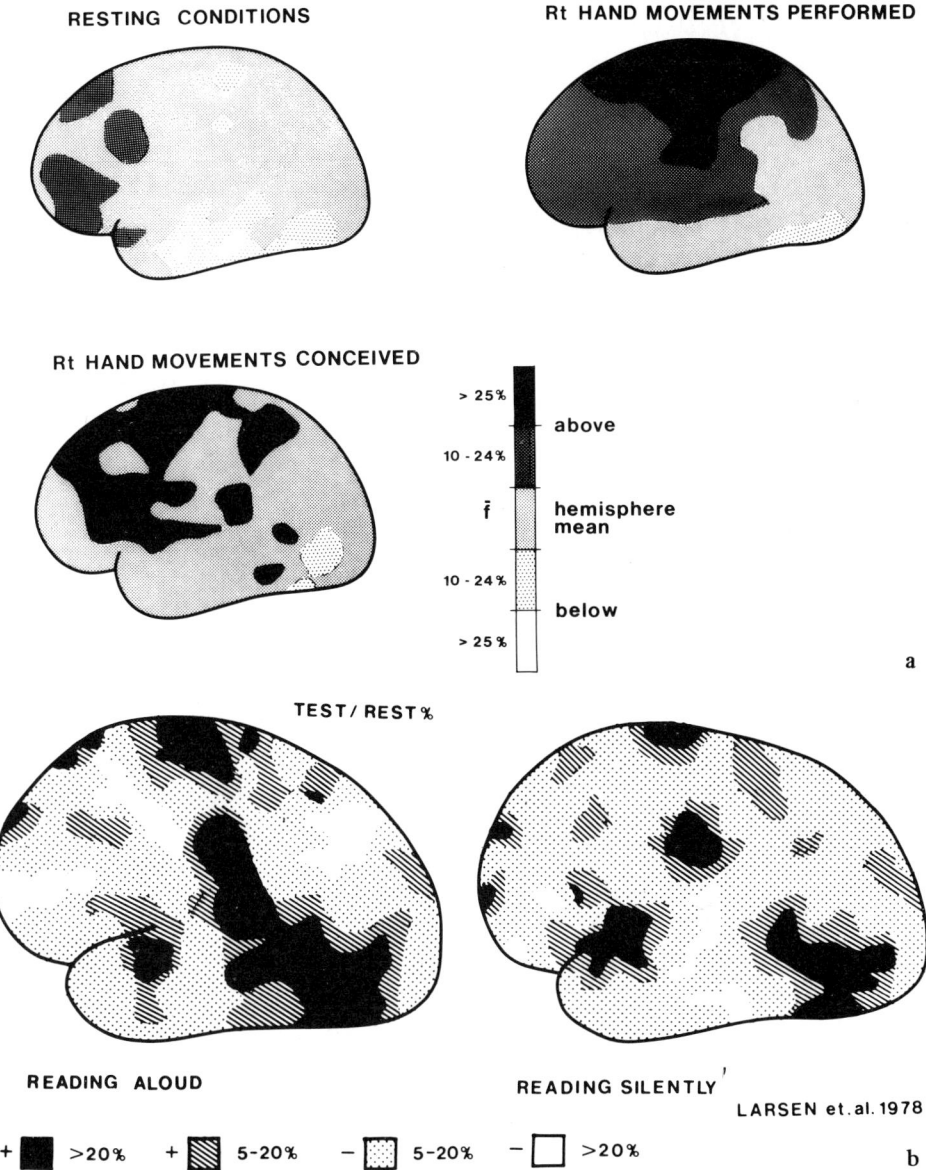

Fig. 8.11a,b. The cerebral blood flow measured under various conditions as indicated. The difference to the mean flow at rest is displayed in per cent of the mean flow at rest. a From Ingvar and Philipson (1977); b From Larsen et al. (1978) (Courtesy Prof. Ingvar)

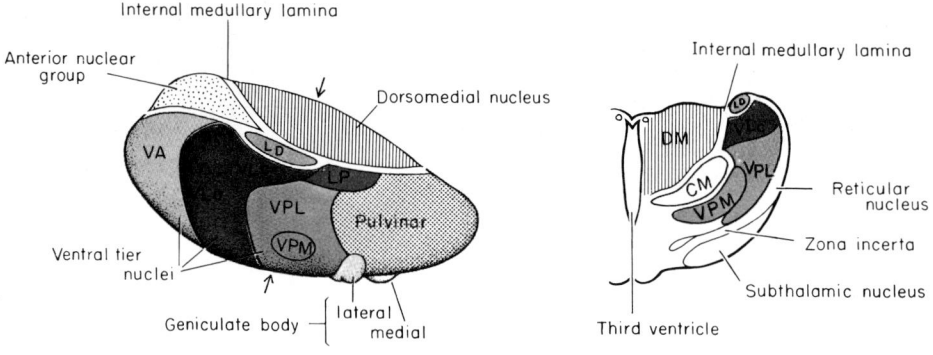

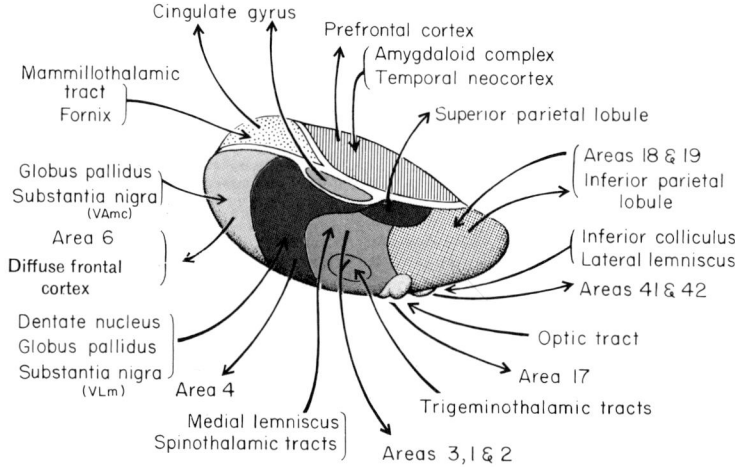

Fig. 8.12a. The principal afferent and efferent projections of particular thalamic subdivisions are indicated. While most cortical areas project fibers back to the thalamic nuclei from which fibers are received, not all of these are shown

Different nuclei of the thalamus seem to be connected in a roughly topographic manner to different regions of the cortex, as indicated in the scheme of Fig. 8.12 (many more details can be found in White 1979).

What can we infer from this arrangement on the dynamics of neuronal activity in this network?

8.4 *The local spread of activity.* Let us disregard for the moment the long-range cortico-cortical fibers passing through the white matter. Then we can try

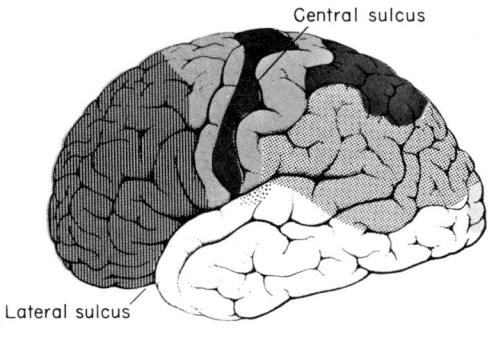

Fig. 8.12b. Diagram of the left cerebral hemisphere showing the cortical projection areas of thalamic nuclei. The color code is the same as in **a**. Information concerning the cortical projection areas of some thalamic nuclei is incomplete (Carpenter 1976)

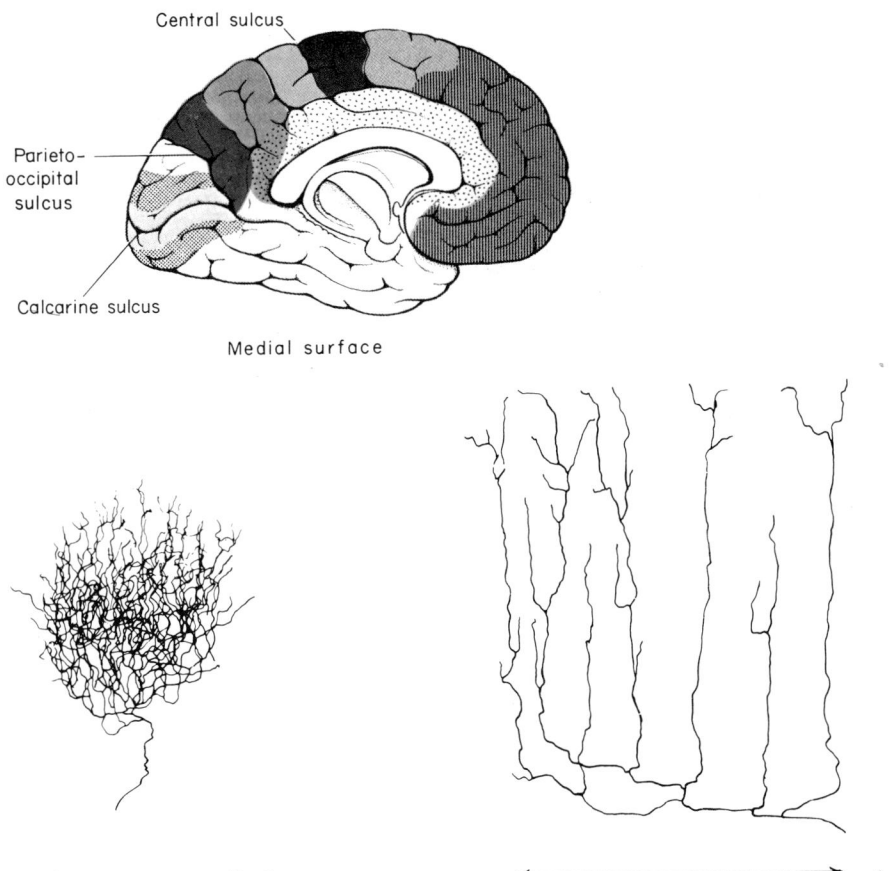

Fig. 8.13. a Terminal axonal plexus generated by specific afferent sensory fiber. **b** Diffuse terminal domain established by nonspecific afferent fiber from brainstem reticular formation of thalamic intralaminar system (Scheibel and Scheibel 1970)

to imagine how a patch of activity will spread through the cortex just by our knowledge of the shape of the input and output trees of the different cell types. This can, however, only be done with some difficulties. First of all we cannot really predict much, if we do not know which synapses are excitatory and which are inhibitory. This question again is very hard to answer experimentally, but the available evidence seems to support the following view (see also Braitenberg 1978a,b, Le Vay 1973, Parnavelas et al. 1977, Peters and Fairen 1978, Shepherd 1974).

a) All the synapses on the axons of pyramidal cells are excitatory,
b) there are inhibitory synapses on the axons of local cells.

Based on this, we can imagine only the average flow of activity, provided that we make some assumptions of a statistical nature about the connectivity between cells of the different types in different areas. We will here use the most naive assumption, namely that there are no preferences for connections between special types. This implies that the probability of a synapse from cell A to cell B only depends on their distance and on the shape of A's and B's dendritic trees or, perhaps more exactly, on the way the presynaptic terminals of A are distributed around A and the postsynaptic terminals of B are distributed around B. Some of these probabilities are calculated approximately from measurements on cells of different types in the mouse cortex (Braitenberg 1978a, 1981, see also Uttley 1955). They are given in Fig. 8.14.

In this way we obviously cannot predict the behavior of any single cell, but we can possibly imagine the average flow of activity, based on the following additional observations (Braitenberg 1961, 1974a,b, 1978a,b).

c) Most cells are pyramidal cells.
d) The axon collaterals of pyramidal cells (those extending locally) reach further than the axons of stellate cells.
e) The axon collaterals of pyramidal cells extend on the average a little below their dendrites.

These observation a) to e) lead to the following qualitative picture.

Let us concentrate on a little patch of cortical grey matter in one moment of time. The axons entering it provide it with a certain amount of excitatory (positive) and inhibitory (negative) postsynaptic potentials, this total amount will be called the *"synaptic excitation"* in that patch of cortex.

Inhibition will be noted as negative excitation. Figure 8.15 shows the evolution of this profile of excitation in time, starting with a little patch of excitation.

To understand this, let us assume that at $t = 0$ in a region of cortex just one pyramidal cell A is active. This cell will distribute excitation into

The Local Spreading of Activity

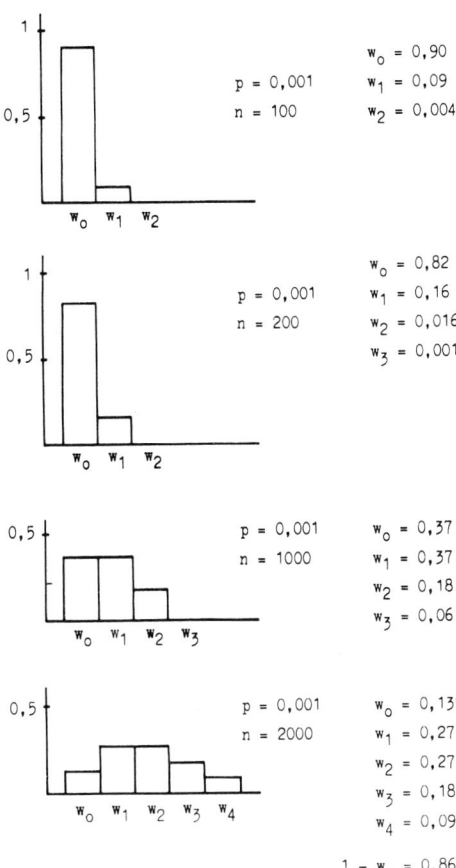

Fig. 8.14. (Braitenberg 1978a)

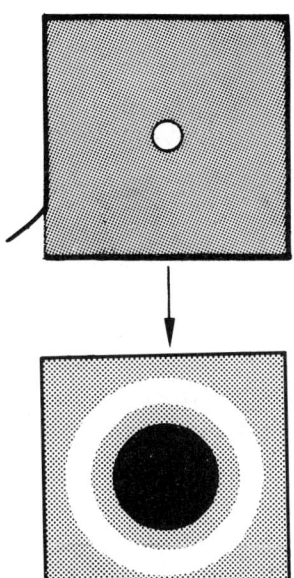

Fig. 8.15. The evolution of a little patch of excitation in time, seen from above. Excitation light, Inhibition dark

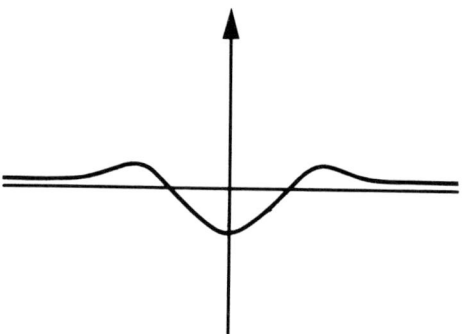

Fig. 8.16. This qualitative picture indicates that excitation is assumed to reach farther than inhibition. *Abscissa* distance from a source of input. *Ordinate* positive values, excitation, negative values, inhibition

its neighborhood. This excitation may cause some cells in the immediate neighborhood of A to fire, and these will be partly excitatory and partly inhibitory. Moreover, it may also happen that very few cells further away from A do fire, if they are (by mechanisms to be discussed in 8.5) in a particularly favorable position. But the average cell at that distance does not by far get enough excitation to fire.

The activity of the cells in the immediate neighborhood of A will at time 1 perhaps lead to a profile of excitation such as in Fig. 8.16.

Here, of course, the absolute strength of inhibition and excitation is not clear. But for reasons of stability, the threshold of the average cell should be high enough to make it improbable that cells of the immediate neighborhood of A (including A) will fire, since otherwise the excited area would steadily grow. Let us suppose now that the inhibition is indeed strong enough. Then only the neurons at about the optimal distance from A (i.e., at the peaks of the curves in Fig. 8.16) would have a reasonably high probability of firing, and we may assume that a certain percentage of these neurons will indeed fire. Which neurons actually fire, will still depend on the details of the wiring and perhaps also on the global state of activity.

8.5 *The global spread of activity*. We may now try to use the impression of the local spread of activity as obtained in 8.4, to understand the global spread of activity. The first observation is that the global spread of activity is mediated essentially by the long axon collaterals and the cortico-cortical fibers of the pyramidal cells. Secondly, the density of the axonal arborizations of a pyramidal cell is usually so low that it is very improbable that a single pyramidal cell will fire another one (see Braitenberg 1978 and Fig. 8.14). Therefore, it will probably take several pyramidal cells whose long-range connections converge on a neuron to fire that neuron. This idea implies that the global spread of activity cannot be under-

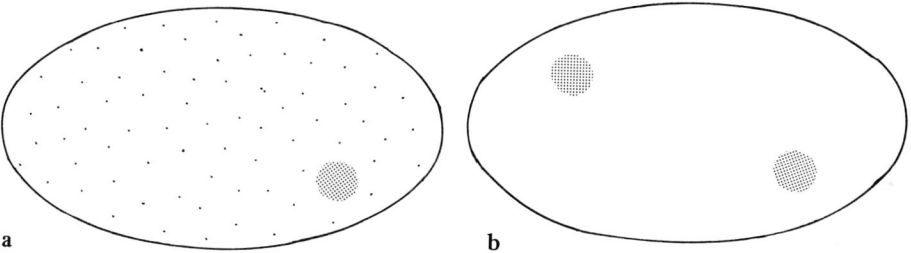

Fig. 8.17. a Where a pyramidal cell gets synaptical inputs from; b where a pyramidal cell gives synaptic inputs to

stood in a statistical way, because it depends entirely on the deviations from the mean. A pyramidal cell will fire either due to strong connection from another pyramidal cell (which has a low probability but will occur now and then) or due to a convergence of long-range connections from a group of other pyramidal cells (which should be about equally improbable all over the cortex).

Figure 8.17a indicates the distribution of those pyramidal cells from which a given pyramidal cell gets excitation, whereas Fig. 8.17b indicates the distribution of those pyramidal cells to which a given pyramidal cell gives excitation.

Of course, we do not know whether in Fig. 8.17a really the whole area should be scarcely but uniformly dotted, or whether it should perhaps look more patchy, maybe even with large empty areas.

This could only be found out by a thorough investigation of all cortico-cortical connections — not only the big fiber bundles (that have been described for example by Bailey and von Bonin 1951, Dusser de Barenne and McCulloch 1938, Dusser de Barenne et al. 1941, and several more detailed anatomical investigations, e.g., Kuypers et al. 1965, Pandya and Kuypers 1969, see also Fig. 8.18).

Still the total length of all cortico-cortical fibers is compatible with the idea that every pyramidal cell can get information from everywhere in the cortex (Braitenberg 1974a, 1978a,b).

The resulting impression is the following: essentially due to the actual distribution of synapses on the long-range connections between pyramidal cells (and on the more distal parts of their axon collaterals) the activity moves from one group of pyramidal cells distributed all over the cortex to another one. This rather vague description will be filled with more life in Chapter 11. In this way the excitation does not die out, due to an interaction of the local and the global connections between pyramidal cells, whereas the local inhibition (of the stellate cells) helps to prevent an explosion of excitation.

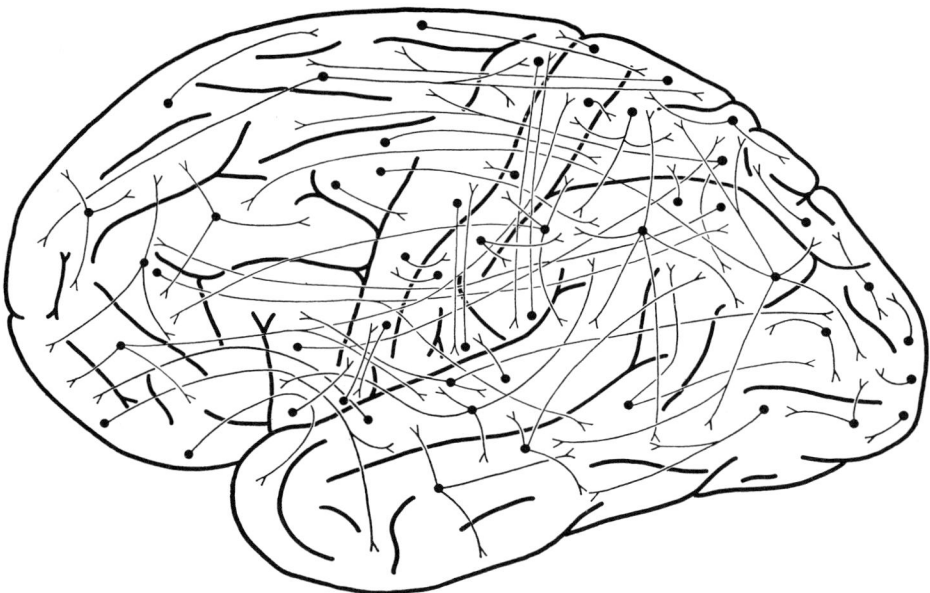

Fig. 8.18. Cortico-cortical connections as revealed by physiological neuronography in the chimpanzee (Bailey and Bonin 1951)

8.6 Let me condense these considerations in some statements and definitions (following Braitenberg 1978 and Palm and Braitenberg 1979):

1. The *"state" of activity* of the cortex is basically determined by the activity of the pyramidal cells.
2. The evolution of cortical activity from state to state is governed by two types of connections: *local* connections and *global* connections.
3. The gobal connections are due to the cortico-cortical fibers, that is, the axons of the pyramidal cells. When re-entering the cortex, these axons make excitatory contacts preferably in the upper layers (cf. Braitenberg 1974a, Heimer et al. 1967, Lund and Lund 1970, Wolff 1976), and therefore mainly to *A*pical dendrites of other pyramidal cells. This system of global connections is called the A-system.
4. The local connections are inhibitory and excitatory. The excitatory local connections are mainly due to axon collaterals of pyramidal cells.
    They spread their excitation on the average a little *below* their input and therefore more often to *B*asal dendrites than to apical dendrites of other pyramidal cells. This system of local connections is called the B-system (see also Palm and Braitenberg 1979).
5. Thus every pyramidal cell has access to global information in the upper layers of the cortex through its apical dendrites and to local information in the lower and middle layers of the cortex through its basal dendrites.

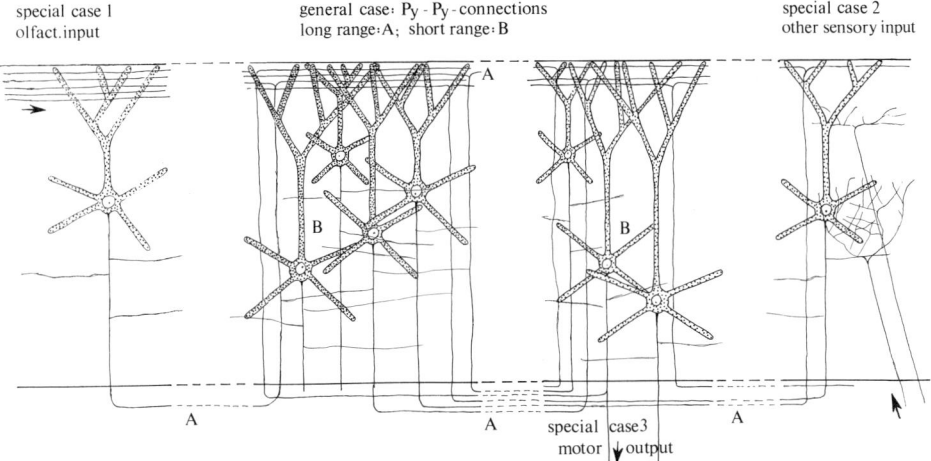

Fig. 8.19. The "skeleton cortex" made only of pyramidal cells (py) and their connections. A system: Apical dendrites, long fibers through the white substance. B system: basal dendrites and axon collaterals. The sensory and motor regions are considered special cases of this general scheme (Braitenberg 1978b)

6. The Martinotti cells gather and distribute excitation locally, but their output is clearly *above* their input. They fit neither into the A-scheme nor into the B-scheme.

8.7 In this first image of the flow of excitation through the cortex we did not yet explicitly account for the specific input and output areas, or for the general influence of the thalamic nuclei on different cortical regions. The general (or nonspecific) thalamic afferents of the cortex seem to distribute a wide-spread excitation into the cortex (see Fig. 8.12).

By these afferents the thalamic nuclei may be used to regulate the total (or average) activity of the entire cortex, and also differentially the average activity of different cortical regions that correspond to different thalamic nuclei. Such a general regulation may be useful to prevent extreme states of excitation (i.e., total fading out or explosion of excitation), it may also correspond for example to different states of attention or arousal. We return to these questions in Chapters 12 and 13.

The cortical output regions are specialized at least by having particularly large pyramidal cells, whose output fibers reach down to the brain stem and the spinal cord, where the control of the muscles is organized.

The cortical input regions are specialized in that they get a strong well organized input from the sense organs through bundles of afferent fibers, that usually spread excitation around the IVth layer, in other words, still in the lower "local" part of the cortex. In this layer of the input regions an unusually high number of stellate cells is commonly found. These considerations are summarized in Fig. 8.19 from Braitenberg (1978b).

8.8 I have to admit that the picture of the flow of activity through the cortex that I have developed is still rather speculative. Moreover, some questions remain unanswered; for example:

How many pyramidal cells are actually "active" in one moment?

How many active excitatory synapses are needed to fire a neuron (on the apical dendrites and/or on the basal dendrites)?

Such questions are hard to answer (although a few attempts to answer them have been made, e.g., Abeles 1981, Creutzfeldt et al. 1964). This is due to limitations of the electrophysiological technique:

First of all, electrophysiologists can only record a few neurons at the same time. Thus it is practically impossible to reconstruct a global picture of activity from their recordings.

Secondly, most electrophysiological preparations include anesthesia of the animal, which may severely alter the general state of activity of the cortex.

Thirdly, my speculations have concentrated on the flow of activity in the general cortex, whereas electrophysiologists (with a few exceptions) stick to the specialized input and output regions, where they have obtained their most convincing results.

The main advantage of doing electrophysiology in the input and output regions is that one can easily correlate neuronal activity to events in the outside world. In this way one can learn a lot about the pre- and post-processing of information on the way to and from the cortex, i.e., on the two outer boxes of Fig. 1.1. Some of the electrophysiological results obtained in the input regions of the cortex are presented in the next chapter.

9 The Visual Input to the Cortex

> *Thus the machinery may be roughly uniform over the whole striate cortex, the differences being in the inputs. A given region of cortex simply digests what is brought to it, and the process is the same everywhere.*   D.H. Hubel and T.N. Wiesel, 1974

Today we have a fairly good idea of the preprocessing of sensory information on its way to the cortex. This chapter is devoted to the most extensively studied example: the visual input. Most of the results presented here are due to electrophysiological investigations (for a review see Hubel and Wiesel 1977).

9.1 Excitation from the retina reaches the cortex in a *topographically* ordered way.

This means that neighboring points in the retina will excite neighboring neurons in the cortex. It is therefore convenient to speak of a *projection* from the retina (via the "geniculate body") into the cortex.

9.2 Neurons in the visual cortex have a *receptive field,* i.e., they respond best to visual stimuli that are located in a small region (called the receptive field) of the whole visual field.

9.3 They have been classified by Hubel and Wiesel into *simple, complex,* and *hypercomplex* neurons on the basis of their responses to little line segments (bars).

   a) Most of the cells in area 17 (the primary visual area) are simple or complex.
   b) Simple cells respond best to bars of a certain dimension and orientation, presented in a certain position (their receptive field).
   c) Complex cells respond well to moving bars of a certain orientation, but at various positions in their larger receptive field.

9.4 The position of the receptive field, the preferred orientation of bars and possibly some other parameters are called the *receptive field properties* of the neuron.

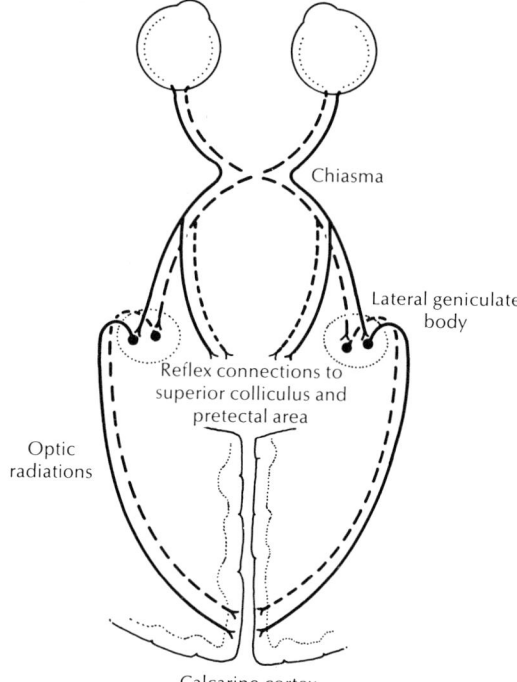

Fig. 9.1. (Matzke and Foltz 1972)

9.5 In cats most neurons in area 17 get inputs from both eyes and their receptive field properties for the right eye are very similar to those for the left eye. Many neurons are not driven equally strongly from the two eyes, i.e., they show a certain degree of *ocular dominance.*

There are a few cells that are responsive to stimuli from only one eye, and these (i.e., their cell bodies) are mainly situated in layer IV, the layer where the input fibers terminate.

9.6 The pathway from the two eyes to the visual cortices is schematized in Fig. 9.1.

9.7 The resolution is not constant over the whole visual field: it is high in the center of gaze (eccentricity 0°) and decreases with increasing eccentricity.

9.8 This is due to the density and shape of the ganglion cells in the retina that send their axons into the optic nerve. The ganglion cells are smaller with correspondingly smaller receptive field and more densely packed in the center, and bigger with correspondingly larger receptive field and less densely packed farther out (Peichl and Wässle 1979). With increasing eccen-

Overlap and Magnification

tricity their packing density decreases inversely proportional to their size, such that their *overlap* is nearly constant over the whole visual field (it is about 70–80 for the cat). The overlap at the point x of the visual field is the number of cells that have that point x in their receptive field.

9.9 This relationship (the constant overlap) is preserved by the projection from the retina into the cortex, i.e., the number of neurons in the visual cortex that receive input from any one ganglion cell does not vary with eccentricity. From anatomical data the overlap in area 17 can be estimated to be 10^5 or more (but of course the physiological overlap depends on the definition of the receptive field).

9.10 The size of the neurons in the cortex also does not vary systematically with the eccentricity of their receptive field. Therefore a neuron situated near the projection of the center of gaze responds to a much smaller part of the visual field than another neuron located at the projection of some place further out in the visual field (cf. Fig. 9.2). This means that the projection of the retina onto area 17 is *magnified* in the center of gaze (see Fig. 9.3).

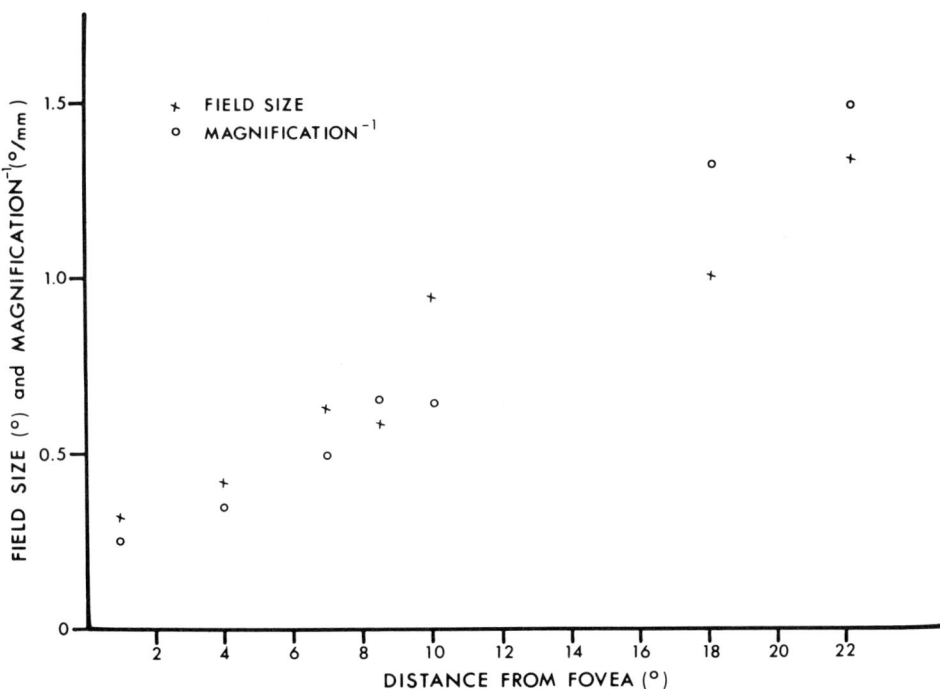

Fig. 9.2. Magnification^{-1} means the visual distance (in °) represented below a certain distance (in mm) on the surface of the cortex (Hubel and Wiesel 1974)

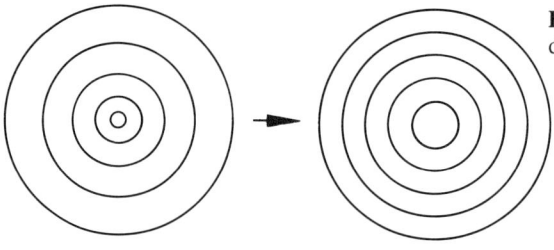

Fig. 9.3. Shows the effect of the data presented in Fig. 9.2

The cortical magnification factor decreases with eccentricity proportionally to the retinal packing density.

9.11 In the tangential direction in the cortex the receptive field properties of neighboring cells vary in a systematic way:

   a) The location of the receptive field in the visual field gradually changes in accordance with the topographic projection from the retina.
   b) The preferred orientation of the cell also changes gradually — apart from a few "jumps". The preferred orientation changes quite fast, namely such that in a cortical area of 1 mm² usually every orientation is present.

   There are more detailed conceptions to describe the changes of preferred orientation and ocular dominance in the tangential direction (e.g., Hubel and Wiesel 1977, a nicely demonstrative picture for the ocular dominance changes can be found in Hubel and Freeman 1977, and an alternative view for the changes of orientation preference is maintained in V. and C. Braitenberg 1979).

9.12 In the vertical direction the location of the receptive field and the preferred orientation of cells do not change — apart from a little scatter. But there is a tendency toward more complex receptive field properties with increasing distance from layer IV.

9.13 Figure 9.4 gives an impression of the number of cells involved in the processing of visual information. Similar data for various animals and also humans have been assembled by Blinkov and Glezer (1968), XIII.7.

Cell Numbers

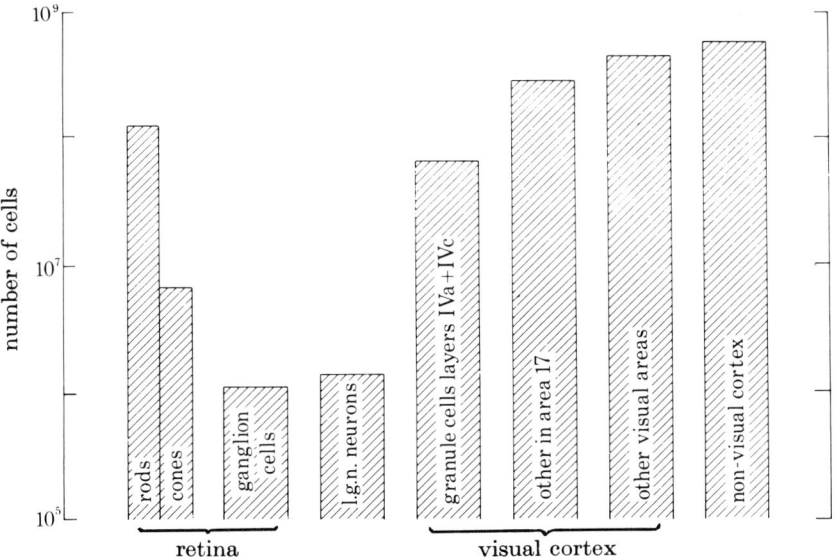

Fig. 9.4. Estimated numbers of cells at various levels in the visual pathway of a monkey (macaque). Note that the scale is logarithmic, and that there are nearly 100 times as many granule cells as retinal ganglion cells. There are even more cells in other layers of the primary visual cortex, and in other visual areas. The last column on the right shows the estimated number of cells in the nonvisual areas of the cortex. (Mainly from Chow et al. 1950.) (Barlow 1981)

10 Changes in the Cortex with Learning

Caminante, no hay camino   *Traveller, there is no path,*
Se hace camino al andar.   *Paths are made by walking.*
A. Machado

When an axon of a neuron x is near enough to help fire a neuron y and does so, some change takes place such that x becomes more effective at exciting y. What is this change and how does it work? This is a question to which we have no final answer. D.O. Hebb, 1958

It is quite clear that a change in an animal's stimulus-response behavior must be reflected in a change in the electrophysiological properties of some neurons in its brain, and such electrophysiological changes have indeed been found after various ways of conditioning the animal (e.g., Doty 1965, 1969).

In this chapter we shall discuss some of these experiments in order to get hints on the mechanism(s) that possibly produce the observed changes in the response properties of neurons.

10.1 The realization of an associative memory in the cortex in terms of neurons and synapses requires changes in the connectivity between neurons during information storage. Therefore it is tempting to look for such changes after learning.

The changes occurring in a normal learning situation can possibly be quite subtle and may therefore be hard to find. Thus many electrophysiologists and anatomists have tried to produce severe changes in the brain by exposing the animal to highly unusual environments, hoping that behavioral adaptation of the animal to such an environment would go together with recognizable changes in the brain.

Young rats and mice have been raised in the dark, leading to some degeneration in their visual cortices (e.g., Cragg 1967, 1968, Globus and Scheibel 1967a,b, Fifkova 1968, 1970, Rosenzweig et al. 1972, Valverde 1971, see also the book by Riesen 1975, and especially the chapter by Globus).

Young cats have been raised in all kinds of visually restricted environments (see Barlow 1975). For example they have been raised with goggles through which they could only see vertical stripes; after that most of the neurons recorded in their visual cortices preferred a vertical orientation (e.g., Hirsch and Spinelli 1970, Stryker et al. 1978).

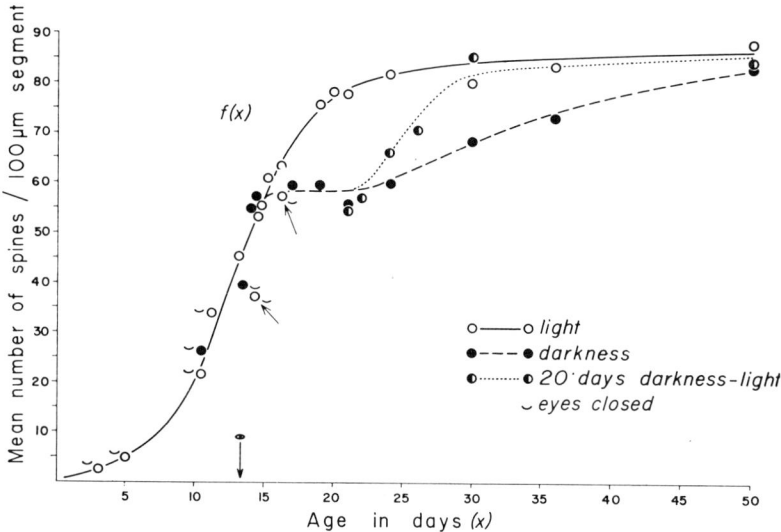

Fig. 10.1. Mean number of dendritic spines per segment in apical dendrites of layer V pyramidal cells of the visual cortex as a function of age. (Valverde 1971)

10.2 The interpretation of these deprivation experiments is controversial and has led to a lot of discussion in the last years. One complication is that people have chosen young animals, since in these much stronger effects can be produced. This is probably due to the fact that in very young animals the influence of the environment interferes with the still very fast development of the brain, which complicates an interpretation of these experiments in terms of learning. For example, one clearly cannot say that the synapses in the visual cortex are produced by visual experience; they probably develop in any case (cf. Figs. 10.1, 10.2).

The total number of synapses, almost certainly, is not an index for the amount of visual information built into the visual cortex, but it could still be that the exact location of the synapses or the variability of their connecting strength indicates that information has been stored.

10.3 A crucial argument that turned up in the discussion of deprivation experiments is the following:

"The observed changes do not really correspond to an active adaptation of the cortex to the environment, but they are just corollaries of the old biological truism that an organ grows with use or degrades with disuse: the cited experiments mean a sensory deprivation to the animal. Therefore the organ handling that sensory information that the animal has been de-

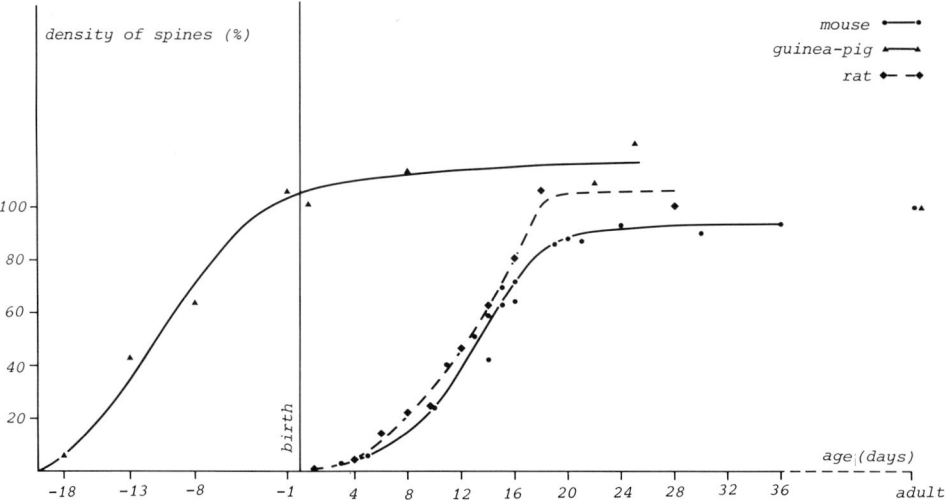

Fig. 10.2. Comparison of spine-growth curves for different animals, adult values of spine density are set as 100% (Schüz 1981)

prived of will degrade, compared to the same organ in a nondeprived animal" (see, for example, the discussion in Lewin 1975).

From this point of view the goggle experiments mainly show that the degradation can be quite specific; i.e., if only vertical stripes are presented all the cells that prefer different orientations will become less vital.

Of course, it could now be argued that such a highly specific degradation can be regarded as a meaningful strategy for adaptation. But still I would not be satisfied with such a strategy, since it works at most on the level of a neuron, whereas a synaptic rule like Hebb's rule (cee Chap. 7.5) should work independently for different synapses on the same neuron, since it requires that the change of the synapse depends on a real interaction of pre- and postsynaptic activity (cf. also Digression 4).

10.4 Let me now present some experiments that provide evidence for a true interaction of pre- and postsynaptic activity at the synapses, and that cannot be interpreted as easily from degradation on the level of the neurons.

Several investigators (Cynader and Mitchell 1977, Rauschecker and Singer 1978, 1979, 1981) have tried to perform deprivation experiments in such a way that it is possible to show that on the whole no strong degradation of the visual cortex has occurred although deviations from the usual receptive field properties can be observed.

Among these kinds of experiments I would, of course, be particularly interested in those where the observed changes can best be interpreted by assuming a law of Hebbian type for the changes in synaptic connectivity.

3 Degrees of Deprivation

What kind of environment should be chosen to avoid too strong a deprivation of the animal?

Let us regard the visual cortex as the organ that is to be studied.

It works on visual input, and there are stronger and weaker ways of depriving an animal of visual input:

1. Deprivation of physical intensity (rearing animals in the dark).
2. Deprivation of information (rearing animals with eyes sutured or with diffusing goggles, so that only diffuse light can be seen).
3. Deprivation of meaning (rearing animals with goggles showing high contrast pictures, which however have no correlation with motions or other experiences of the animal).

From the last chapter it is quite clear that the physical as well as the information deprivation will render most neurons in the visual cortex inactive and will therefore mean a severe deprivation to it.

For the deprivation of meaning this is not so clear, although the behavioral effects can be strong (Held 1966, 1970). If we compare, however, different kinds of goggle experiments, we can get a hint in that direction.

It is possible to construct goggles with cylindric lenses that blur all contours except vertical ones (Freeman and Pettigrew 1973, Cynader and Mitchell 1977, Rauschecker and Singer 1978). Kittens raised with these goggles are in fact deprived visually but they can still make use of the vertical contours that they can see, since these correspond to edges of objects in their environment.

In many cases it had indeed been possible to show that the total degradation of the visual cortex of these kittens (as far as could be measured electrophysiologically) was minimal [the percentage of visually unresponsive neurons was below 25% in the experiments of Figs. 10.5, 10.6, 10.7, for example (Rauschecker and Singer 1981)], especially if compared to the total degradation in kittens raised with goggles showing a fixed picture of vertical lines (cf. Stryker et al. 1978).

One series of experiments with these cylindric lenses seems of particular interest to me, since their results can really be interpreted best by a Hebbian type of synaptic rule, and will be in fact hard to interpret by other mechanisms, such as pure axonal competition of the afferents for the postsynaptic cells in the visual cortex. For a better understanding of these experiments I should first report some earlier experimental results.

10.5 Hubel and Wiesel (1965) produced artificial squint in kittens, which leads to a disappearance of binocular cells in the visual area 17 (Fig. 10.3). Alternating closure of the left and right eye with a period of about one day

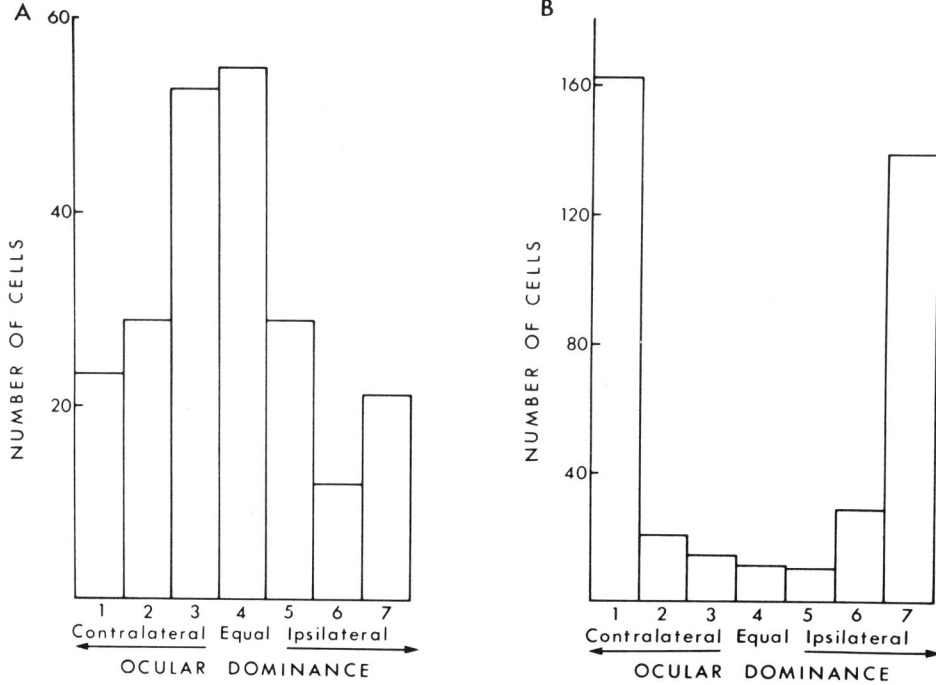

Fig. 10.3A. Occular dominance distribution in normal adult cats. Cells of group *1* were driven only by the contralateral eye; for cells of group *2* there was marked dominance of the contralateral eye, for group *3*, slight dominance. For cells in group *4* there was no obvious difference between the two eyes. In group *5* the ipsilateral eye dominated slightly, in group *6*, markedly and in group *7* the cells were driven only by the ipsilateral eye. **B** Ocular dominance distribution in cats with artificial squint (**A,B** from Hubel and Wiesel 1965)

for several weeks produces the same effect in kittens (see also Hubel and Wiesel 1965).

These experiments can be easily explained by a Hebb-like synaptic rule in the neurons of the visual cortex, which potentially receive input from afferents of both eyes. Only in normal vision will the signals of the afferents from the left and right eye coincide (roughly) and therefore lead to a sufficiently strong postsynaptic activity which will in turn enhance these connections.

These experiments alone, however, can still be explained as well by mere presynaptic competition for the postsynaptic terminals. The more detailed experiments of Blakemore and Van Sluyters (1974) and Movshon (1976) (Fig. 10.4) are much harder to explain by pure presynaptic competition alone, if this can be done at all.

Evidence for Hebb's Rule

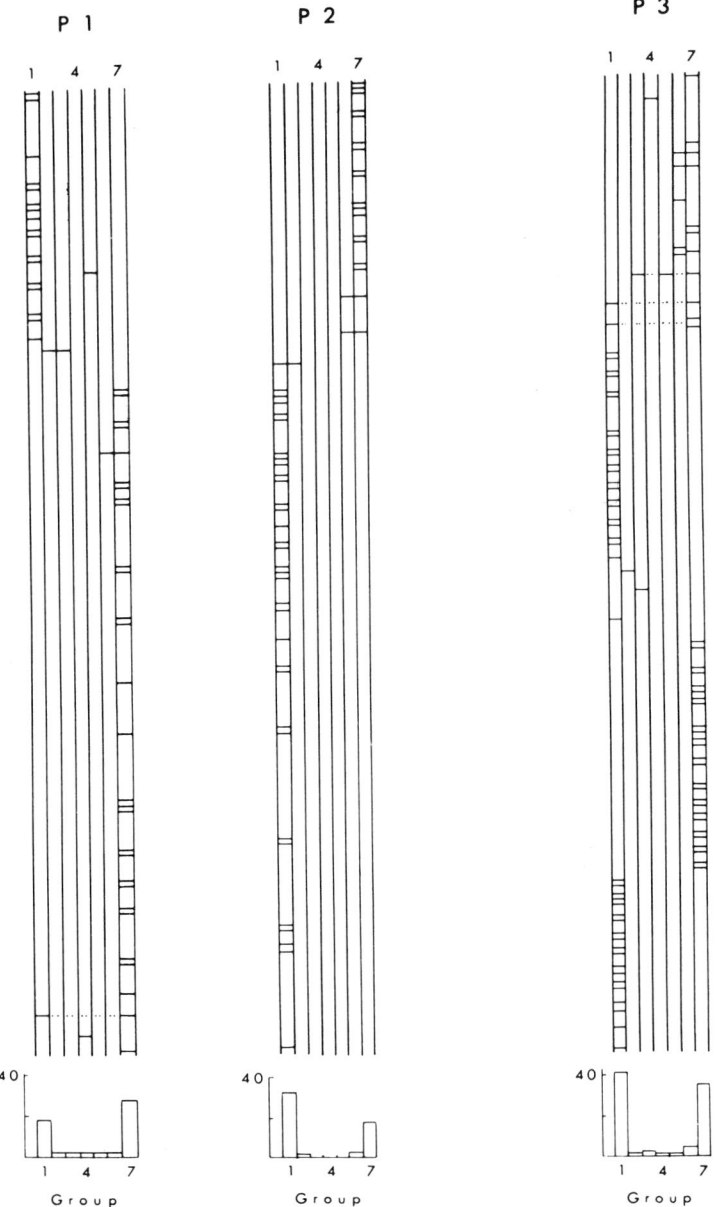

Fig. 10.3C. Schematic reconstruction of three penetrations in the striate cortex of two 10-week-old kittens raised from the time of normal eye opening with an opaque contact occluder covering one eye one day, and the other eye the next. Each penetration extended into cortical gray matter for about 1.5 mm (Hubel and Wiesel 1965)

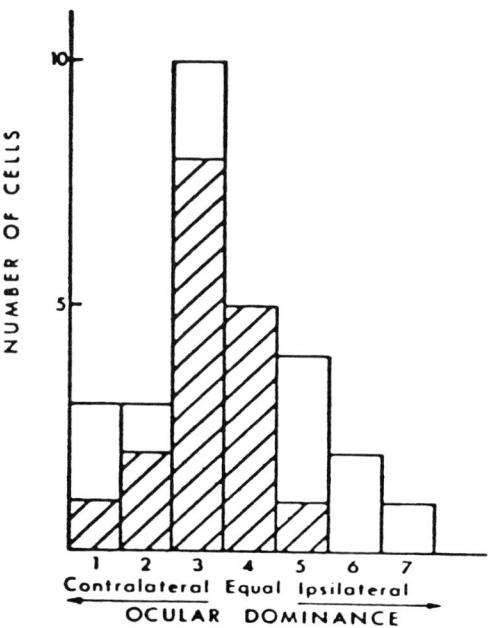

Fig. 10.3D. Ocular dominance distribution in kittens with no or very little visual experience (Hubel and Wiesel 1963)

In particular, it is hard to explain why in Fig. 10.4 the ocular dominance distribution cannot be brought back to the initial configuration, i.e., why only very few binocular units reappear again. Assuming a Hebb-like synaptic rule, however, exactly this would be expected. Moreover, the monocular eye closure experiments (which can as well be done with opaque goggles) do not severely disturb the activity in the visual afferent fibers from the deprived eye to the cortex (Singer et al. 1977, Eysel et al. 1979).

These arguments can perhaps be made more convincing by studying the interaction between monocular and orientational deprivation (Rauschecker and Singer 1981, Rauschecker 1979), compare Figs. 10.5 and 10.6.

For example, Fig. 10.7 shows that neurons that prefer a roughly vertical orientation remain binocular, whereas other neurons are no longer driven equally strongly from the right eye which had been deprived of all orientations except vertical ones. This already implies that axonal competition cannot be the whole story, but that the postsynaptic cortical neuron actively enters the decision through its preferred orientation (remember that this orientation is defined only in the cortex; the afferent axons do not yet have a clear idea of orientation).

In these experiments the observed bias in ocular dominance could be produced by competition of the geniculo-cortical afferent axons alone (i.e., by a mechanism that is governed only by *presynaptic* activity to the

Evidence for Hebb's Rule

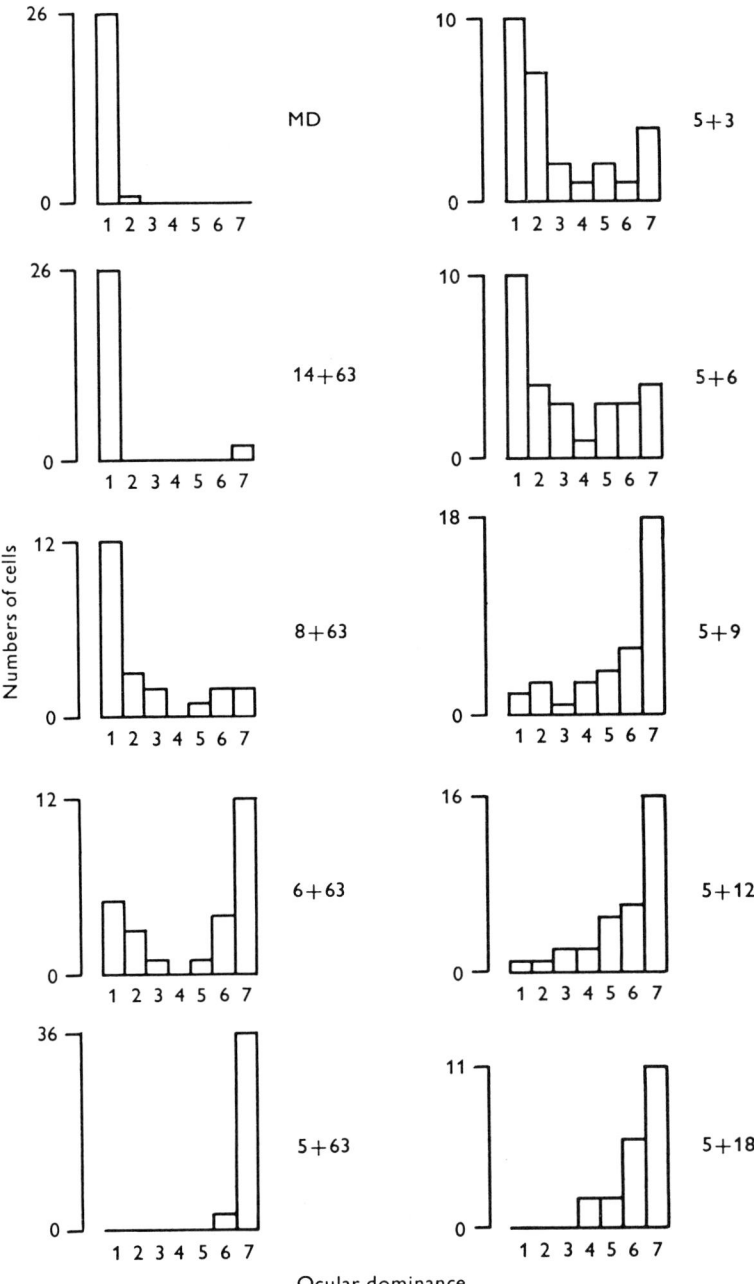

Fig. 10.4. Ocular dominance histograms of 286 visually responsive neurones from ten kittens with one eye sutured from birth followed by a reversed suture. The age (in weeks) at reverse-suturing and the duration (in days) of the reversed suture are indicated beside each histogram. All recordings were made from the right hemisphere, so cells on the left-hand side of each histogram were driven primarily or totally from the initially experienced left eye, while cells on the right-hand side of each histogram were driven primarily or totally from the initially deprived right eye. The ocular dominance classification is that of Hubel and Wiesel (from Blakemore and Van Sluyters 1974, and Movshon 1976) (Dürsteler et al. 1976)

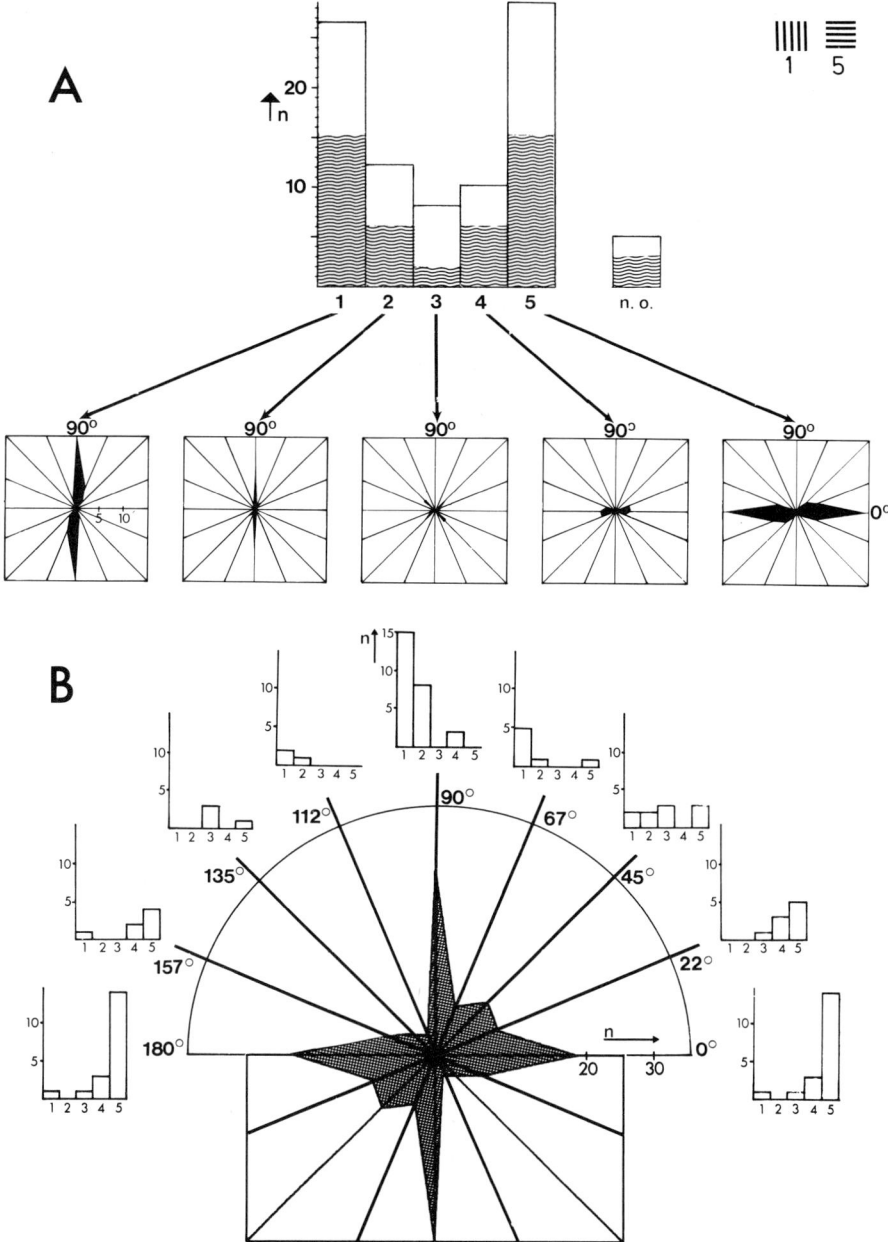

Fig. 10.5A,B. Results of single-unit recording from the striate cortex of two kittens whose visual experience was restricted simultaneously to vertical contours in one eye and to horizontal contours in the other eye by means of cylindrical lenses. The raising condition is displayed symbolically at the upper right corner. Since the eyes which experienced vertical and horizontal contours were different in the two kittens, ocular dominance classes *1* and *5* in this case correspond to the eye with vertical and horizontal experience respectively, and classes *2–4* accordingly. **A** Polar histograms of preferred orientation as a function of the ocular dominance of the particular neurones. The ocular dominance diagram on top comprises all orientation selective neurones; the number of nonoriented neurones is shown in a separate column to the right. The distributions of the individual kittens are indicated by different shading. **B** Ocular dominance distributions as a function of the orientation preference of the particular neurones. Number of neurones is shown on the ordinates. The polar plot of all orientation selective neurones is given in the centre (Rauschecker and Singer 1981)

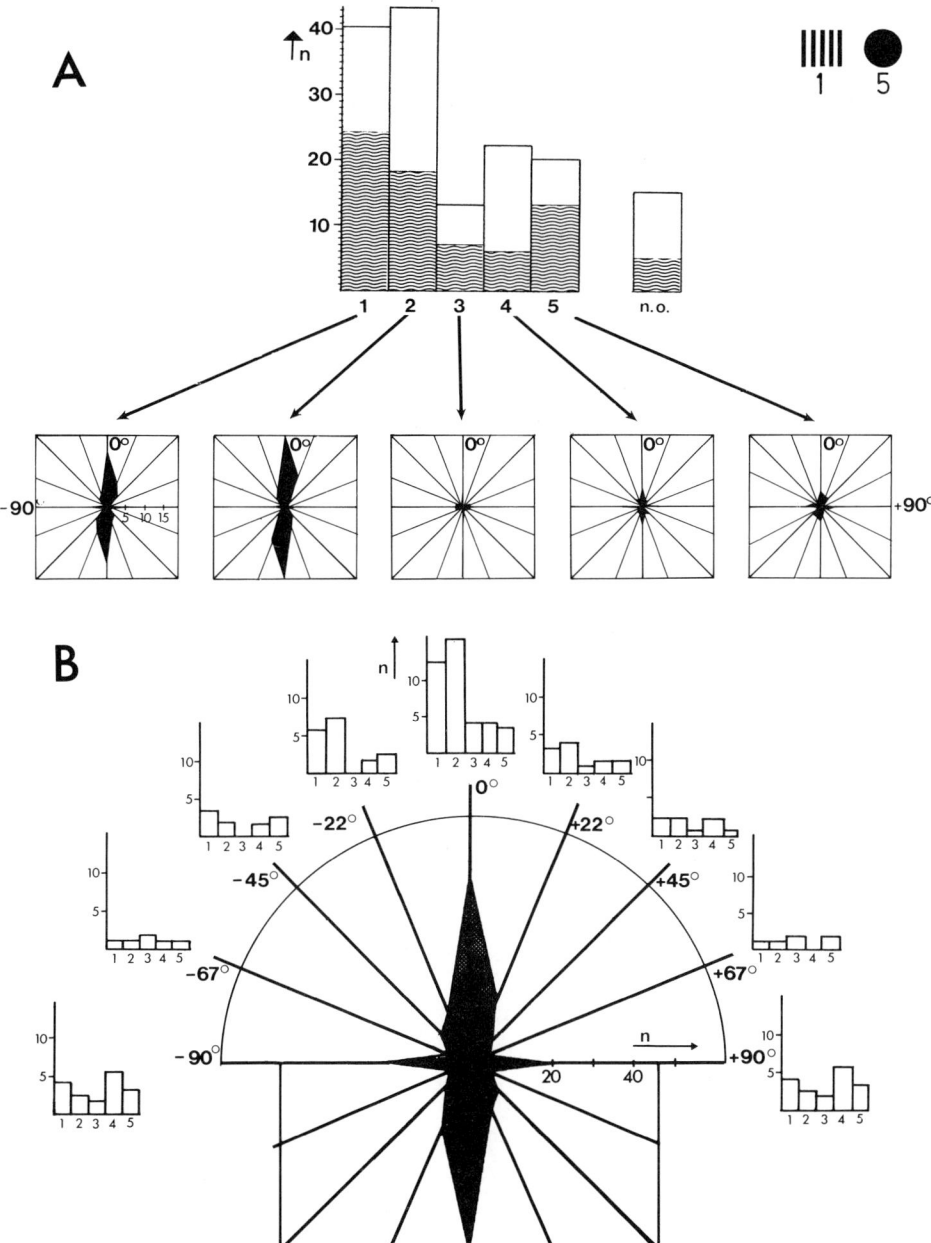

Fig. 10.6A,B. Results from two kittens, litter-mates, with visual experience restricted to either vertical or horizontal contours in the right eye and no experience in the left eye. Since the experienced orientation was different in the two kittens, orientation preference is given as the difference between experienced orientation and preferred orientation. 0° corresponding to no difference. **A** Polar histograms of preferred orientation as a function of ocular dominance. **B** Ocular dominance distributions as a function of orientation preference (Rauschecker and Singer 1981)

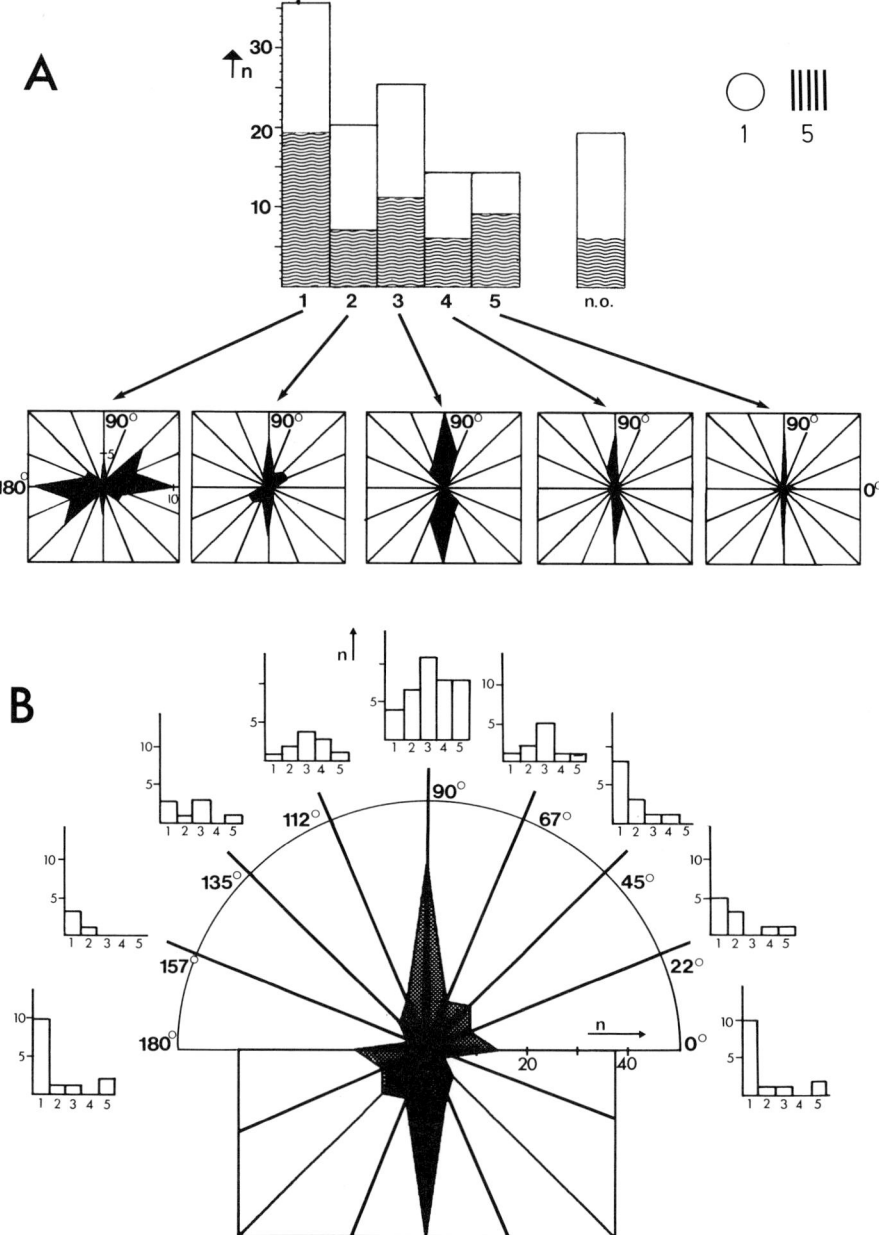

Fig. 10.7 A,B. Results from three kittens, litter-mates, with visual experience restricted to vertical contours in the left eye and normal experience in the right eye. **A** Polar histograms of preferred orientation as a function of ocular dominance. In the ocular dominance diagram (on top) of all orientation selective neurones, the *shaded part* comprises the units from the two kittens in which only one hemisphere was recorded from. **B** Ocular dominance distributions as a function of orientation preference (Rauschecker and Singer 1981)

recorded cortical neuron), whereas the observed orientation bias could be due to a mechanism in which the cortical neuron changes its reactivity to all its afferent synapses in the same way (i.e., by a mechanism that is governed only by *postsynaptic* activity in the recorded neuron itself). We may, for example, assume that a neuron that "likes" a certain orientation becomes inactive if it does not "see" this orientation during the deprivation (cf. Stryker et al. 1978).

The data of Fig. 10.5, however, clearly show that there must be a true interaction between these two mechanisms, i.e., the postsynaptic neuron reduces its reactivity only to those afferents which did not contribute to its activity. This speaks for a Hebbian mechanism (see Chap. 7.5 and Digression 4).

11 From Neural Dynamics to Cell Assemblies

> *Common events in the baby's experience repeatedly excite groups of neurons in the cortex. The neurons that are excited when one of these things happens are not the same every time, but there is a common core of ones that are excited every time. The core neurons therefore tend to become connected with one another in a single system that we will call a* cell-assembly. *Many of these neurons are in closed self-re-exciting circuits and so . . . the system can continue to be active after outside stimulation has ceased.*
>
> D.O. Hebb, 1958

In this chapter I want to introduce a certain type of mathematical brain model. Such models arise from the desire to understand the dynamics in a large network of interconnected neurons. Thus they study the flow of activity through a neuronal network on the basis of comparatively simple assumptions on the dynamics of the individual neurons (and synapses) and on the pattern of their connectivity. The results are usually interpreted in comparison with introspective, psychological, or psychophysical experiences. This kind of interpretation, of course, tends to be very speculative, especially since usually not the whole brain is modeled but just some part of it (e.g., the cortex, the hippocampus, the visual cortex, the cerebellum), and it remains unclear to what degree other parts of the brain contribute to the experiences referred to.

Nevertheless, I think these brain models are quite important, since they provide images for the possible flow of activity in the brain. These images are usually obtained from computer simulations of the flow of activity in an artificial neuronal network. In this way computer simulations can serve as a quasi-experimental approach to the understanding of the flow of activity in neuronal networks.

In this chapter I shall show some of these simulations and discuss the ideas about the flow of activity in our brains that we can draw from them. But in order to understand these simulations properly, we should first get a good idea about the general framework into which these models have been built.

11.1 By *neural dynamics* we understand rules governing the change of the *state* of the brain in time.

The concept of a *state* stems from physics and implies that from complete knowledge of the state at some time t_o and the rules governing the change of state, the state of any later time $t > t_o$ can be determined.

The State

The rules themselves are usually determined from assumptions on the dynamics of a single neuron and from the connectivity scheme of the network. In many models also the connectivities between neurons (i.e., the strength of synapses) may change, again according to given rules.

Let me use a simple neuronal network model to illustrate the concepts of "state" and "rules" governing the change of "state" more clearly.

11.2 The *state of activity* of the network can be described by the activity of every neuron in the network. The activity of one neuron n is usually viewed as a real valued function of time $a_n(t)$. The activity of a neuron at time t can, for example, be measured as the "instantaneous spike frequency" of that neuron, i.e., the inverse of the interspike time interval between the two spikes around t.

If we number the N neurons in the network, we can describe the state of activity by a "vector" $(a_1(t), a_2(t), \ldots, a_N(t)) = A(t)$. In many models the state of activity alone is not enough to describe the state of the brain, since the connectivity of the synapses also changes. By a synapse we mean a connection between two neurons n, n'. Thus we can denote the strength of this synapse by $c_{n\,n'}$.

11.3 Then the *state of connectivity* at time t is given by the matrix $(c_{n\,n'}(t)) = C(t)$.

If $c_{n\,n'}(t) = 0$, there is no actual synapse from n to n',
$c_{n\,n'}(t) > 0$, there is an excitatory synapse from n to n',
$c_{n\,n'}(t) < 0$, there is an inhibitory synapse from n to n'.

The matrix $C(t) = \begin{pmatrix} c_{11}(t) & \ldots & c_{1N}(t) \\ c_{21}(t) & \ldots & c_{2N}(t) \\ \vdots & & \\ c_{N1}(t) & \ldots & c_{NN}(t) \end{pmatrix}$

is called the *connectivity matrix*.

In other words, the following arrangement of formal neurons is expressed by the matrix C (see Fig. 11.1).

The appearance of the connectivity matrix C depends on the numbering of the neurons in N, although the concept of connectivity itself is not in any way dependent on the actual ordering of neurons in the cortex nor on the artificial ordering of the neurons obtained by numbering them. An alternative way of expressing the connectivity of the network is to construct a graph whose points represent the neurons and whose joining arrows represent the connecting synapses (see also Appendix 4).

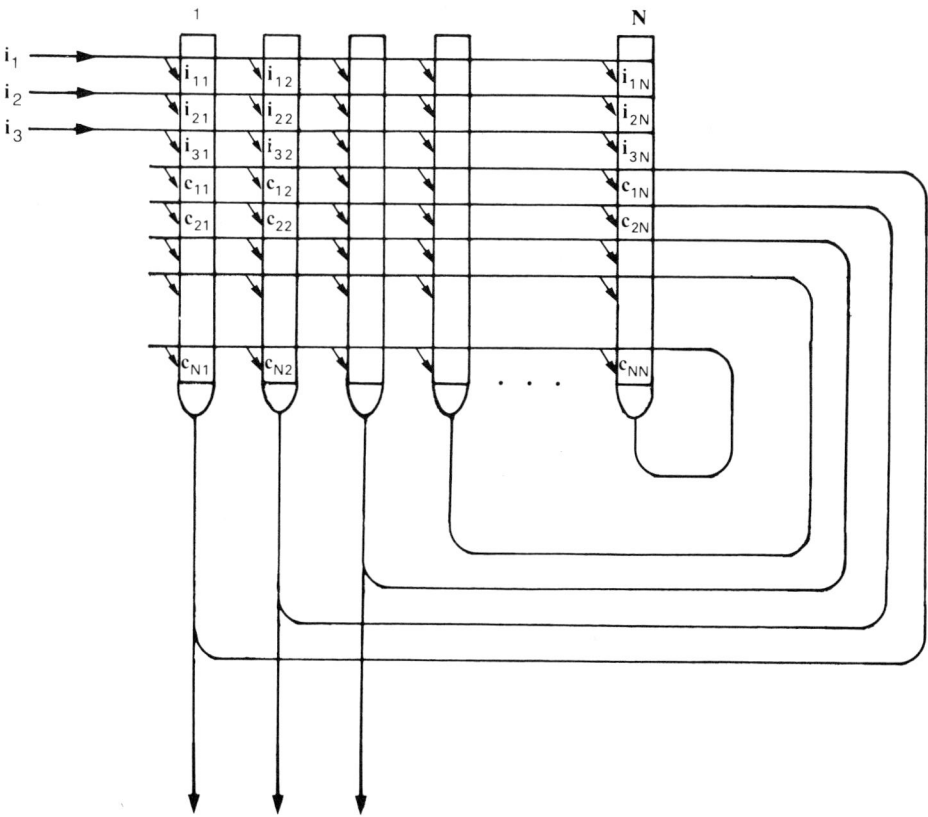

Fig. 11.1. The matrix C describes the internal connectivity of a neural network. Input to the network may be modeled by additional input fibers ($i_1, \ldots, i_k$) with fixed connections i_{jn} ($j = 1, \ldots, k, n = 1, \ldots, N$). Output from the network may be modeled by declaring certain neurons as output neurons. In the diagram (and in the cortex as well) this is realized by providing these axons with output branches

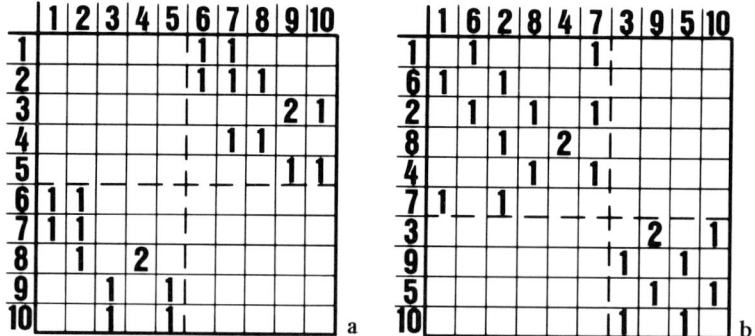

Fig. 11.2a,b. The two matrices **a** and **b** represent the same connectivity between ten neurons

The Flow

Let me give an example of the possible variations of the matrix C, that can be obtained just by renumbering the neurons (Fig. 11.2).

11.4 To analyze the flow of activity, the *initial state* of the brain has to be given, from which the development in time starts. Here usually different initial states of activity are used, whereas the initial state of connectivity is not varied in one model, since it corresponds to the genetically predetermined connectivity of the immature brain. The initial connectivity can be described by the matrix C. This matrix is either given explicitly or determined statistically.

11.5 The state of the network at time t is given by the vector A(t) and the matrix C(t). The rules have to define the "next" state A(t + 1), C(t + 1) from A(t) and C(t).

The next state of activity A(t + 1) is determined from A(t) and C(t) by the assumptions that are made about the dynamics of every single neuron in the network. For example, if we assume that the network consists simply of threshold neurons, then we get for the n-th neuron

$$a_n(t+1) = \begin{cases} 0 & \text{if } \Sigma_i a_i(t)\, c_{i\,n}(t) < \theta_n \\ 1 & \text{if } \Sigma_i a_i(t)\, c_{i\,n}(t) \geq \theta_n \end{cases}$$

(cf. Fig. 3.4). This is true for every neuron, i.e., for $n = 1, \ldots, N$.

We can use the matrix notation to write these equations in one. Defining $f_\theta(B)$ for any vector $B = (b_1, \ldots, b_N)$ by

$$(f_\theta(B))_n = \begin{cases} 0 & \text{if } b_n < \theta \\ 1 & \text{if } b_n \geq \theta \end{cases} \quad (n = 1, \ldots, N),$$

we get $A(t+1) = f_\theta(A(t) \cdot C(t))$.

To determine C(t + 1) from C(t) and A(t), let us now simply assume that the change in connectivity between two neurons n and n' depends only on the activity in these two neurons. This means that $c_{n\,n'}(t+1) = c_{n\,n'}(t) + f(a_n(t), a_{n'}(t))$. The function f determines the amount of change in the connectivity $c_{n\,n'}$ from the activity values $a_n(t)$ and $a_{n'}(t)$ in the two neurons that are concerned. For example, we could use $f(a_n(t), a_{n'}(t)) = a_n(t) \cdot a_{n'}(t)$. This corresponds exactly to Hebb's rule, as stated in Chapter 7.5.

Any such function f is said to represent a *local synaptic rule*, and these local synaptic rules are treated more extensively in Digression 4 and Appendix 2.

11.6 Given an initial state and the rules governing the change of state, more or less in the way described above, one can use the resulting equations to analyze the dynamics in this model network, i.e., the evolution of the state of activity and of the state of connectivity in time. This is usually done by computer simulations, and I will now show some examples.

11.7 First of all, one may be interested in the general time evolution of activity in a randomly interconnected neuronal network. Some interesting results in this direction have been obtained by Anninos et al. (1970) and Harth et al. (1970), who simulated and studied the dynamics of the average activity α (i.e., the total number of active neurons divided by the total number of neurons) for different parameters, such as

 h = percentage of inhibitory cells
 μ^+ = average number of synapses of an excitatory cell
 μ^- = average number of synapses of an inhibitory cell
 η = threshold of all neurons in terms of synapses, i.e., number of excitatory synapses needed to fire a neuron.

Three basic types of dynamics are obtained (see Fig. 11.3):

Type A: there is one stable value of α, which is reached from every initial value.
Type B: 0 is also a stable value for α, and below a certain threshold value α' for α the activity goes down to 0, above α' it approaches the nonzero stable value.
Type C: $\alpha = 0$ is the only stable value, and every initial activity finally dies out.

It is a pity that the concrete parameter values chosen in Anninos et al. (1970) are far from those values which I believe to be true for the real cortex, since all of the parameters used are very relevant and it would be important to make inferences on the actual values of h and η for example. In any case, it is important to know the basic types of dynamics that can occur in randomly connected neuronal networks. These more general results are confirmed and refined by statistical investigations on neurodynamics (see Amari 1974, Amari et al. 1977).

But of course, these statistical inferences only concern rather global parameters like the average activity in the network, which are important for the stability of the dynamics, but only of marginal interest for the analysis of the information processing that can be performed by such a network. In this respect, these investigations on randomly connected neuronal networks correspond more to the rough image of the flow of activity in the cortex which I sketched in Chapters 8.4 and 8.5, than to the more de-

3 Types of Dynamics

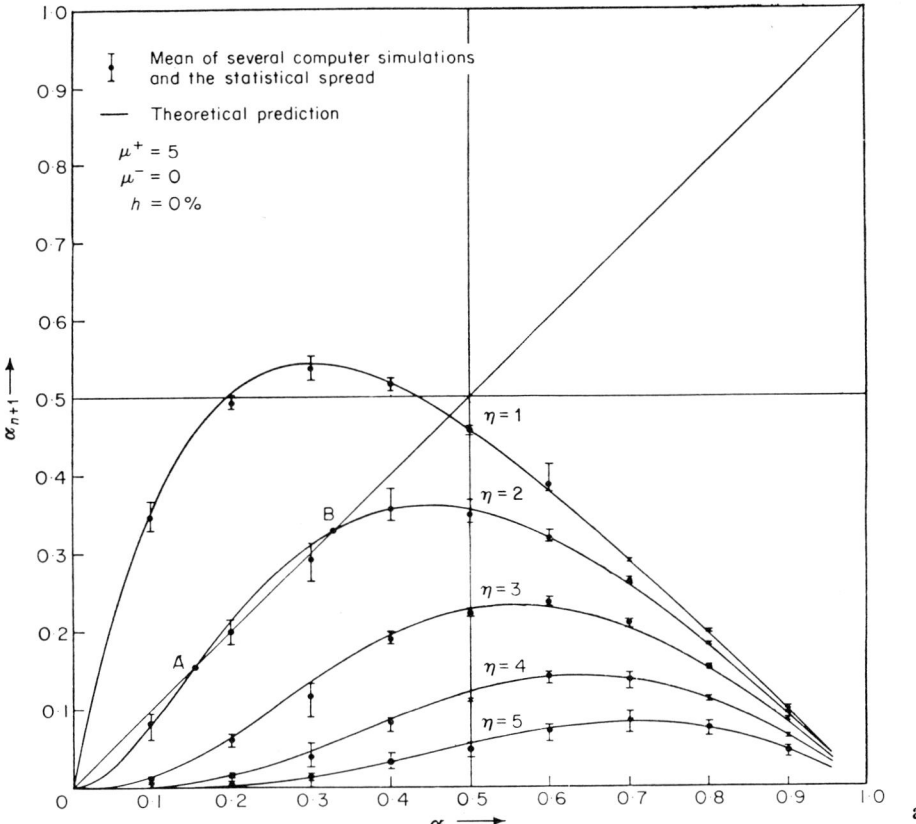

Fig. 11.3a–c. Time evolution of the mean activity in neuron networks with random connectivity (Anninos et al. 1970). **a** Expectation value of neural activity $\langle \alpha_{n+1} \rangle$ vs. preceding activity $\langle \alpha_n \rangle$. The netlet is characterized by the parameters $h = 0, \mu^+ = 5$. Curves are the theoretical values. Points were obtained by computer simulation of a netlet of 1000 neurons.

Using one of these curves one can reconstruct the evolution of mean activity in time: starting from an initial value α_0 one can look up α_1, from this one can look up α_2, and so on. The result is shown in **b**

tailed considerations on information processing in the first part of this book. In the following I want to discuss neuronal network models that show interesting information processing capabilities.

11.8 As a guideline for presenting the information processing possible in such networks, I will again use the improved matchbox algorithm of Chapter 5. As you remember, apart from simple logical networks, this algorithm needed two main associative memories:

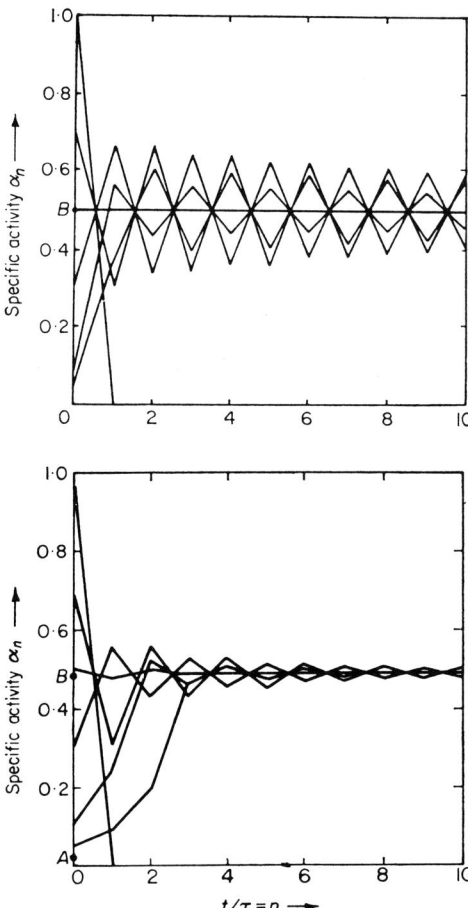

Fig. 11.3 b. Legend see p. 109

— a matrix P to predict the most probable "next" situation from a given situation (see Chap. 7.2),
— a matrix C to complete a pattern from which only parts are given (see Chap. 7.3).

It finally needed some more, but probably smaller, matrices like C to "hold" information for a comparatively short time during operation of the look-ahead algorithm. The learning possibilities of matrices arranged as in Fig. 11.1 or as in Figs. 7.2, 7.8 and 7.9 are nicely illustrated in Kohonen's simulations (see Figs. 11.4 and 11.5).

11.9 But the look-ahead algorithm might indeed require a little more. For example, it may sometimes become necessary to proceed from the most probable next move to the second-most probable next move, or to asso-

Information Processing

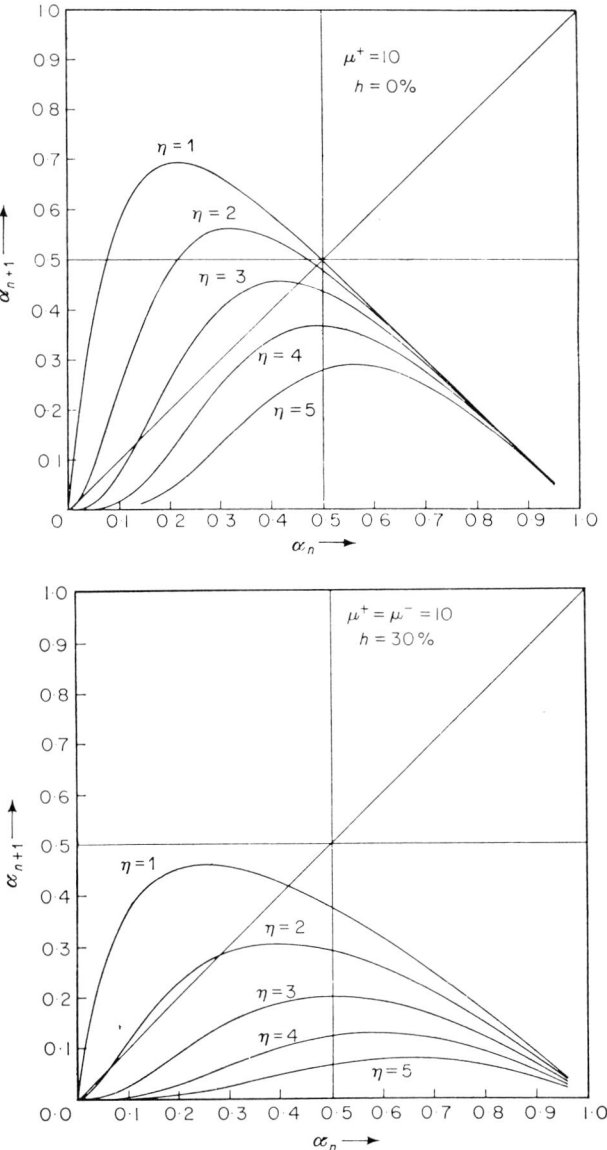

Fig. 11.3c. The same as **a** for different parameters (Anninos et al. 1970)

ciate a valuation that is obtained by looking ahead with the position at hand. To do the first, one should have a way of "holding" part of a pattern, while changing other parts in a correlation matrix with feedback. To do the second, one would like to switch on (and off) different inputs into such a matrix.

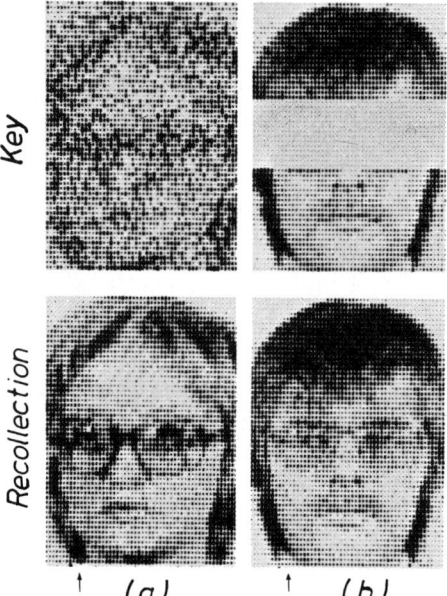

Fig. 11.4. The recall performance of an associative memory in which several patterns have been stored by auto-association (cf. Chap. 7.3) (Kohonen 1981)

This "steering" of associations can indeed be done in such a network by using "threshold control", i.e., an additional parameter that works uniformly on all excitatory neurons in the network and is used to control the average activity.

This is nicely demonstrated in the simulations of Willwacher (Fig. 11.6).

By changing the parameter SHE that governs the threshold of the model neurons, one can obviously change the mode of operation of the whole network between "holding" and "changing". It is easily conceivable that independent regulation of that threshold in different regions of the network would make it possible to hold one part of a pattern while changing another. Of course, it is tempting to compare these remarks with my remarks in Chapter 8, on the probable influence of the thalamus on the cortex.

11.10 In Willwacher's model, threshold regulation is even used to switch between temporal succession of events and completion of events; i.e., the two basic operations performed in the matrices P and C could be performed in one matrix (cf. Figs. 11.6 and 11.7).

There is, however, a slight problem here. Namely, association through forced temporal succession, i.e., through projection from one pattern to another, as in Fig. 11.7, cannot be distinguished from association through

Threshold Regulation

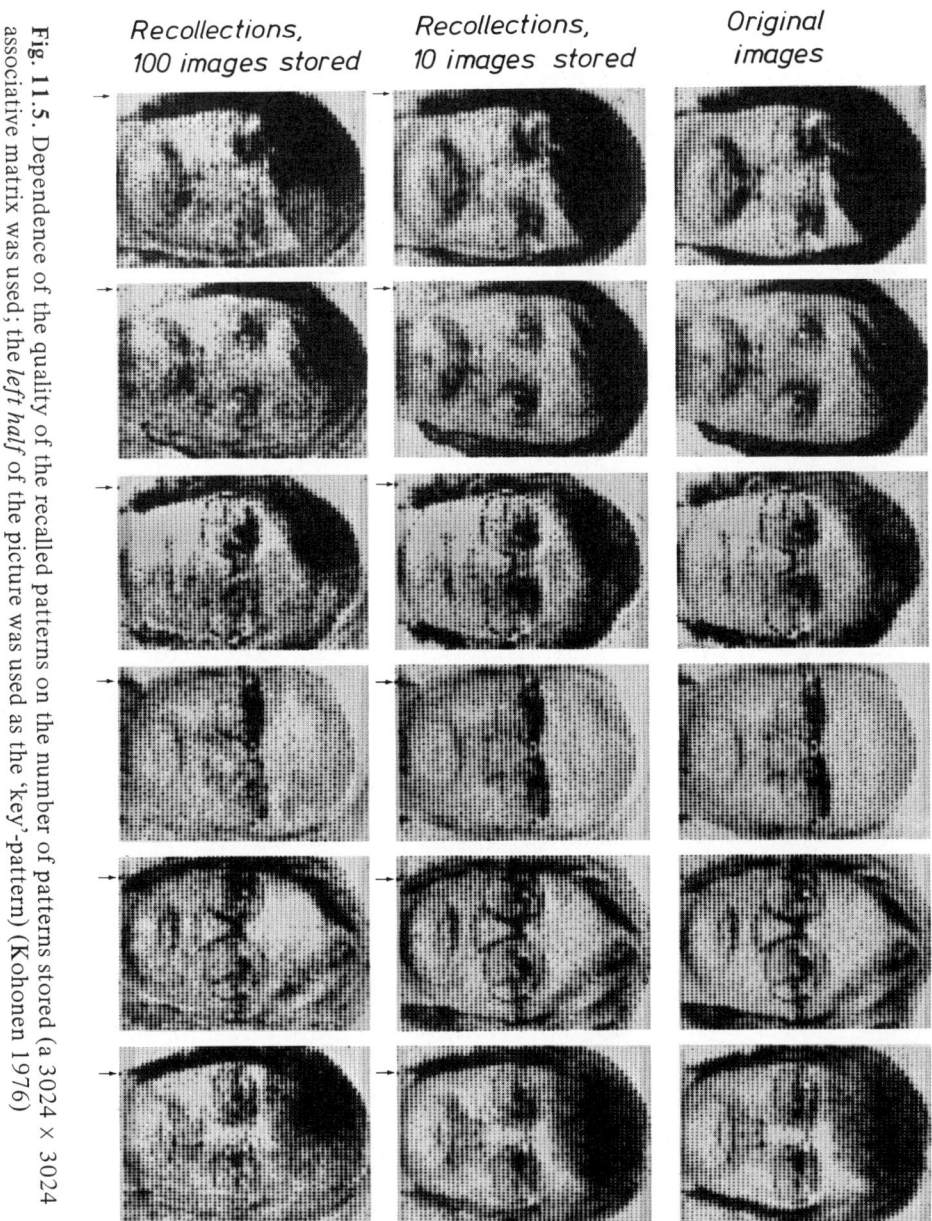

Fig. 11.5. Dependence of the quality of the recalled patterns on the number of patterns stored (a 3024 × 3024 associative matrix was used; the *left half* of the picture was used as the 'key'-pattern) (Kohonen 1976)

overlap of patterns, as in Fig. 11.6, since they are both done by the same change in threshold (decreasing).

One can avoid this problem simply by using two different matrices P and C, but there may be still another way. Willwacher assumes in his simulations that a sequence X → Y is stored by a weak connection from every

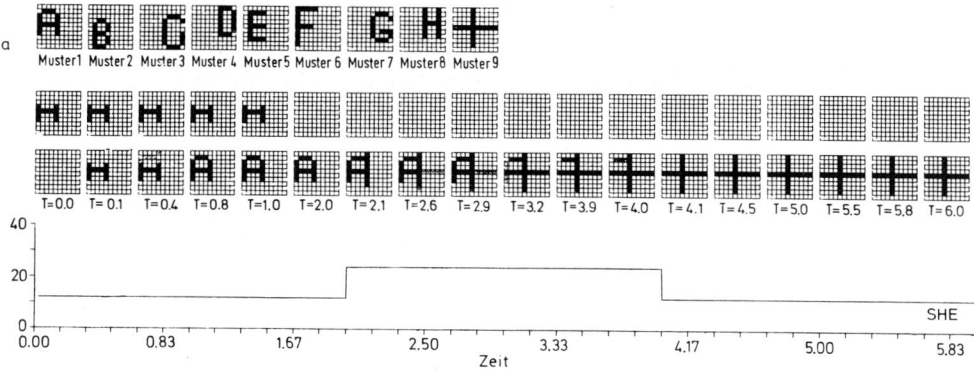

Fig. 11.6a. The patterns (*letters*) were stored in a 100 × 100 connectivity scheme, that contained strong connectivity between all the points of each of the patterns (1–9), and somewhat weaker connectivities from the points of each pattern to the point of the next pattern in the sequence. **b** Association obtained by changing the parameter SHE in time. A higher value of the parameter SHE corresponds to a lower value of the threshold θ. The first line of patterns shows the input patterns, the second line the output patterns (Willwacher 1976)

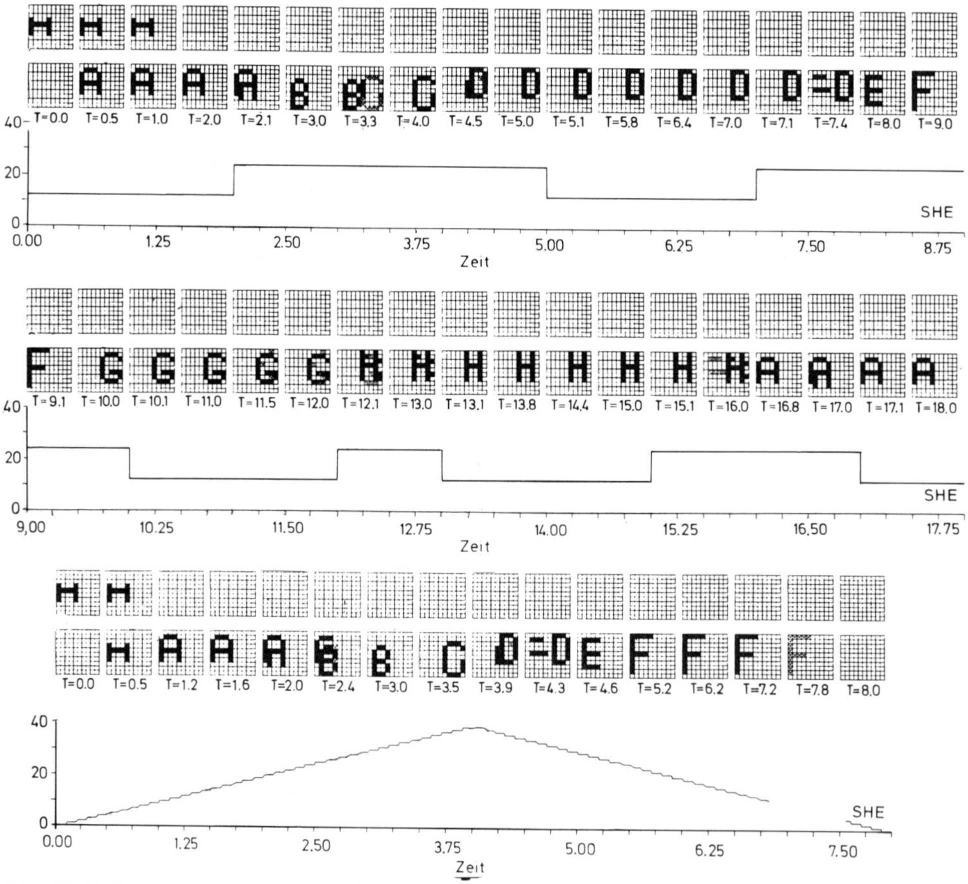

Fig. 11.7. Sequence of patterns obtained by changing the parameter SHE in time. For further explanation see Fig. 11.6 (Willwacher 1976)

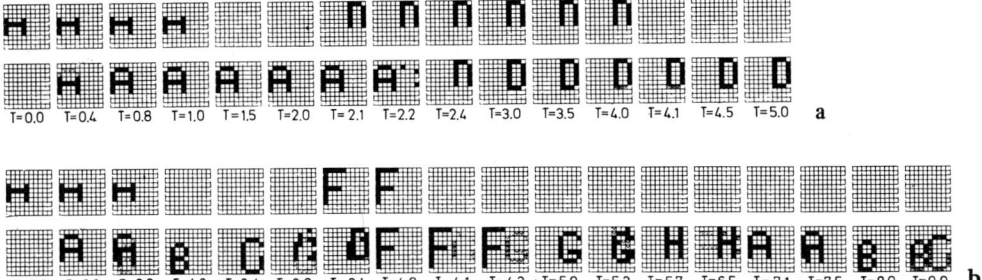

Fig. 11.8a. SHE = 120, b SHE = 240; for further explanation see Fig. 11.6 and the text (Willwacher 1976)

element of X to every element of Y. If, however, such a sequence were stored by somewhat stronger connections from only a "characteristic" part of X to a part of Y, then it would perhaps be possible to switch to temporal succession by increasing the threshold so that X dies out, but its characteristic part remains for the longest time and induces the forming of Y, if the threshold is now lowered again.

How an additional input may interact with the usual flow of activity can also be demonstrated in Willwacher's model: see Fig. 11.8.

11.11 But how can an input channel from sensory organs or from another matrix to an association matrix be switched on and off — remembering that these channels have to contain quite a large number of fibers (cf. Chap. 7.6)? One simple way of doing this would be to concentrate the input fibers in a comparatively high density in one region — which would then be called an input region — and to use independent threshold control for that region.

Of course, for the output of such a matrix, one could use the same idea — concentration in one region and threshold control — to switch it on and off. Again it is tempting to compare this idea with the anatomy of input and output regions of the brain. It could perhaps also be used to identify nonsensory input and output regions where the switching between different matrices is done. But I think it will require a very detailed knowledge of the anatomy to identify these regions and to speculate about the "number of matrices in our brain" (cf. also Chap. 7.6).

In any case, I think the reader will now have enough material to imagine the dynamics of a neural implementation of our improved matchbox algorithm at work.

Digression 5 gives one more concrete model of the improved matchbox algorithm in terms of a flow diagram.

11.12 Finally, I want to put down some terms which I consider to be useful to describe neural and synaptical dynamics locally and globally, and which are in accordance with most of the models cited in this section and in Appendix 2.

1. A *cell assembly* is a set of neurons that fire together because the activity of some of them is sufficient to excite the whole set. This notion goes back to the psychologist D.A. Hebb (1949). It is important to notice that two different assemblies do not have to be disjoint. In fact there should usually be a considerable *overlap,* in the sense that the average single neuron belongs to many assemblies. Appendix 4 deals with the problem of defining cell assemblies in the set-up of mathematical graph-theory.
2. Neural dynamics can be described globally as
   a) forming (ignition) and diminishing of cell assemblies (probably through threshold control),
   b) temporal sequence of cell assemblies (through projection from one assembly to another), this may occasionally lead into cycles,
   c) "holding" of one assembly for some time.
3. The type of dynamics in a neural network is mainly determined by the *connectivity matrix* (that gives the connectivity $c_{n\,n'}$ between any two neurons n, n' in the network).
4. To a certain degree the connectivity is determined through learning.
5. The basic mechanism for this is a *local synaptic rule,* like *Hebb's rule:* The amount of excitation a synapse will transmit is enhanced by the coincidence of pre- and postsynaptic activity.
   This rule has several consequences:
6. The connectivity matrix can be regarded as the matrix of an associative matrix memory with feedback connections.
7. The main global characteristic of such a memory is that it performs *pattern completion.* The completion of a pattern corresponds to the ignition of a cell assembly.
8. In the dendritic tree of a single neuron, Hebb's rule enhances the effectivity of synapses that are activated at the same time: neurons become *detectors for coincident* (or correlated) *activity* in their dendritic tree. This idea can most easily be understood in the input regions where correlated presynaptic activity directly stems from correlated events in the outside world (cf. the simulations of von der Malsburg 1973, and Nass and Cooper 1975).

12 Introspection and the Rules of Threshold Control

> *All ideas which are different are separable.*   David Hume, 1739
>
> *... Nature in a manner pointing out to every one those simple ideas, which are most proper to be united into a complex one. The quantities, from which this association arises and by which the mind is after this manner conveyed from one idea to another, are three, viz.* resemblance, contiguity *in time or place, and* cause and effect.   David Hume, 1739

In the first section we have seen that we are not aware of all the information that reaches our brain through the sensory channels.

We know this since at any moment we can concentrate on some aspect of our sensory input and perceive it very accurately, whereas other parts we just assume to remain constant — or to evolve as they usually would. In this way we have a feeling of getting a rich image of our surroundings at any moment, although only less than 40 bits/s of new information can really enter our consciousness.

In other words, we are always aware of just a small segment of our surroundings, our "view" is restricted by a "window", but we can move this window around by concentrating on various things.

In the following I will try to describe how I can control the movement of the location of that window, i.e., of what I concentrate on or am aware of. And I can only hope that the reader will share these introspections.

12.1 First of all, the window moves automatically to where something new and surprising happens.

   a) But I can control the strength of this tendency, i.e., I can make it move to everything that is moderately surprising, if I want to be very alert, and I can make it ignore all that, although I still cannot prevent it from moving to something very surprising.
   b) I can control this degree of alertness independently for the different senses. For example, I can be "all ears" or "all eyes", if I want to.
   c) I can also rule down the degree of alertness for all senses at the same time. In this case, I concentrate on some mental events or images; one would say that I "think"; right now when I am writing I am also in that state.
   d) But how can I control what I concentrate on, in this case? Let me take an example. If I try to remember something that does not come to my mind immediately, I will usually try to "hold on" to some details that

I believe to be correct and try to associate to them the right answer. If I still do not get the desired answer, I might at least get some more hints, i.e., some more details that I believe to be most probably correct. I can then hold on to these, too — perhaps in turn — and keep on trying to let more associations come up. Finally, I am usually lucky and I get the answer I believe to be correct. I believe that this answer now is correct, since it all fits: the answer fits with the hints I started from and with most of the intermediate hints I obtained on the way. Systematizing this kind of description, I think I always use a few basic mechanisms:

e) I can selectively "hold on" to something that I have in mind.
f) I can unselectively associate something else to it. I can let associations "come up".
g) Perhaps I can also "combine" two things I had in mind very recently, that is I can "hold on" to both of them.
h) Finally, I need a mechanism that tells me that *it all fits*.

12.2 I think that I use these mechanisms not only when I try to remember something, but whenever I am thinking. For example, if I have a problem to solve, this usually consists of finding a way from the present situation to a desired situation. In this case I can use a strategy of the type described above. I can combine (g) the characteristic picture of the desired situation with the situation at hand, hold on (e) to this and associate (f) intermediate steps to it. Then I can selectively hold on to some of these and associate again. This way, I proceed exactly according to the above description, until I hopefully come to a pattern where it all fits (h), i.e., a pattern that combines the two situations and contains many of the intermediate steps or hints obtained on the way (and probably also some restrictive conditions).

One may think at this point that these mechanisms cannot be enough, and indeed one can easily think of some more mechanisms that would be convenient to guide awareness or thoughts, but — at least for me — the ones I mentioned are the only ones I am quite sure of.

12.3 Why do I describe these introspections at this point? I believe that they reflect the dynamics that goes on in my brain in some metaphoric may. When I speak about "strategies" and "mechanisms" that "I" use to steer that "window of awareness", I use these metaphors to state principles that are derived from all I can introspectively — and therefore rather indirectly — observe of the dynamics in my own brain. And I do not want to discard this information; in fact, it can be interpreted rather well in terms of the mechanisms used by the "survival algorithm", as examplified in the simula-

Introspection

tions shown in the last chapter. It should be clear by now that I do not use these metaphors to re-introduce the "little man" into the brain (who now uses the strategies described above instead of simply looking at preprocessed pictures and controlling muscles). In fact, I believe that the "algorithm" that would have to be performed by this "little man" is so simple that we do not need a man for it (one version of this algorithm is given in Digression 5). It is the basic algorithm that is built into the survival robot (or even into a chess-playing machine) and that has been continuously refined throughout the first part of this book.

At this point the reader may have two questions:

If this book has been written by a realization of a "survival algorithm" at work,

a) how can a survival robot report about his own mechanisms?
b) how seriously should such a report be taken?

I will return to the first question in the last two chapters. As for the second question, I can only warn the reader to be very cautious in the interpretation of any kind of introspection. Nevertheless, in the following most speculative part of this book I shall try to use the language of "cell assemblies" to describe the dynamics in our brains in terms that can be interpreted physically *and* introspectively at the same time.

12.4 *Thinking in terms of cell assemblies* (Hebb 1949, 1958) *and threshold control* (Braitenberg 1978)

1. In the cortex we have an associative memory, more exactly, an association matrix with feedback, where pattern completion is performed (the main memory of a survival robot, e.g., as specified in Digression 5).

2. Such a completed pattern of activity is called a *cell assembly* (cf. Chap. 11.12). Every cell assembly corresponds to a specific content of our consciousness, i.e., what we are aware of momentarily, namely the situation $s = (cs,a,v)$ combined of circumstances, (planned) activities and (expected) values (as in Chap. 7.3). The pattern has been stored by learning (as in Chap. 5); this means that a new cell assembly can be formed by holding a "new" input to the matrix constant for some time. There can be a considerable overlap between different assemblies (see also Appendices 1 and 3).

3. At any moment there is always only one assembly active, since there is always one pattern in the memory. But the different patterns may, of course, overlap, i.e., the same neuron may belong to different assemblies.

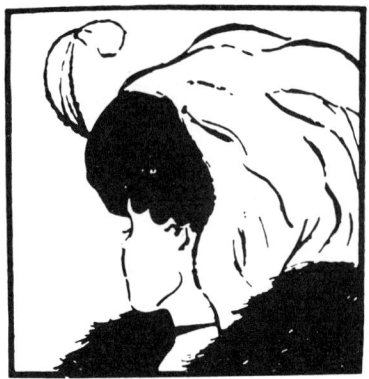 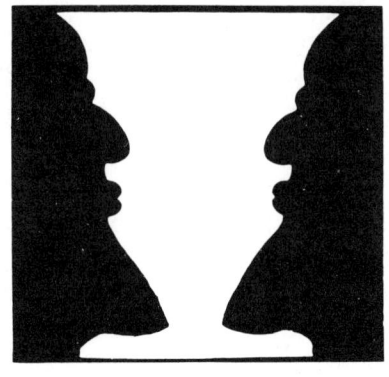

Fig. 12.1 a,b. Two ambiguous figures: in **a** one can see either a young or an old woman, in **b** one can see either two faces or a vase (Szentagothai and Arbib 1974)

We notice this, introsepctively, when on the one hand two imaginations can have many things in common, and on the other hand, we usually cannot concentrate on two different things at once (unless we can embed both of them into one consistent situation), and if we try, the two imaginations tend to inhibit each other until one of them "wins". For example, look at Fig. 12.1.

The inhibition between cell assemblies may well be due to local unselective inhibition in the cortex (cf. Chap. 8).

4. An assembly (A) usually has an inner structure: it contains subassemblies that hold at different thresholds; some subassemblies may even hold at the same or higher threshold than A. Of course, a subset B of a cell assembly A can only be regarded as a sub*assembly,* if it can hold at some threshold. This means that the neurons in B have to be connected together more strongly than in an average subset of A. These problems of connectivity are discussed in Appendix 4.

5. A movement from assembly to assembly can occur for two reasons: a) "surprising" sensory inputs, b) "association" through *"threshold control".*

If this does not happen, an activated assembly has the tendency to stay active, we say that it *holds.*

6. We have a simple immediate prediction mechanism that is directly connected to the sensory inputs and motor outputs (Fig.12.2). The deviation between predicted and actual sensory data determines the degree of surprise of the sensory input, as used for (5a). This mechanism lowers the threshold in those sensory areas where something surprising has occurred.

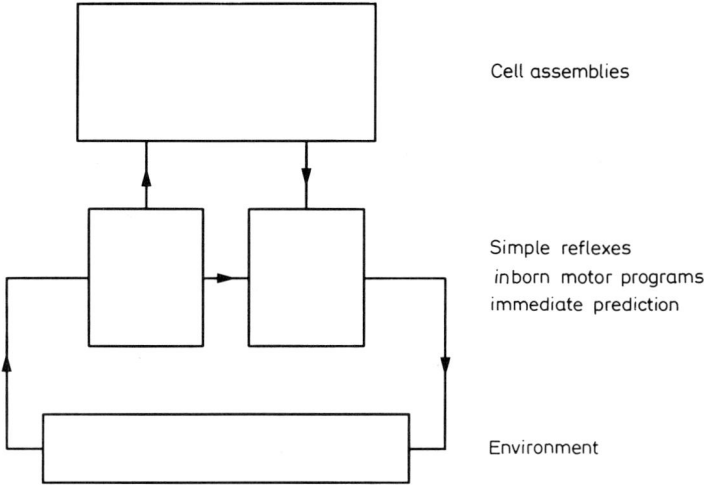

Fig. 12.2. This figure is nearly identical with Fig. 1.1

7. Threshold control (5 b) is performed through diffuse influence on the activity of whole areas of cortex. Probably, this is done by the diffuse nonspecific thalamo-cortical fibers (cf. Chap. 8.5). The heights of threshold in the various regions define the "state of mind":

"Alert": low threshold in sensory and motor areas, high threshold in associational areas.

"Absent-minded", thinking: vice versa.

"All eyes": low threshold in primary visual area. Etc.

One assembly may have a different "loudness" in different areas, according to different amplitudes in the threshold control.

8. Associations are performed through threshold control as in Fig. 12.3 (Braitenberg 1978a, and cf. Fig. 11.6):

These changes in threshold can be performed independently in different areas, although there seems to be a basic rhythm of threshold control,

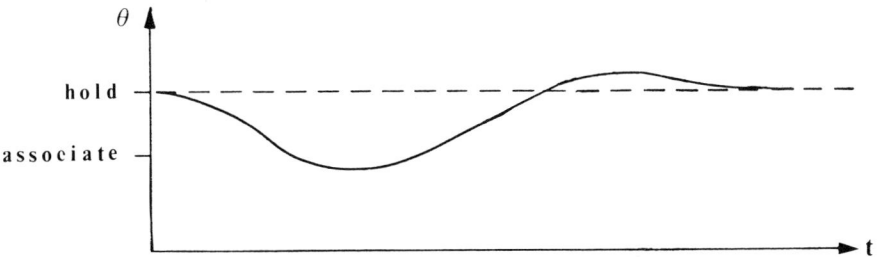

Fig. 12.3. Association from one assembly to another one can be performed by lowering the threshold temporarily (from the usual "holding level" of threshold)

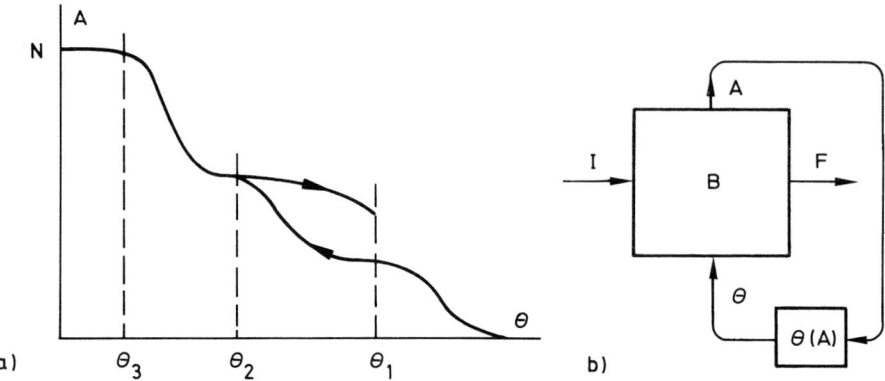

Fig. 12.4. a The relationship between activity (A) or number of active neurons (N) and threshold (θ). A hysteresis-effect can be observed, if the threshold is lowered from θ_1 to θ_2, and then raised again. **b** The brain B with its sensory input I and motor output F and the additional threshold-control mechanism, that regulates θ as a function of A (Braitenberg 1978a)

probably for the whole cortex. This idea seems plausible, since it is very hard for us to produce two movements at the same time that have different basic rhythms (strictly, this argument applies only to the motor regions).

9. How do we detect that "it all fits" and how can we test the "reliability of ideas"? Usually the average activity decreases monotonically in a certain way with increasing threshold, and it increases monotonically with decreasing threshold (see Fig. 12.4).

Thus, we expect a certain average activity at a given threshold. If a number of details are given and, by adding one more detail, we suddenly see that they fit into a scheme, by which they all belong together, this is reflected in an unusually high amount of recurrent excitation between the neurons belonging to the corresponding pattern of activity in our brain – or, in other words, in the firing of a large cell assembly. This is detected by a mechanism that counts the number of active cells and compares it with the usual average activity at the momentary threshold. It can be tested further by increasing the threshold again. If the activity pattern survives this, it is more "reliable" as a cell assembly and we can take the maximal threshold which this assembly can sustain as a measure of to what degree it all fits.

Some simple simulations of this type of threshold control in a very small network are given in Fig. 12.5.

The first detection of a large assembly gives us a good feeling and I think it is that what happens if we suddenly have an idea, or if we laugh at a joke.

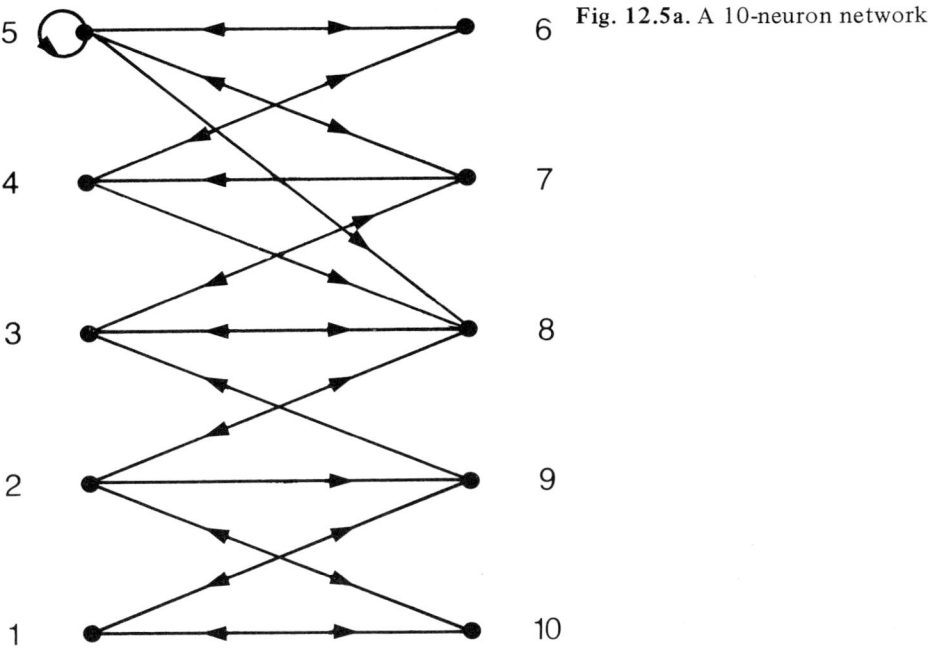

Fig. 12.5a. A 10-neuron network

10. The threshold control is carried out according to an inborn search algorithm, like the minimax algorithm of Chapter 5, or rather like the search strategy described in Chapter 12.1d or in Digression 5. This algorithm changes the thresholds of the main memory using the assembly detection mechanism of (9) and the strategy described in (8). It may be built into some subcortical structure.

The end to which the algorithm works is genetically determined: it tries to find strategies leading to "good" situations. The search algorithm is "switched on" only in particular situations, where, for example, a drastic change in the current evaluation of the situation is predicted. Normally it is switched off.

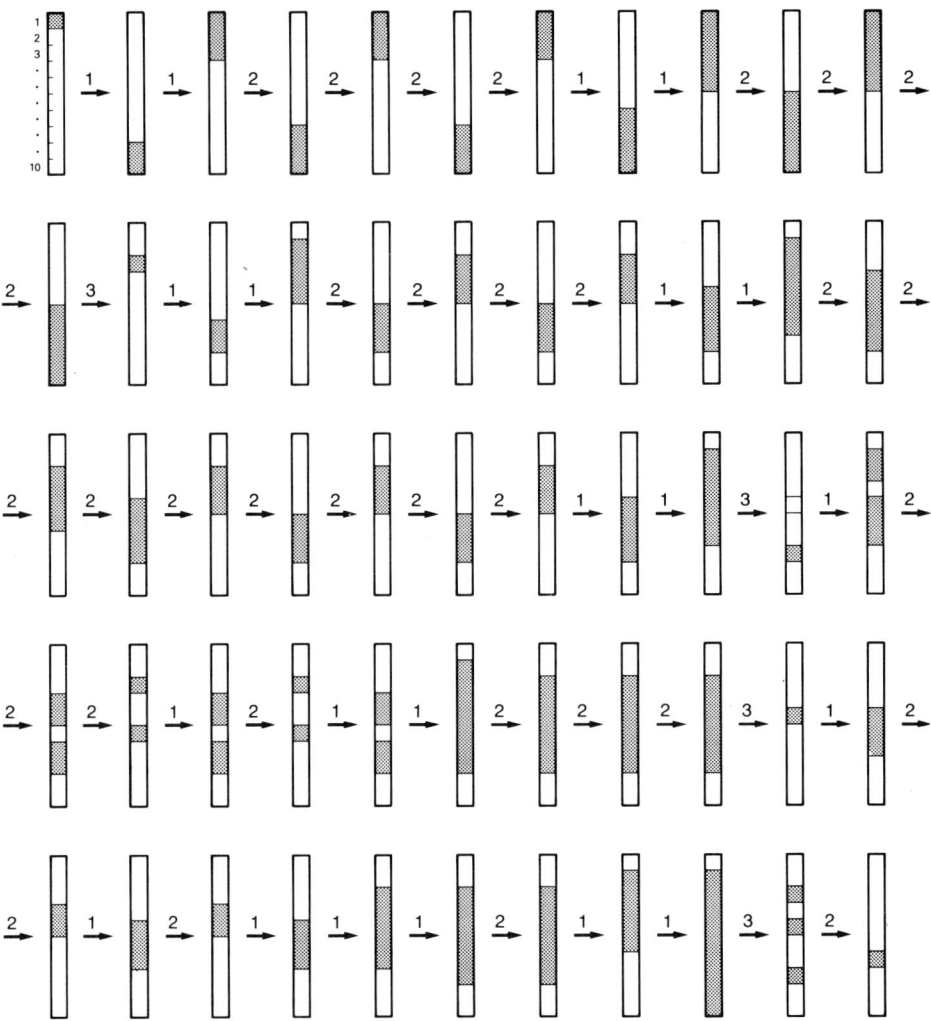

Fig. 12.5b. Activity in this network. At the beginning only neuron no. 1 is active. The *numbers on the arrows* signify the threshold level at which the next state is obtained. For example at threshold 1 the second state is reached with neurons 9 and 10 active

13 Further Speculations

It is absurd to deny the role of fantasy in even the strictest science.
K.I. Lenin

This chapter contains some rather wild speculations that are meant to fill out the rough image sketched in the last chapter.

13.1 In Chapter 12.4.6 we postulated a simple immediate prediction mechanism. I believe that this mechanism is part of the preprocessing of sensory inputs that has to be performed before these inputs enter the main memory. As I mentioned in Chapter 6, a good preprocessing is very important to make the memory itself more effective; it has probably been optimized during evolution and contains a lot of knowledge about our usual natural environment. This preprocessed sensory information tends to give the more excitation into the sensory cortical areas, the more "surprising" (from the point of view of this inborn knowledge about our environment) it is.

But certainly it would be good also to incorporate some "learned" (i.e., not inborn) knowledge into this simple prediction mechanism. This could be done by providing the general prediction mechanism (Section 13.2) with an additional possibility of regulating the sensory input. This kind of regulatory function has been attributed to the specific sensory thalamic nuclei, which receive inputs from the cortical "prediction areas" (see the next Section).

13.2 In the search strategy of the improved matchbox algorithm as well as in the search strategy described in Chapter 12.2, we need not only associative pattern completion, but also a kind of prediction. Such a prediction mechanism can also be realized in an associative matrix (cf. Chap. 7.2). Moreover, it could be realized in the same matrix where the associative pattern completion takes place (see Chap. 11.10 and especially Figs. 11.6 and 11.7).

As I already mentioned in the last chapter, a cell assembly could contain a special part where the corresponding neurons project quite strongly to a subpart of the temporally next assembly. If this special part survived an increase of the threshold a little longer than the rest, one could detect

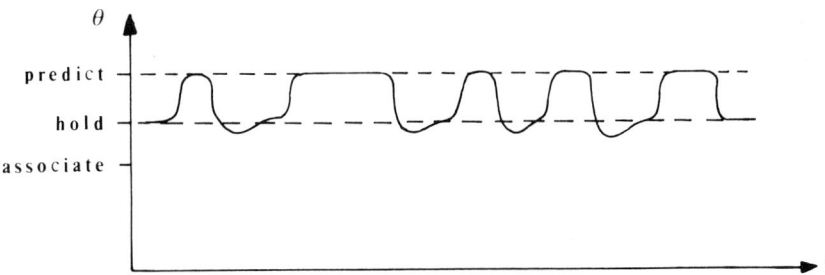

Fig. 13.1. For explanation see text and Fig. 12.3

a highly probable temporal succession of assemblies by the threshold control of Fig. 13.1.

For this mechanism it would be convenient if, in addition, the "temporal projection" parts of different assemblies were all concentrated mainly in certain regions of the cortex. Then one could produce temporal succession of assemblies by keeping the threshold at "holding level" in these regions and increasing it (as indicated in Fig. 13.1) only in the remaining regions. I shall call those areas where the threshold is kept at "holding level" (cf. Figs. 12.3 and 13.1) during prediction, the *P-areas*. The remaining areas, where the threshold is increased during prediction, are called *C-areas*. The sensory areas do not quite fit into this scheme, see Chapter 12.4.6. In the following we divide the cortex into associative pattern completion, C-, associative pattern prediction, P-, and perhaps, sensory, S-areas.

Up to now I have mostly concentrated on the C-areas. Now I want to speculate a little more about the P-areas. Basically the P-areas should contain the associative prediction mechanism of Chapter 7.2 (see especially Fig. 7.4), and therefore upon increase of the threshold in the C-areas the activity should move from situation to situation (like a movie) in the P-areas. But of course it will often happen that in a sequence of patterns a certain part remains constant for some time (representing something like the common context of this part of the sequence). Let me illustrate this by an example. Perhaps the simplest predictions can be made about the mechanisms that are built into the organism itself, for example all the reflexes involved in movement control, lead to fairly constant relations between the neurons initiating a movement, and the proprioceptors reporting the execution of this movement. These causal relationships inside the body should be reflected in a highly probable succession of patterns in the cortex (that is triggered from P-areas), and therefore the motor cortex (that contains neurons that initiate movements) should belong to the P-areas. Moreover, there should be a strong connection from the motor cortex to the somatosensory cortex (that gets a lot of motoric

Motor Programs

feedback information), in order to facilitate the detection of those causal relationships. Other secondary or tertiary motor areas can probably trigger inborn motor programs like "walking", "orienting", "standing" etc. that have been prewired genetically into some subcortical structures. These areas should also belong to the P-areas and they should contain those parts of the patterns that remain constant for some time. This would make it possible to predict (for example in the somatosensory cortex) the internal feedback resulting from standard inborn programs (and later perhaps also from new, acquired programs that have been built from the inborn programs). Such a prediction would mean that a comparatively constant activity in a group of P-neurons that represent a program like "walking", triggers a chain of activities in the neurons of the motor cortex (a P-area) and of the somatosensory cortex (an S-area).

This could be pictured as follows (Fig. 13.2).

Thus an assembly may have a certain temporal inner structure that reflects the temporal structure of the corresponding program.

13.3 How can we program new sequences of movements? On a rather fast time scale this means that we have to create new cell assemblies with a certain temporal inner structure. One way of doing this would be to try combinations of the inborn motor programs, i.e., to use the already existing assemblies with a temporal inner structure in the P-areas, and to combine them (or parts of them) to new assemblies. This means that we learn new movements as certain combinations or superpositions of (parts of) our inborn motor programs. Moreover, a learning capacity of the cerebellum (see Marr 1969, Albus 1971, Ito 1981) may also help in shaping these fast newly learned movements.

On a slower time scale we can program sequences of actions by establishing directed connections between cell assemblies through threshold control. For example, if we can produce a certain sequence of assemblies by using threshold control as a "steering" mechanism, then we can also re-

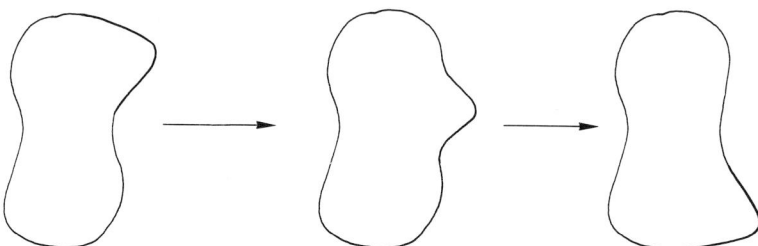

Fig. 13.2. A cell assembly with temporal structure

peat this sequence several times and thus introduce a weak connection from one assembly to the next in this sequence.

13.4 We have defined a state of "absent-mindedness" or "thinking", as a state where the thresholds are high in the sensory areas and low in the "associational" areas, i.e., nonsensory C-areas. But what about the P-areas? It is clear that thinking will often involve predictions and therefore we should require the P-areas to be able to have a low threshold in this state. But for example, when I am thinking about a complicated action while I am sitting, the program of sitting has to be carried out, whereas its representation in the P-areas should not interfere with my imagination of other actions, and also the actions I am imagining should not interfere with the action of sitting that I am carrying out. The problem is that on one hand the motor parts of the P-areas are used to trigger motor programs that are to be actually carried out, whereas on the other hand they are used to evoke predictions in sensory-motor and perhaps also other sensory areas, even when I am only imagining actions.

This problem can be solved by a double representation of certain motor programs and their sensory counterparts, which makes it possible to perform certain tasks or reactions, while the main part of the cortex is rather "disconnected" from these tasks and is used to think about something else (see also Section 13.5). This necessity of a double representation may be the reason for the existence of secondary (and perhaps tertiary) motor and sensory areas with comparatively strong connections to the corresponding primary areas.

13.5 The distinction between P- and C-areas, as introduced here, can perhaps be clarified further by relating it to the distinction of "plan" and "image", made by Miller et al. (1960). Generally speaking, plans should correspond to (parts of) assemblies in the P-areas and images should correspond to (parts of) assemblies in the C-areas. But here we have the problem that a plan can be part of an image, and the prediction of a sequence of images can be part of a plan (as I tried to explain in Fig. 13.2), therefore plans may be partly represented also in the C-areas and images may be partly represented in the P-areas. In general, a cell assembly should always contain neurons in both the P- and C-areas; and if a cell assembly represents something like a situation, it should contain both aspects: plan and image.

Furthermore we may have "metaplans" or higher-level plans that contain a sequence of lower-level plans (in the sense of Fig. 13.2). To describe this it seems reasonable to view the cortex as a hierarchy like Fig. 13.3a.

1. In such a hierarchy, a high-level plan can be fixed (it can "hold"), for example in P_2, and this high-level plan can trigger a sequence of lower-level plans, for example in P_3, which still are "comparatively fixed", compared to the sequences of movements which they trigger. At this point I do not want to spell out in detail the meaning of a "comparatively fixed" plan; obviously such a plan should "hold" for a certain, operatively defined time (this can be realized by conceiving a plan as a TOTE unit, see Miller et al. 1960).
2. A higher-level plan may also contain a conditional command: "If A happens, do B". In other words, in addition to a constant input from the higher level, a certain input A from a C-area (or a certain sensory input) may be required to trigger the response B (cf. the phenomenon of "set"). Therefore it is perhaps more reasonable to conceive a hierarchical organization of the cortex as in Figs. 13.3b or 13.3c.

These two hierarchical mechanisms correspond to the distinction between chaining (1) and concatenation (2) of plans or reactions in Miller et al. (1960).

Note that all the conceptual organization schemes of Fig. 13.3 do not impose any severe restriction on the flow of information (or the connectivity), and therefore cannot be distinguished anatomically (or electrophysiologically) from the simple scheme of Fig. 12.2.

13.6 The distinction between C- and P-areas (as expressed in Fig. 13.3b) probably fits quite well with the distinction between frontal and occipital parts of the cortex (cf. Fig. 8.10) and with the saying that the front of the head contains the future (the plans) whereas the back contains the past (the image) (cf. Luria 1973, Miller et al. 1960).

13.7 Another important point concerning the P-areas is the speed of prediction. To understand how much the speed of prediction can probably be increased compared to real time, we have to discuss the usual time needed to build up a cell assembly. I think that this usually takes around 50–250 ms, since a cell assembly corresponds to what we are aware of, and the "time unit" of awareness seems to be in that range (see Chap. 1). Thus the change of assemblies follows a much slower time course than, for example, unconscious eye movements. On the other hand, a simple projection from a rudiment of one cell assembly to a rudiment of another one only requires a series of 1–3 synapses, i.e., around 3–12 ms. Therefore the speeding up can well be done by a factor of 10. This way, however, the prediction would become quite imprecise with increasing speed, for no

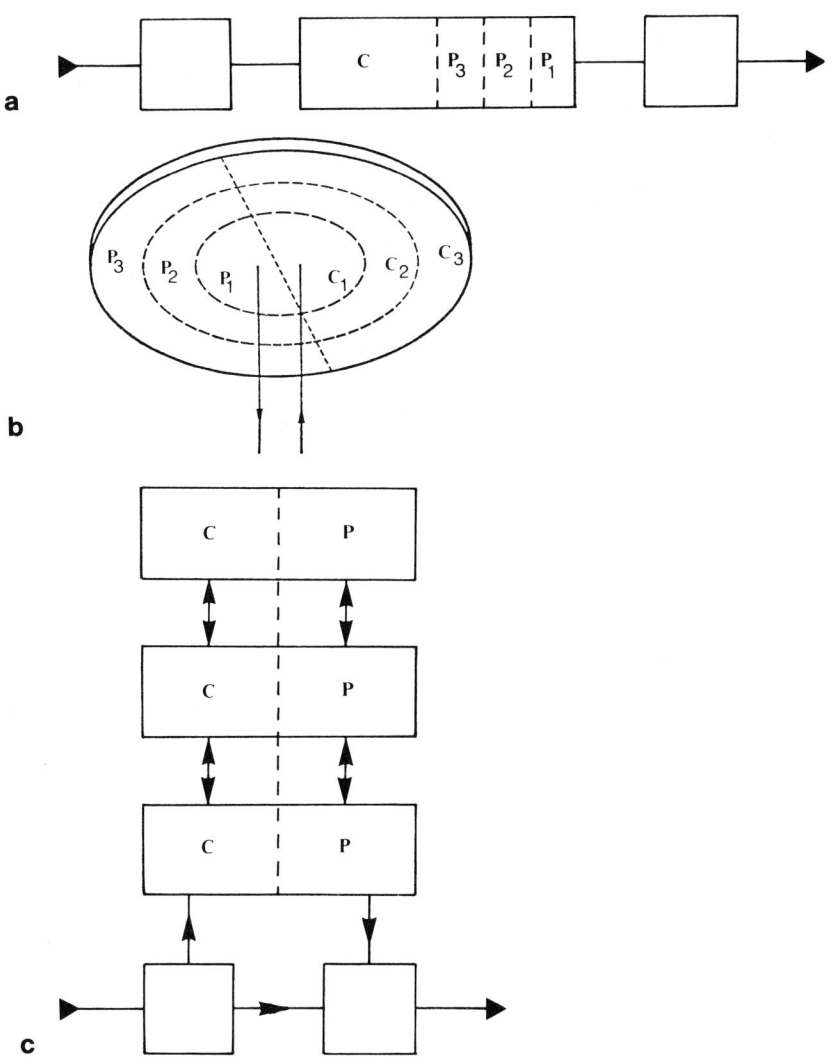

Fig. 13.3. a See text. **b** In this diagram the hierarchical organization is expressed as a gradient from lower levels (of plan and image) to higher levels, which is directed from the center of the flattened cortex (cf. Fig. 8.3) towards the boundary (i.e., the hippocampus in the back and the limbic cortex in the front). **c** This is quite a common scheme for the hierarchical organization of the brain and we can find it in several variations (see, for example, Albus 1979, Fig. 22, for a somewhat restricted and slightly skewed version of it)

cell assemblies are really formed, but just rudiments are following each other, always in danger of a complete dying-out of activity.

This kind of prediction should be used only for a few steps at a time, allowing a full assembly to build up every now and then, i.e., the threshold should be regulated in the C-areas somewhat like Fig. 13.1.

As in Section 13.5, here again the use of different levels of prediction may be helpful: in this case it could further increase the speed and length of prediction by taking larger, but less precisely defined steps at higher levels of prediction.

I do not believe that this type of prediction is used for ballistic movement control, e.g., in playing table tennis, since here a high precision seems to be required. I believe that ballistic prediction is part of the motor-control part of the brain and is carried out in a specialized organ, like the cerebellum (see also Pellionisz and Llinas 1979, Braitenberg and Onesto 1962).

13.8 In the framework of the improved matchbox algorithm, the threshold control is carried out by the search algorithm in order to find sequences of moves or strategies what to do, or sequences of motor programs which are in the end temporarily stored in the main memory as a cell assembly and connected to the motor servo-mechanism to be actually carried out (see also Digression 5). In the higher sensory-motor and motor regions of the cortex, motor programs like "walking" are probably represented. One of these programs might be the search algorithm itself, that threshold-controls the cortex. In this way, the "state of mind" may also be represented in the cortex. It may even be possible to learn new "metastrategies" concerning the search algorithm itself, i.e., the use of threshold control.

13.9 The mechanism that detects the average activity over wide parts of the brain, as postulated in Chapter 12.4.9, could for example be located in the "caudate nucleus", a part of the striatum that extends beyond the cortex from front to back, and thus could diffusely gather excitation from all over the cortex (I owe this suggestion to V. Braitenberg).

13.10 For an actual animal a diary might be of great help to speed up its learning.

Normally the animal will just react through its reflexes in the P part of the cortex. It would perhaps also continuously run a short-time prediction of the future in its P part, while an assembly is forming in the C part. Only rarely does something unusual happen and is noted as a difference between real-time prediction and actual input.

Perhaps even more rarely the short-time prediction will yield an evaluation that is significantly below the value of the present situation. This event, however, means that something has to be done to prevent the unpleasant situation that is predicted. At this point the animal will somehow have to change its normal reflexes and probably it will have to make a plan. If these rare occasions were stored in a diary this would be a great step toward improving behavior.

Indeed, if something bad happens to me, I try to look back into the past for a reason for it. What have I done wrong that might have caused this trouble? If I find a doubtful act in the near past, I will test some alternatives and if one of these allows me to avoid the trouble (according to my prediction), I will give this alternative a higher value than the one I had previously preferred. To do this I do not have to store all the events of the past, but just the "important" ones (in the sense defined above). I believe that at least people possess this kind of diary memory (and that it might be located in the hippocampus). This idea turned up after I had read an article of Rozin (1976). It is also consistent with the idea expressed in Fig. 13.3b, that there is a gradient toward higher level plans and images toward the border of the cortex of which the hippocampus is a large part.

13.11 What about sleeping and dreaming? Up to now I have not mentioned these phenomena since I was mainly concerned with that intelligent behavior of humans which I believe to be the hardest to produce artificially. Of course, the periodic changes in general activity (sleeping and waking) that occur in most animals and also in humans [with an internally determined period of about a day, usually a little longer (Aschoff 1965, Enright 1980, Ward 1971)], also affect the brain and the cortex. This can be seen most directly from a change in the EEG (Creutzfeldt and Houchin 1974, Andersen and Andersson 1968). It is known that subcortical centers (especially the so-called "reticular formation") have an influence on the cortical activity that corresponds to their influence on the different states of alertness (Magoun 1963).

These facts should fit with the ideas developed here. I believe that these subcortical "activation" or "arousal" centers contain certain programs according to which they threshold-control the cortex. In other words: there are different basic programs for the threshold-control mechanism, that are genetically determined, and that correspond to the different states of mind or states of alertness. In this book I try to concentrate on those programs that are used when we are awake.

But two side remarks may be allowed here.

1. If we really have cortical access to these programs for threshold control (Sect. 13.8), then it may be possible to combine some of these inborn programs to create new programs for the threshold control of the cortex [just as we may create new movements from inborn motor programs (Sect. 13.3)]. These would correspond to new "states of mind". Maybe it is this that some people do when they meditate.

2. When we report a dream, we probably report something that reflects the flow of cortical activity during the last dreaming phase, i.e., under a threshold control program that is different from the ones we "know" from our waking state, but we try to report the dream in "usual" terms, that correspond to a flow of activity in the waking state. Therefore I believe that inferences from this kind of introspection on the flow of activity in the cortex during dreaming are impossible, whereas it may be possible to make inferences on the state of connectivity, i.e., on the contents of the memory, since under any kind of threshold control, the flow of activity will have to follow the existing paths of connectivity.

13.12 Let me stop my speculations at this point. I guess the reader may now be eager to know some more facts that confirm or disconfirm the picture I gave. Especially, he might be interested in the following questions:

a) Are there secondary areas for all primary sensory and motor areas with strong projections from primary to secondary sensory and motor areas? (The primary motor areas might have projections both ways, since they may also be regarded as proprioceptive sensory areas — and there are indeed projections from primary motor to secondary, so-called sensory motor areas).
b) What about the synchronization of the threshold control rhythm in different areas? Can it be correlated with EEG waves?
c) What does the striatum and especially the nucleus caudatus look like anatomically? Why is it believed to provide motor programs, and how could these be embodied there?
d) How can novelty be detected and enhanced in an interplay between primary sensory cortex and thalamus? Is that really the case?

I cannot provide answers to these questions here. I can only state that my speculations are consistent with what I have read about these subject so far.

I hope these speculations will motivate the reader to gather further facts about subjects such as:

the EEG, the striatum, special cortico-cortical projections, the thalamus, the hippocampus, experiences with brain lesions, etc.

More generally, these speculations hopefully raise the reader's interest in experimental and theoretical work on adaptive information processing, in psychological investigations, since they should be interpretable in the language of cell assemblies, and of course, in the latest experimental evidence concerning Hebb's synaptic rule, which is the basic hypothesis for all the speculations presented here.

The literature concerning these subjects is extensive and often boring to read, therefore it is essential to have some concrete questions in mind, at least when you start reading: they will get muddled up early enough.

In Digression 6 I have listed some books on these issues that I enjoyed reading.

14 Men, Monkeys, and Machines

Er funktioniert wie eine Uhr, und ist doch bloß ein Uhu nur.
C. Morgenstern

Now we come back to the question that has clearly emerged from the construction given in the first part of this book, and that may have lingered in the back of the reader's mind most of the time. Can we regard ourselves as robots?

14.1 In a way we cannot: the robots we have built are machines built for a certain purpose, i.e., they are built to be of a certain use for us. They are complicated tools of their possessor. But are we (as well as animals) built by somebody just for his purpose? We could argue that we are built by our genes for the pupose of their proliferation (cf. Dawkins 1976), but the usual point of view is that an organism works for its own purpose, that is, for its own survival.

In a way we can: most people will agree that the laws of physics also hold for what goes on inside their heads, and that the physical mechanisms there determine what they are thinking. Therefore their thinking can be an object of physical study in the same way as the functioning of a robot.

14.2 In Chapter 2 we have changed the question slightly:

Can we regard each other as robots?

In other words: is there anything in the behavior of other human beings that we can observe and that could not be produced by a robot?

We have answered the last question in the negative, in principle (Chap. 3), and throughout this book we have worked on the construction of a robot for intelligent human behavior.

Here we have concentrated on the information-handling aspects and, for example, not on the problem of producing something that can walk on human-like legs etc.

Moreover, we have neglected some very hard problems of proper input coding and output organization. We have tried to design a machine that solves the problems faced by a biological organism, and we have shown that the appropriate pre- and post-coding can be done (in an inflexible way).

Furthermore, we have assumed that in actual beings, evolution has by now provided a reasonable, if not excellent pre- and post-coding for biological organisms. The special tricks used in the actual pre- and post-coding of many different species are investigated in many laboratories today.

14.3 But can the algorithm we have finally developed really display human behavior?

We shall approach this question by trying to find the proper place for the "survival robot" on the evolutionary scale.

The main point in the construction was to build a flexible prediction and association mechanism that controls a pure reflex mechanism according to genetically determined goals. This idea puts the algorithm probably somewhere in the family of mammals, for example we could imagine it simulating a quite clever fox. But what makes the difference from a fox to a monkey and from a monkey to a human? (Their brains at least have a highly similar structure, although the human brain is one of the larger mammalian brains).

Let us examine the traditional answers to this question.

14.4 Eye-hand coordination and the human hand itself have been mentioned, but these could certainly be constructed. They also do not present a problem for the information-handling point of view taken here.

Certain instincts, like curiosity, imitation, empathy, and playing have been mentioned, but these we share with many other mammals. It is, however, very important to incorporate these into our algorithm, e.g., as genetically predetermined goals or valuations. It is "good" to perceive something new, to imagine the situation another similar animal is in (our input-precoding makes this possible since it usually involves an objective as well as a self-centered representation of the sensory inputs), or to run certain motor programs. Also our interest in dangerous situations (suspense), close to the point of bad experiences, can be produced by such a valuation.

Man differs from animals in that he more often encounters situations, where his inborn reflexes and drives do not automatically produce his behavior. In such a situation we can (and in some sense have to) make plans for the near future (see also Fromm 1973, p. 219–236). This faculty is further enhanced by the possibility of detaching the "plan-making" or "thinking" part of our brains to a certain degree from the sensory-motor reflex mechanisms. This possibility was inherent in the design of the survival algorithm, since we began with the problem of chess-playing; it is reflected again in the last two Chapters (and in the flow diagram of Digression 5).

Acquisition of Language

14.5 The main feature that remains to be considered is language. The acquisition of language in the child is closely interrelated with the development of intelligence. Let us describe this development in some more detail. It starts with the so-called babbling phase. In this phase probably the child learns the correlation between certain motor acts (concerning mouth, tongue, and throat) and the noises that are produced. In this way the child learns to form many different syllables (Braitenberg 1980). This learning is probably facilitated in humans by a special fiber bundle between the acoustic- and speech-regions of the cortex, which yields a higher than average connectivity between these two regions. The babbling itself can be regarded as an inborn motor program. Later the child's ability to distinguish and imitate spoken syllables is probably reduced (and adapted) to the syllables that are used by his parents (see for example Eimas et al. 1971, Eimas 1978, Lasky et al. 1975).

Based on this ability the child learns to use these syllables for communication with other humans (usually at first the parents and perhaps brothers and sisters).

Of course, from the moment of birth there is a nonverbal kind of communication between the child and his mother and later also other persons. The child is dependent on his parents to take care of his most vital needs, and he has ways to communicate these to them, i.e., there are inborn ways to say "I'm fine", "I need food", "something is bothering me".

When the child starts to use his fingers (hands) to specify objects he wants by pointing (grasping) at them, this gesture can be easily understood from the inborn grasping mechanism and the tendency of the parents to hand certain things to the child, when they see that he tries to grasp them. Later objects and also persons are specified by simple nouns. For the child this has the obvious advantage of not depending on sight-contact between himself and his parents, and still makes it possible for him to specify his needs to some degree of precision. To do this the child has to acquire two things:

a) the correlation between the one or two syllables of a noun and the object or person meant by it;
b) the idea of specifying something in order to get it from the parents (this he may have learned before by unsuccessful trials of grasping where the parents helped).

These associations then have to be used in order to reach the goal of getting the desired object. (This is what a planning algorithm does).

After this stage ofe "one-word sentences", the stages of two- and more-words sentences are described (cf. Braine 1963, Weir 1962, Wolff 1973, Moskowitz 1978).

In this way the communication between the child and his parents (and later also other children) is steadily refined.

After some time, language can be understood not only in the context of the present situation, for example when the child is told or read a fairy-tale or given rules for his proper behavior by his parents. These "teleological" rules in turn are the prototypes at first for all kinds of moral and physical laws, which are made by God or Nature and told to the child by his parents. Only at school age, in games with other children does the child begin to formulate his own rules.

I do not want to go into the details at this point; they are described very accurately, for example, by Piaget (1954, 1955), Spitz (1965), Brown (1973) and Luria and Yudovich (1971). In any case, a more detailed study of the stages of the development of intelligence and language in the child that breaks down this development into sufficiently small steps can only contribute more evidence to the general impression that at any stage this development can be explained in terms of quite simple mechanisms, namely a combination of

1. inborn motor programs (like grasping, babbling),
2. inborn drives or valuations (like imitating, first playing — i.e., experimenting with the own body, with objects),
3. the general mechanism of learning correlations and forming associations,
4. a planning or look-ahead algorithm.

It has to be noted, however, that all this is only possible with the (often unconscious) help of the parents.

Therefore one can say that the developing of language in the child depends very strongly on the existence of language in his surrounding.

14.6 Therefore one could speculate that the historical development of language might have started with the *invention* of the use of syllables for certain specifications in some tribe. This, giving the obvious advantages, would be inherited not genetically but socially in this tribe, in the same way we still inherit our language today. From this kind of invention onward the evolution of men might even have taken another, faster form. I think it is probably this phenomenon that Dawkins (1976) means, when he talks about the final evolution of "memes" instead of genes.

I want to stop these considerations here, since they begin to involve the next higher level of organization above the organization of the individual from cells.

In conclusion I may say that the main difference between monkey and man most probably lies in the human culture that has developed in the last 10,000 years, and not so much in specific differences in their brains.

This book is not the place to describe and understand the development of human cultures, since this belongs to a still higher level of organization; I have only tried to show in this chapter that the prerequisites necessary for a cultural development are provided by the mechanisms described in this book. Perhaps even a Neanderthal baby, if raised in our culture, would not be immediately distinguishable by its intelligence from our children. We could imagine the same to be true for a survival robot with a sufficiently big associative memory that has been patiently trained by us for 12 years, as we would a child.

15 Why All These Speculations?

> *I simply believe that some part of the human self or soul is not subject to the laws of space and time.*
> C.G. Jung
>
> *There is no separate soul or life-force to stick a finger into the brain now and then and make neural cells do what they would not otherwise.*
> D.O. Hebb, 1949

Motivated by the question how our brain might work, we have gone a long way through the design of our "improved matchbox algorithm" that finally even served as a model for human behavior. But this whole construction is only a speculation, it is not a fact (although en route we learned some "real" facts about the brain). So what do we get out of all these constructions?

15.1 First of all, we have seen that it is indeed possible to design and understand the design of an algorithm that can in principle produce human behavior. This is a strong argument against those who still believe that this is impossible in principle.

15.2 Secondly, such a construction may serve to organize known facts about the brain (as for example in Chaps. 8, 9, 10), it may generate interest in specific questions that may even be experimentally accessible (as in Chaps. 13 and 14), and it provides a new viewpoint for the reading of the vast literature on the brain. Thus it may help the experimenter in choosing what to investigate from the infinite amount of possibilities, and it may help the newcomer in this field to direct and select his reading of papers and books on the brain.

In fact, it is impossible today to read everything, and there is generally a lack of organization and motivation in the literature, thus selection is inevitable.

15.3 The problem of brain theory is a well known and difficult one in science.
We have acquired knowledge on the brain on different levels. First of all on the behavioral or psychological level. Secondly on the level of neurons, and basically on the level of the organic molecules composing the neurons. We know that the neurons are composed of molecules, that the brain is composed of neurons, and that our behavior is determined by the physical processes that happen on the level of the neurons — or even on the level of the molecules.

The theory now has to form the connection between these levels.

The classical analogy to this problem is the problem of thermodynamics, where the known laws of the "theory of heat" were based on the known laws of the Newtonian mechanics and the laws of collision. What was gained by this?

At first sight not much actual knowledge was gained, since on both levels the effects were known. But it simplified the theory in the sense that the laws of the theory of heat could now be deduced from the laws of mechanics. Moreover, this new correspondence could lead to predictions in both fields, which could be tested later.

15.4 In brain theory the task is much harder for two reasons:

a) On the level of neurons and synapses the investigations are far from complete, in the sense that we do not even yet have all the knowledge that we know we could have from molecular biology. Even the basic picture of the working of a single neuron can still be at least refined, if not changed. In particular, the way in which the axonal activity around the dendritic tree of a neuron contributes to its axonal output certainly is much more complicated than our common simplifying descriptions, where we disregard local changes of the ionic concentration, possible nonlinear interactions of different synapses close together on the dendrite, the role of glia cells, in short all that today goes by the name of "microcircuitry" and is one of the main subjects of contemporary research. But all this can only add to the information-processing power of the neuron model used here, and therefore I believe that these investigations cannot be critical for the picture sketched in this book, although they may add a lot to our biophysical knowledge.

b) On the level of behavior the investigations have not even let to *one* framework of description, in other words: today there exist many phenomenological theories on behavior, that are even partly conflicting with each other.

Therefore, a serious attempt to connect both levels may help to clarify problems and motivate investigations on both the neuronal and the behavioral level.

15.5 I think that historically this particular situation is quite new. Today we have indeed reached the point where we begin to have specific ideas as to how to connect the two levels (we have accumulated a considerable amount of knowledge on how the brain is composed of neurons and how these work), whereas we have no clear-cut "phenomenological" theory of what to predict at the higher level, and there certainly are still many details to be settled at the lower level.

The great demand in this new situation is today felt by many scientists and has led to some understandable "escape reactions" that do not offer much help to solve it:

1. To analyze simpler systems, where the phenomenological theory is easier to accomplish.
2. To maintain that the solution is impossible, since human behavior can *never* be understood on a purely physical basis. This position is not only metaphysical but antiphysical; it is rather pessimistic, if it is meant to imply that human behavior is unpredictable in principle. On the other hand, it is certainly doubtful whether physical methods of measurement should be applied directly on the behavioral level.
3. To maintain that a good phenomenological theory is enough. This position can be understood as a reaction to (2), since it makes it possible at least to use a "scientific" methodology (i.e., to mimic physics); it often comes together with an overestimation of one specific phenomenological theory, which is rather dangerous. I think, either from the exposition in this book or from the history of psychological and behavioral theories, the difficulty of the problem of understanding human behavior should be clear enough to be cautious with generalizations of experiments on the behavioral level.

The dispute between positions (2) and (3) has also led to a rather fruitless revival of the old discussion about "what is science".

In any case, both positions will not bring the desired relief for the neurologist or psychiatrist, that after all he has a sound "scientific" basis for what he is doing. He still has to make his decisions on a rather shaky basis where it is perhaps the best strategy to use all possible sources of information (or "knowledge") he can get hold of.

15.6 There is an additional guideline in brain theory, compared to thermodynamics, namely the use of teleological arguments. In physics it is regarded as nonsense to talk about the purpose of molecules or the purpose of the universe; when dealing with biological organisms, however, we may do this, since we believe that they have developed ways of achieving the purpose of staying alive (through evolution), and we can try to derive other subpurposes from this general purpose.

It is perhaps the basic idea of cybernetics (as "founded" by N. Wiener in his book *Cybernetics,* 1948) to use teleological arguments or engineering methods of design as a *heuristic* guideline for the analysis of biological systems. This idea has proved to be fruitful and stimulating for the analysis of biological systems, and it has led to the discovery of many similarities in the way engineers and biological organs solve their problems.

Purpose

15.7 Recently, this idea of using teleological arguments has been stressed again by a branch of science or engineering, called Artificial Intelligence. I think today it is even overstressed a little sometimes in Artificial Intelligence, for example when the goal (or computation that has to be done) is put as a top level of analysis above the biophysical and the behavioral level[1]. This in itself speaks for a certain epistemological confusion. After all, the "lower" two levels are levels of description or analysis of the system which are experimentally accessible, whereas the "top level" of computation is not. I think the goal or purpose can be used to "understand" the "system"; as for its analysis, it can only be regarded as a heuristic guideline; and indeed, I have used the guideline of purpose for the presentation of facts and ideas in this book.

Furthermore, in Artificial Intelligence it is often maintained that one has to do nothing but find algorithms solving well-defined (so-called computational) problems. These algorithms can then be regarded as solutions to technical as well as biological questions.

Here usually the "relative independence" of different levels is used as an argument for the imputation of technical algorithms in (the analysis of) biological organisms[2] (although the ultimate motive for the research usually is to connect levels).

I think that this view is influenced by the every-day experience of the universality of modern computers and that this approach is clearly promising as far as technical applications are concerned. Moreover, the historical

---

1 "The core of the problem is that a system as complex as a nervous system or a developing embryo must be analyzed and understood at several different levels. For a system that solves an information-processing problem, we may distinguish four important levels of description. At the lowest, there is basic component and circuit analysis — how do transistors, neurons, diodes, and synapses work? The second level is that of particular mechanisms: adders, multipliers, and memories accessed by address or by content. The third level is that of the algorithm, and the top level contains the theory of the overall computation!" (Marr and Poggio 1977, p. 470)

2 "Each of these four levels of description has its place in the eventual understanding of perceptual information processing and it is important to keep them separate. Of course, there are logical and causal relationships among them, but the important point is that these levels of description are only loosely related.... More disturbingly, although the top level is the most neglected, it is also the most important. This is because the structure of the computations that underlie perception depends more upon the computational problems that have to be solved than on the particular hardware in which their solutions are implemented." (Marr and Poggio 1977, p. 470–471, see also Harmon 1970)

development of this view can be easily understood by the early successes of Artificial Intelligence[3].

But for the application to biological questions — as in brain theory — the hardest part may actually consist in formulating the problem, and here one may have to take into account information obtained at *all* levels, in particular on the building blocks that are biologically available to "implement" the algorithm.

15.8 The language of cell assemblies may serve as a framework for behavioral or psychological descriptions of behavior (i.e., phenomenological models), and at the same time can be interpreted as a rough and simplified description of the underlying biophysical neural events. This language should (of course after an intensive discussion with psychologists) finally make it possible to talk about associations, etc., with a mechanistic picture in mind which is not just a phenomenological model but relates to neural activity. The consequence of this would (hopefully) not be just a simple mechanistic description of human "subjects", but a picture that, although mechanistic in principle, always keeps us aware of the uncertainties and complexities that in every single case have to be solved in order to interpret the picture unambiguously on the biophysical level. Therefore I think it will rather lead to *more* caution in the administration of psychic drugs and other "psycho-chemical" means of "controlling" the subject's mind; for example it keeps us aware of how far we still are from understanding the effects of alcohol or aspirin.

---

3 "A common interest in model-making, particularly of CNS function, drew together participants from the diverse disciplines of mathematics, engineering, neurophysiology, molecular biology, biophysics, and psychology. There were, however, significant differences of approach and emphasis.

In the course of the development of the mathematical science of the brain over the last twenty years, the attempt has been made, especially with computers in mind, to create a mathematical theory, description, or model of the central nervous system. Such a model would perform general intelligence functions in the same manner as the brain. This accomplishment is still distant. Some individuals have tried to model total brain behavior and have so convinced themselves of their efforts that they have published their mathematical models. Other scientists have wisely specified intermediate goals and by means of this self-imposed discipline, have achieved some substantial results, particularly in the areas of artificial intelligence and engineering models.

The artificial intelligence group, constructing mathematical programs for computing machinery which do not resemble the brain in any detail, have obtained satisfactory performance of general intelligence functions such as proving theorems, playing chess and checkers, recognizing patterns, and translating languages." (Stark and Dickson 1965, p. 7, see also p. 6)

15.9 A common argument against the reduction of human behavior to physics and chemistry is that it implies predictability of our behavior, which may be a cause for fatalism.

The situation can be sketched as follows:

1. A vital requirement for doing physics is the general predictability of the events that are objects of physical investigation.
2. A reduction of behavior to physics would make behavior also an object of physical investigation.
3. We believe that our own behavior obeys the same rules as the behavior of other members of our species (i.e., other humans).
4. From the introspective experience of our own "freedom of will", we infer that our own behavior is not completely predictable.

(1)–(4) together yield a contradiction, therefore we have to abandon at least one of these statements, and in fact, today we can find any of the four resulting opinions. I personally indeed tend to abandon the last assumption, although of course I still experience my own "freedom of will"; and I do not think that I am particularly fatalistic. Clearly, (1), (2), and (3) together imply that my own behavior is predictable, in principle. But after all, what does it matter that it is in principle predictable what I will do in the next minute or the next year, when no one on earth can actually predict it? I believe that I share this position with many scientists and philosophers (for example with Ryle 1949), maybe just because I have not taken much care to define it from other similar positions.

To abandon the third assumption leads to the following rather strange position: you may believe that you are free yourself, but all other men are robots. This may be a sound position to believe in, but it would perhaps be unwise to state it in a discussion with somebody else.

To abandon the second assumption leads to a position which I have called "antiphysical" above. This position implies that the laws of physics do not always apply to men. It is for example expressed by Eccles (in Popper and Eccles 1977). He assumes the existence of another world besides the world of physics, which interacts with it (through some kind of "interface"). Such an assumption implies that sometimes there will occur events in the world of physics that cannot be explained by the laws of this world alone, but only through the interaction with this "other world".

Surprisingly enough, it is in physics itself that some physicists today believe to find reasons to abandon the first assumption. Many modern physicists believe that in quantum mechanics not every event is stricly predictable (in connection with the Heisenberg uncertainty principle). This book is not the place to discuss this belief. It is sometimes used as an argument for our "freedom of will", but an argument based on quantum mechanical uncertainty or probability certainly does not fit introspectively with such a noble feeling as that of freedom of will. This is pointed out by Hassenstein (1979), and it is illustrated in the following anomymous German poem which I have translated into English.

> A quantum flies along the lane
> in search of Mr von Korff's brain,
> since there inside the cortex tissue
> a certain molecule 's at issue:
> Von Korff is not at all at ease,
> "Do I want bacon, ham, or cheese?"
> The quantum speaks with boasting lust:
> "You think you want, in fact you must.
> That freedom you will never gain,
> it's me who's free, your will 's in vain".
> Electron 9 begs "Jump on me!";
> The quantum wavers leisurely.
> Electron 8 is not a frump;
> so she gets the acausal jump.
> Just whereupon spontaneously
> von Korff decides to take the Brie,
> and contemplates in peace that still
> he has the freedom of his will.
> This was too much for our poor quantum
> he died at (free) will, albeit wanton.

References

Abeles M (1981) The role of the cortical neuron: integrator or coincidence detector. Reprint
Abeles M, Goldstein MH (1977) Multispike train analysis. Proc IEEE 65:762
Abeles M, Lass Y (1975) Transmission of information by the axon: II. The channel capacity. Biol Cybern 19:121
Addams C (1957) Nightcrawlers. Simon and Schuster, New York
Albus JS (1971) Theory of cerebellar function. Math Biosci 10:25
Albus JS (1979) Mechanisms of planning and problem solving in the brain. Math Biosci 45:247
Amari S-I (1974) A method of statistical neurodynamics. Kybernetik 14:201
Amari S-I (1977) Neural theory of association and concept-formation. Biol Cybern 26: 175
Amari S-I, Yoshida K, Kanatani K (1977) A mathematical foundation for statistical neurodynamics. SIAM J Appl Math 33:95
Andersen P, Andersson SA (1968) Physiological basis of alpha thythm. Appleton, New York
Andersen P (1981) In: Advances in physiological sciences, vol 30. Neural communication and control. Academici Kiado, Budapest
Anderson AR (ed) (1964) Minds and Machines. Prentice Hall, Englewood Cliffs NJ
Anderson JA (1972) A simple neural network generating an interactive memory. Math Biosci 14:197
Anderson JA (1973) A theory for the recognition of items from short memorized lists. Psychol rev 80:417
Anninos PA, Beek B, Csermely TJ, Harth EM, Pertile G (1970) Dynamics of neural structures. J Theor Biol 26:121
Arbib MA, Kilmar WL, Spinelli DN (1976) Neural models and memory (in: Rosenzweig and Bennett, p 109)
Aschoff J (1965) Circadian rhythm in man. Science 148:1427
Ash R (1965) Information theory. Interscience, New York London Sidney
Attneave F (1959) Applications of information theory to psychology. Holt & Co, New York
Bailey PA, Bonin von G (1951) The isocortex of man. Univ. Illinois Press, Urbana
Barlow HB (1975) Visual experience and cortical development. Nature (London) 258: 199
Barlow HB (1981) Critical limiting factors in the design of the eye and visual cortex. Proc Soc London Ser B 212:1–34
Bennett EL, Diamond MC, Krech D, Rosenzweig MR (1964) Chemical and anatomical plasticity of brain. Science 146:610
Berliner HJ (1978) A chronology of computer chess and its literature. Artif Intell 10: 201
Beurle RL (1956) Properties of a mass of cells capable of regenerating pulses. Proc R Soc London Ser B 240:55
Blakemore C, Cooper GF (1970) Development of the brain depends on visual environment. Nature (London) 228:477

Blakemore C, Sluyters Van RC (1974) Reversal of the physiological effects of monocular deprivation in kittens: further evidence for a sensitive period. J Physiol 237: 195

Blakemore C, Sluyters Van RC (1975) Innate and environmental factors in the development of the kitten's visual cortex. J Physiol 248:663

Blinkov SM, Glezer II (1968) The human brain in figures and tables. Basic books. Plenum Press, New York

Bloch A (1977) Murphy's law. Price Stern Sloan Publ, Los Angeles

Bloch V (1970) Facts and hypotheses concerning memory consolidation. Brain Res 24:561

Bohn G (1978) A structure for associative information processing. Biol Cybern 29: 193

Botwinnik MM (1970) Computers, chess and long-range planning. Springer, Berlin Heidelberg New York

Braak H (1980) Architectonics of the human telencephalic cortex. Springer, Berlin Heidelberg New York

Braine MDS (1963) The ontogeny of English phrase structure: the first phrase. Language 39:1

Braitenberg V (1961) Funktionelle Deutung von Strukturen in der grauen Substanz des Nervensystems. Naturwissenschaften 14:489

Braitenberg V (1974a) Thoughts on the cerebral cortex. J Theor Biol 46:421

Braitenberg V (1974b) On the representation of objects and their relations in the brain (see ref. Güttinger et al., p 290)

Braitenberg V (1977) On the texture of brains. Springer, Berlin Heidelberg New York

Braitenberg V (1978a) Cell assemblies in the cerebral cortex (in: Heim and Palm, p 171)

Braitenberg V (1978b) Cortical architectonics: general and areal (in: Brazier and Petsche, p 443)

Braitenberg V (1980) Alcune considerationi sui meccanismi cerebrali del linguaggio. In: Braga G, Braitenberg V, Cipolli C, Coserin E, Crespi-Reghizzi S, Mehler J, Titone R (eds) Laccostamento interdisciplinare allo studio del linguaggio. Franco Angeli, Milano, p 96

Braitenberg V (1981) Anatomical basis of divergence, convergence and integration in the cerebral cortex, p 411. In: Grastyan E, Molnar P (eds) Sensory Functions. Akademiai Kiado, Budapest (Advances in physiological sciences, vol 16)

Braitenberg V, Atwood RP (1958) Morphological observations on the cerebellar cortex. J Comp Neurol 109:1

Braitenberg V, Braitenberg C (1959) Geometry of orientation columns in the visual cortex. Biol Cybern 33:179

Braitenberg V, Onesto N (1962) The cerebellar cortex as a timing organ. In: Atti 1 Congr Int Med Cibern. Giannini, Napoli

Brazier MAB, Petsche H (eds) (1978) Architectonics of the cerebral cortex. Raven Press, New York

Breese BB (1909) Binocular rivalry. Psychol Rev 16:410

Brodal A (1969) Neurological anatomy. Oxford Univ Press, New York London Toronto

Brodmann K (1909) Vergleichende Lokalisationslehre der Großhirnrinde in ihren Prinzipien, dargestellt auf Grund des Zellenbaues. Barth, Leipzig

Brown R (1970) Psycholinguistics. Free Press, New York

Brown R (1973) A first language: the early stages. Harvard Univ Press, Cambridge Mass

Brown RW, Bellugi-Klima U (1964) Three processes in the child's acquisition of syntax. Harv Educ Rev 34, also in Brown (1970)

Caianiello ER (1961) Outline of a theory of thought processes and thinking machines. J Theor Biol 1:204

Caianiello ER, Grimson WEL (1976) Methods of analysis of neural nets. Biol Cybern 22:1

References

Caianiello ER, Luca de A, Ricciardi LM (1967) Reverberations and control of neural networks. Kybernetik 4:10—18
Cajal SR (1911) Histologie du systeme nerveux de l'homme et des vertebres. Maloin, Paris
Carpenter MB (1976) Human neuroanatomy. Williams & Wilkins, Baltimore
Cherry C (ed) (1956) Information theory. 3rd London Symposium. Butterworths, London
Chow K, Blum JS, Blum RA (1950) Cell ratios in the thalamo-cortical visual system of macaca mulatta. J Comp Neurol 92:227
Coleman BD (1971) A mathematical theory of lateral sensory inhibition. Arch Rat Mech Anal 43:79
Coleman BD, Renninger GH (1974) On the integral equations of the linear theory of recurrent lateral interaction in vision. Math Biosci 20:155
Colonnier M (1968) Synaptic patterns on different cell types in the different laminae of the cat visual cortex. An EM Study. Brain Res 9:268
Conrad M, Güttinger W, Dal Cin M (eds) (1974) Physics and mathematics of the nervous system. Springer, Berlin Heidelberg New York
Cooper LN, Liberman F, Oja E (1979) A theory for the acquisition and loss of neuron specificity in visual cortex. Biol Cybern 33:9
Cowan JD (1970) A statistical mechanics of nervous activity. In: Gerstenhaber M (ed) Lecture on mathematics in the life sciences. Am Math Soc, Providence RI
Cowan JD (1976) Are there modifiable synapses in the visual cortex. In: Rosenzweig and Bennett, p 133
Cowan JD, Ermentrout GB (1978) Some aspects of the 'Eigenbehavior' of neural nets (in: Levin, p 67)
Cragg BG (1967) The density of synapses and neurons in the motor and visual areas of the cerebral cortex. J Anat 101:639
Cragg BG (1968) Are there structural alterations in synapses related to functioning? Proc R Soc London Ser B 171:319
Creutzfeld OD, Houchin J (1974) The neuronal basis of EEG waves. In: Creutzfeldt O (ed) Handbook of EEG and clinical neurophysiology, vo II, part C, p 5. Elsevier, Amsterdam
Creutzfeld OD, Lux HD, Nacimiento AC (1964) Intracelluläre Reizung corticaler Nervenzellen. Pflügers Arch 268:129
Cynader M, Mitchell DE (1977) Monocular astigmatism effects on kitten visual cortex development. Nature (London) 270:177
Dal Cin M (1976) Fehlertolerante Systeme. Teubner, Stuttgart
Dal Cin M (1978) Self-diagnosis of interactive systems (in: Heim and Palm, p 229)
Daniel PM, Whitteridge D (1962) The representation of the visual field on the cerebral cortex in monkeys. J Physiol (London) 159:203—221
Dawkins R (1976) The selfish gene. Oxford Univ Press, New York Oxford
Diamond MC, Krech D, Rosenzweig MR (1964) The effects of an enriched environment on the histology of the rat cerebral cortex. J Comp Neurol 123:111
Dijkstra N (1968) Cooperative sequential processes. In: Genuys F (ed) Programming languages. Raven Press, New York
Doty RW (1965) Conditioned reflexes elicited by electrical stimulation of the brain in macaques. J Neurophysiol 28:623
Doty RW (1969) Electrical stimulation of the brain in behavioral context. Annu Rev Psychol 20:289
Doty RW (1973) Ablation of visual areas in the central nervous system (in: Jung, p 483, part B)
Dürsteler MR, Garey LJ, Movshon JA (1976) Reversal of the morphological effects of monocular deprivation in the kitten's lateral geniculate nucleus. J Physiol 261:189
Dusser de Barenne JG, McCulloch WS (1938) Sensorymotor cortex, nucleus caudatus and thalamus opticus. J Neurophysiol 1:364

Dusser de Barenne JG, Garol HW, McCulloch WS (1941) Physiological Neuronography of the corticostriatal connections. Assoc Res Nerv Ment Dis 21:246
Eccles JC (1957) The physiology of nerve cells. Johns Hopkins Press, Baltimore
Eccles JC (1964) The physiology of synapses. Springer, Berlin Heidelberg New York
Eckhorn R, Grüsser O-J, Kröller J, Pellnitz K, Pöpel B (1976) Efficiency of different neuronal codes: information transfer calculations for three different neuronal systems. Biol Cybern 22:49
Eimas DE (1978) Developmental aspects of speech perception (in: Held et al., p 357)
Eimas DE, Siqueland ER, Jusczyk P, Vigorito J (1971) Speech perception in infants. Science 171:303
Enright JT (1980) The timing of sleep and wakefulness. Springer, Berlin Heidelberg New York
Ernst GW, Newell A (1969) GPS: a case study in generality and problem solving. Academic Press, London New York
Ervin FR, Anders TR (1970) Normal and pathological memory: data and a conceptual scheme (in: Schmitt et al, 2nd Study program, p 163)
Eysel UTh, Grüsser O-J, Hoffmann K-P (1979) Monocular deprivation and the signal transmission by x- and y-neurons of the cat lateral geniculate nucleus. Exp Brain Res 34:521
Feldman JL, Cowan JD (1975) Large scale activity in neural nets I: Biol Cybern 17: 29–38, II: Biol Cybern 17:39–51
Fichte JG (1794) Grundlage der gesamten Wissenschaftslehre (als Handschrift für seine Zuhörer). Gabler, Jena Leipzig
Fichte JF (1800) Die Bestimmung des Menschen. Voß'sche Buchhandlung, Berlin
Fifkova E (1968) Changes in the visual cortex of rats after unilateral deprivation. Nature (London) 220:379
Fifkova E (1970) The effect of monocular deprivation on the synaptic contacts of visual cortex. J Neurobiol 1:285
Fischer B (1973) A neuron field theory: mathematical approaches to the problem of large numbers of interacting nerve cells. Bull Math Biophys 35:345
Frank H (1962a) Pawlows bedingte Reflexe und Steinbuchs Lernmatrizen (see ref. Frank, p 125)
Frank H (ed) (1962b) Kybernetik. Umschau-Verlag, Frankfurt
Freeman RD (ed) (1979) Developmental neurobiology of vision. Plenum Press, New York London
Freeman RD, Pettigrew JD (1973) Alteration of visual cortex from environmental asymmetries. Nature (London) 246:359
Freeman W (1975) Mass action in the nervous system. Academic Press, London New York
Frey PW (1977) Chess skill in man and machine. Springer, Berlin Heidelberg New York
Fromkin V, Rodman R (1974) An introduction to language. Holt Rinehart and Winston, New York
Fromm E (1973) The anatomy of human destructiveness. Holt Rinehart and Winston, New York
Fukushima K (1973) A model of associative memory in the brain. Kybernetik 12:58
Fukushima K (1975) Cognitron: a self-organizing multilayered neural network. Biol Cybern 20:121
Fukushima K, Miyake S (1978) A self-organizing neural network with a function of associative memory: feedback-type cognitron. Biol Cybern 28:291
Gabor D (1969) Associative holographic memories. IBM J Res Dev 13:156
Gardner M (1969) The unexpected hanging and other mathematical diversions. Simon and Schuster, New York
Gilbert CD, Wiesel TN (1979) Morphology and intracortical projections of functionelly characterised neurones in the cat visual cortex. Nature (London) 280:120–125
Globus A (1975) Brain morphology as a function of presynaptic morphology and activity (in: Riesen, p 9)

References

Globus A, Scheibel AB (1967a) The effect of visual deprivation on cortical neurons: a Golgi study. Exp Neurol 19:331
Globus A, Scheibel AB (1967b) Pattern and field in cortical structure: the rabbit. J Comp Neurol 131:155
Gluhbegovic N, Williams TH (1980) The human brain, a photographic guide. Harper and Row, Cambridge New York London
Gödel K (1931) Über formal unentscheidbare Sätze der Principia Mathematica und verwandter Systeme I. Monatsh Math Phys 38:173
Griffith JS (1963) A field theory of neural nets I. Bull Math Biophys 25:111
Griffith JS (1965) A field theory of neural nets II. Bull Math Biophys 27:187
Griffith JS (1966) A theory of the nature of memory. Nature (London) 211:1160
Hadeler KP (1974) On the theory of lateral inhibition. Kybernetik 14:161
Halmos P (1960) Naive set theory. Van Nostrand, Princeton NJ
Harari F (1969) Graph theory. Addison-Wesley, Reading Mass
Hammarberg C (1895) Klinik und Pathologie der Idiotie. Akad Buchdruckerei Berling, Upsala
Harmon LD (1970) Neural subsystems: an interpretive summary (in: Schmitt et al, 2nd Study program, p 286)
Harth EM, Csermely TJ, Beek B, Lindsay RD (1970) Brain functions and neural dynamics. J Theor Biol 26:93
Hassenstein B (1979) Willensfreiheit und Verantwortlichkeit. Naturwissenschaftliche und juristische Aspekte (in: Hassenstein et al, p 202)
Hassenstein B, Mohr H, Osche G, Sander K, Wülker W (1979) Freiburger Vorlesungen zur Biologie des Menschen. Quelle & Meyer, Heidelberg
Hebb DO (1949) The organization of behaviour. John Wiley, New York
Hebb DO (1958) Textbook of psychology. Sanders, Philadelphia London Toronto
Heiden an der U (1980) Analysis of neural networks. Springer, Berlin Heidelberg New York
Heim R, Palm G (eds) (1978) Theoretical approaches to complex systems. Springer, Berlin Heidelberg New York
Heimer L, Ebner FT, Nauta WJH (1967) A note on the termination of commissural fibers in the neocorex. Brain res 5:171
Held R (1966) Plasticity in sensory-motor systems. Sci Am, p 84
Held R (1970) Two modes of processing spatially distributed visual stimulation (in: Schmitt et al, p 317)
Held R, Leibowitz HW, Teuber H-L (eds) (1978) Handbook of sensory physiology, vol VI: Perception. Springer, Berlin Heidelberg New York
Hirsch HVB, Spinelli DN (1970) Visual experience modifies distribution of horizontally and vertically oriented receptive fields in cats. Science 168:869
Hoffstaedter DR (1979) Gödel, Escher, Bach. Basic books. Plenum Press, New York
Holden AV (1976) Models of the stochastic activity of neurons. Springer, Berlin Heidelberg New York
Hubel DH, Freeman DC (1977) Projection into the visual field of ocular dominance columns in macaque monkey. Brain Res 122:336
Hubel DH, Wiesel TN (1963) Receptive fields of cells in striate cortex of very young, visually inexperienced kittens. J Neurophysiol 27:994
Hubel DH, Wiesel TN (1965) Binocular interaction in striate cortex of kittens reared with artificial squint. J Neurophysiol 28:1041
Hubel DH, Wiesel TN (1974) Uniformity of monkey striate cortex: a parallel relationship between field size, scatter and magnification factor. J Comp Neurol 158:295
Hubel DH, Wiesel T (1977) Functional architecture of macaque monkey visual cortex. (Ferrier Lecture) Proc R Soc London Ser B 198:1
Hume D (1739) A treatise of human nature. John Noon, London
Hume D (1938) An abstract of a treatise of human nature 1740 by David Hume. Univ Press, Cambridge

Ingvar DH (1976) Functional landscapes of the dominant hemisphere. Brain Res 107: 181
Ingvar DH, Philipson L (1977) Distribution of cerebral blood flow in the dominant hemisphere during motor ideation and motor performance. Ann of Neurology 2: 230
Ito M (1981) In: Advances in physiological sciences, vol 30: Neural communication and control. Academici Kiado, Budapest
Jasper HH (1969) Mechanisms of propagation: extracellular studies (in: Jasper et al, p 421)
Jasper HH, Ward AA, Pope A (eds) (1969) Basic mechanisms of the epilepsies. Little Brown, Boston
John ER (1972) Switchboard versus statistical theories of learning and memory. Science 177:850–864
Julesz B (1971) Foundations of cyclopean perception. Univ Press, Chicago
Jung R (ed) (1973) Handbook of sensory physiology, vol VII/3. Central processing of visual information. Springer, Berlin Heidelberg New York
Katchalsky AK, Rowland V, Blumenthal R (1974) Dynamic patterns of cell assemblies. NRP Bull 12 No 1
Katz B (1966) Nerve, muscle and synapse. McGraw-Hill, New York
Klaczko-Ryndziun S (1975) Systemanalyse der Selbstreflexion. Birkhäuser, Basel Stuttgart
Kleist K (1934) Gehirnpathologie. Barth, Leipzig
Kohler I (1964) The formation and transformation of the perceptual world. Psychol Issues III: Monogr 12
Kohonen T (1974) An adaptive associative memory principle. IEEE Trans. on Computers 23:444
Kohonen T (1977) Associative memory. Springer, Berlin Heidelberg New York
Kohonen T (1981) Recent approaches to the theory of biological associative memory. (Preprint)
Kohonen T, Oja E (1976) Fast adaptive formation of orthogonalizing filters and associative memory in recurrent networks of neuron-like elements. Biol Cybern 21:85
Kohonen T, Reuhkala E, Mäkisara K, Vainio L (1976) Associative recall of images. Biol Cybern 22:159
Kohonen T, Oja E, Kortekangas A, Mäkisara K, Lehtiö P (1977a) Demonstration of pattern processing properties of the associative mappings. Proc 7th Int Conf Cybern and Soc, Washington, p 581
Kohonen T, Lehtiö P, Rovamo J, Hyvärinen J, Bry K, Vainio L (1977b) A principle of neural associative memory. Neuroscience 2:1065–1076
Koschmieder EL (1974) Benard Convection. Adv Chem Phys 26:177
Kuffler SW, Nichols JG (1976) From neuron to brain. Sinauer Associates, Sunderland Mass
Kuhn TS (1962) The structure of scientific revolutions. Univ Press, Chicago
Kuypers HGJM, Szwarcbart MK, Mishkin M, Rosvold HE (1965) Occipitotemporal corticocortical connections in the rhesus monkey. Exp Neurol 11:245
Larsen B, Skinhoj E, Lassen NA (1978) Variations of regional cortical blood flow in the right and left hemispheres during automatic speech. Brain 101:193
Lashley KS (1931) Mass action in cerebral function. Science 73:245
Lashley KS (1950) In search of the engram. In: Physiological mechanisms in animal behaviour. Academic Press, London New York
Lashley KS (1951) The problem of serial order in behaviour. In: Cerebral mechanisms in behaviour. John Wiley, New York
Lasky RE, Syrdal-Lasky A, Klein RE (1975) VOT discrimination by four- to six-and-a-half month old infants from Spanish environments. J Exp Child Psychol 20:215
Lassen NA, Ingvar ES (1978) Brain function and blood flow. Sci Am Oct, p 62
Lefrancois GR (1972) Psychological theories and human learning: Kongors report. Wadsworth Publ Comp, Belmont

References

Legendy CR (1967) On the scheme by which the human brain stores information. Math Biosci 1:555
Legendy CR (1968) How large are Hebb's cell assemblies? In: Oestreicher HL, Moore DR (eds) Cybernetic problems in bionics. Gordon and Breach, New York
Legendy CR (1975) Three principles of brain function and structure. Int J Neurosci 6:237
Lettvin JY, Maturana HR, McCulloch WS, Pitts W (1959) What the frog's eye tells the frog's brain. Proc IRE 47:1940
Le Vay S (1973) Synaptic patterns in the visual cortex of the cat and monkey. Electron microscopy of golgi preparations. J Comp Neurol 150:53
Levin SA (ed) (1978) Studies in mathematical biology. Math Assoc America
Lewin R (1975) Cat's brain are controversial. New Sci Nov: 457
Loguet-Higgins HC, Willshaw DJ, Buneman OP (1970) Theories of associative recall. Q Rev Biophys 3:223
Lopes de Silva FH, Storm van Leeuwen W (1978) The cortical alpha rhythm in dog: the depth and surface profile of phase (in: Brazier and Petsche, p 319)
Luce RD, Raiffa H (1957) Games and Decisions. Wiley, New York
Lund JS (1973) Organization of neurons in the visual cortex, area 17, of the monkey. J Comp Neurol 147:455
Lund JS, Lund RD (1970) The termination of callosal fibers in the paravisual cortex of the rat. Brain Res 17:25
Lund JS, Henry GH, MacQueen CL, Harvey AR (1979) Anatomical organization of the primary visual cortex (area 17) of the cat. A comparison with area 17 of the macaque monkey. J Comp Neurol 184:599–618
Luria AR (1973) The working brain. Penguin, New York
Luria AR, Yudovich FIa (1971) Speech and the development of mental processes in the child. Penguin, New York
MacGregor RJ, Lewis ER (1977) Neural modelling. Plenum Press, New York
Magoun HW (1963) The waking brain. Thomas, Springfield
Malsburg von der C (1973) Self-organization of orientation sensitive cells in the striate cortex. Kybernetik 14:85
Mark R (1974) Memory and nerve cell connections. Clarendon Press, Oxford
Marr D (1969) A theory of cerebellar cortex. J Physiol 202:437
Marr D (1970) A theory of cerebral neocortex. Proc R Soc London Ser B 176:161
Marr D (1971) Simple memory. Philos Trans R Soc London Ser B 262:23
Marr D (1981) Vision. Freeman, San Francisco
Marr D, Poggio T (1977) From understanding computation to understanding neural circuitry (in: Pöppel et al)
Marr D, Palm G, Poggio T (1978) Analysis of a cooperative stereo algorithm. Biol Cybern 28:223
Massaro DW (1975) Experimental psychology and information processing. Rand McNally, Chicago
Matzke HA, Foltz FM (1972) Synopsis of neuroanatomy. Oxford Univ Press, New York
McCulloch WS (1965) Embodiments of minds. MIT Press, Cambridge Mass
McCulloch WS, Pitts W (1943) A logical calculus of the ideas immanent in nervous activity. Bull Math Biophys 5:115
Mesarovic MD, Macko D, Takahara Y (1970) Theory of hierarchical, multilevel systems. Academic Press, London New York
Miller GA (1951) Language and communication. McGraw-Hill, New York Toronto London
Miller GA, Galanter E, Pribram KH (1960) Plans and the structure of behavior. Holt, New York
Milner PM (1970) Physiological psychology. Holt, New York
Minsky M (ed) (1968) Semantic information processing. MIT Press, Cambridge Mass

Minsky M, Papert S (1969) Perceptrons. MIT Press, Cambridge Mass
Mitra NL (1955) Quantitative analysis of cell types in mammalian neo-cortex. J Anat 89:467
Mitzdorf U, Singer W (1978) Prominent excitatory pathways in the cat visual cortex (A 17 and A 18): a current source density analysis of electrically evoked potentials. Exp Brain Res 33:371
Moskowitz BA (1978) The acquisition of language. Sci Am, p 47
Mountcastle VB (ed) (1968) Medical physiology. CV Mosby Company, Saint Louis
Movshon JA (1976) Reversal of the physiologic effects of monocular deprivation in the kitten's visual cortex. J Physiol 261:125
Muroga S (1971) Threshold logic and its applications. Wiley-Interscience, New York
Nass MM, Cooper LN (1975) A theory for the development of feature detecting cells in visual cortex. Biol Cybern 19:1
Nathanson JA, Greengard P (1977) Second messengers in the brain. Sci Am, p 108
Nelson K (1973) Structure and strategy in learning to talk. Monogr Soc Res Child Dev 149
Neumann von J (1958) The computer and the brain. Yale Univ Press, New Haven
Newell A, Simon H (1972) Human problem solving. Prentice Hall, Englewood Cliffs NJ
Newell A, Shaw JC, Simon H (1957) Empirical explorations with the logic theory machine. Proc West Joint Comp Conf 218
Nilsson NJ (1965) Learning machines. McGraw-Hill, New York
Nilsson NJ (1971) Problem solving methods in artificial intelligence. McGraw-Hill, New York
Noback CR, Demarest RJ (1967) The human nervous system. McGraw-Hill, New York
Palm G (1979) On representation and approximation of nonlinear systems, part II: discrete time. Biol Cybern 34:49–52
Palm G (1980) On associative memory. Biol Cybern 36:19
Palm G (1981a) On the storage capacity of an associative memory with randomly distributed storage elements. Biol Cybern 39:125
Palm G (1981b) Towards a theory of cell assemblies. Biol Cybern 39:181
Palm G, Braitenberg V (1979) Tentative contributions of neuroanatomy to nerve net theories. In: Trappl R, Klir GJ, Ricciardi L (eds) Progress in cybernetics and systems research, vol III. Wiley, New York, p 369
Pandya DN, Kuypers HJM (1969) Cortico-cortical connections in the rhesus monkey. Brain Res 13:13
Parnavelas JG, Sullivan K, Liberman AR, Webster KE (1977) Neurons and their synaptic organization in the visual cortex of the rat. Cell Tissue res 183:499
Peichl L, Wässle H (1979) Size, scatter and coverage of ganglion cell receptive field centres in the cat retina. J Physiol 291:117
Pellionisz A, Llinas R (1979) Brain modeling by tensor network theory and computer simulation. The cerebellum: distributed processor for predictive coordination. Neuroscience 4:323
Perkel DH, Bullock TH (1968) Neural coding. Neurosci Res Program Bull 6: No 3
Peters A, Fairen A (1978) Smooth and sparsely-spined stellate cells in the visual cortex of the rat: a study using a combined golgi-electron microscope technique. J Comp neurol 181:129–172
Peters A, Feldman ML (1976) The projection of the lateral geniculate nucleus to area 17 of the rat cerebral cortex. I. General description. J Neurocytol 5:63–84
Peters A, Feldman ML (1977) The projection of the lateral geniculate nucleus to area 17 of the rat cerebral cortex IV. Terminations upon spiny dendrites. J Neurocytol 6:669–689
Peters A, Saldanha J (1976) The projection of the lateral geniculate nucleus to area 17 of the rat cerebral cortex III. Layer VI. Brain Res 105:533–537

Peters A, Feldman M, Saldanha J (1976) The projection of the lateral geniculate nucleus to area 17 of the rat cerebral cortex. II. Terminations upon neuronal perikarya and dentritic shafts. J Neurocytol 5:85–107

Peters A, Proskauer CC, Feldman ML, Kimerer L (1979) The projection of the lateral geniculate nucleus to area 17 of the rat cerebral cortex. V. Degenerating axonterminus synapsing with Golgi impregnated neurons. J Neurocytol 8:331–357

Piaget J (1954) The construction of reality in the child. Basic books. Plenum Press, New York

Piaget J (1955) The language and thought of the child. Meridian books. Plenum Press, New York

Pitts W, McCulloch WS (1947) How we know universals. Bull Math Biophys 9:127

Pöppel E, Held R, Dowling JE (eds) (1977) Neuronal mechanisms in visual perception. Neurosci Res Program Bull 15: No 3

Poggio T (1975) On optimal nonlinear associative recall. Biol Cybern 19:201

Polya G (1949) How to solve it. Univ Press, Princeton

Popper KR, Eccles JC (1977) The self and its brain. Springer, Berlin Heidelberg New York

Powell TPS, Guillery RW, Cowan MM (1957) A quantitative study of the fornix-manillo-thalamic system. J Anat 91:419

Quastler H (1956) Studies of human channel capacity (in: Cherry, p 361)

Rall W (1962) Electrophysiology of a dendritic neuron model. Biophys J 2:145

Rall W (1967) Distinguishing theoretical synaptic potentials computed for different soma-dendritic distributions of synaptic input. J Neurophysiol 30:1138

Rall W (1970) Cable properties of dendrites and effects of synaptic location. In: Anderson P, Jensen JKS (eds) Excitatory synaptic mechanisms. Univ Forlaget, Oslo

Rauschecker JP (1979) Orientation-dependent changes in response properties of neurons in the kitten's visual cortex (in: Freeman, p 121)

Rauschecker JP, Singer W (1978) Experience-dependent modification of response properties in striate cortex: instructive versus selective mechanisms. Neurosci Lett Suppl 1:395

Rauschecker JP, Singer W (1979) Changes in the circuitry of the kitten's visual cortex are gated by postsynaptic activity. Nature (London) 280:58

Rauschecker JP, Singer W (1981) The effects of early visual experience on the cat's visual cortex and their possible explanation by Hebb synapses. J Physiol 310:215

Riesen AH (ed) (1975) The developmental neuropsychology of sensory deprivation. Academic Press, London New York

Rinzel J (1978) Integration and propagation of neuroelectric signals (in: Levin)

Rosenblatt F (1962) Principles of neurodynamics. Spartan Books, Macmillan, New York

Rosenzweig MR, Bennett EL (eds) (1976) Neural mechanisms of learning and memory. MIT Press, Cambridge Mass

Rosenzweig MR, Bennett EL, Diamond MC (1972) Brain changes in response to experience. Sci Am, p 22

Rozin P (1976) The psychobiological approach to human memory (in: Rosenzweig and Bennett, p 3)

Ryle G (1949) The concept of mind. Hutchinson, London

Sampson JR (1976) Adaptive information processing. Springer, Berlin Heidelberg New York

Samuel AL (1959) Some studies in machine learning using the game of checkers. IBM J Res Dev 3:210

Samuel AL (1967) Some studies in machine learning using the game of checkers II – Recent progress. IBM J Res Dev 11:601

Sanders AF (1971) Psychologie der Informationsverarbeitung. Hans Huber, Bern Stuttgart Wien

Schapiro S, Vukovich KR (1970) Early experience effects upon cortical dendrites: a oposed model for development. Science 167:292

Scheibel AB, Scheibel ME (1970) Elementary processes in selected thalamic and cortical subsystems – the structural substrates (in: Schmitt et al, p 443)

Schmitt FO, Melnechuk T, Quarton GC, Worden FG (eds) (1967, 1970, 1974, 1979) The neurosciences. 1st, 2nd, 3rd and 4th Study program. Rockefeller Univ Press, New York

Schüz A (1981) Pränatale Reifung und Postnatale Veränderung im Cortex des Meerschweinchens: Mikroskopische Auswerung eines natürlichen Deprivationsexperimentes I, II. J Hirnforsch 22:93–127

Scott AC (1977) Neurophysics. Wiley, New York

Shannon CE (1948) A mathematical theory of communication. Bell Syst Tech J 27: 379, 623 (Reprinted in Shannon and Weaver 1949)

Shannon CE (1950) Programming a digital computer for playing chess. Philos Mag 41: 356

Shannon LE, McCarthy I (eds) (1956) Automata studies. Univ Press, Princeton NJ

Shannon CE, Weaver W (1949) The mathematical theory of communication. Univ Illinois Press, Urbana Ill

Shepherd GM (1974) The synaptic organization of the brain. Oxford Univ Press, New York London Toronto

Sholl DA (1967) The organization of the cerebral cortex. Hafner Publ Comp, New York London

Simon HA (1969) The sciences of the artificial. MIT Press, Cambridge Mass

Singer W, Ruaschecker JP, Werth R (1977) The effect of monocular exposure to temporal contrasts on ocular dominance in kittens. Brain Res 134:568

Smith A (1740) An abstract of treatise of human nature (see ref. Hume 1938)

Smullyan R (1978) What is the name of this book? Prentice-Hall, Englewood Cliffs NJ

Sperry RW (1947) Cerebral regulation of motor coordination in monkeys following multiple transection of sensorimotor cortex. J Neurophysiol 10:275–294

Sperry RW, Miner N (1955) Pattern perception following insertion of mica plates into visual cortex. J Comp Physiol Psychol 48:463–469

Spitz RA (1965) The first years of life. Int Univ Press, New York

Stark L, Dickson JF (1965) Mathematical concepts of central nervous system function. NRP Bull 3: No 2

Steinbuch K (1961) Die Lernmatrix. Kybernetik 1:36

Stent GS (1973) A physiological mechanism for Hebb's postulate of learning. Proc Nat Acad Sci USA 70:997

Strypker MP, Sherk H, Leventhal AG, Hirsch HVB (1978) Physiological consequences for the cat's visual cortex of effectively restricting early visual experience with oriented contours. J Neurophysiol 41:896

Szentagothai J (1968) Structuro-functional considerations of the cerebellar neuron network. Proc IEEE 56:960

Szentagothai J (1969) Architecture of the cerebral cortex (in: Jasper et al, p 13)

Szentagothai J, Arbib MA (1974) Conceptual models of neural organization. NRP Bull 12: No 3

Terrace HS, Petitto LA, Sanders RJ, Bever TG (1979) Can an ape create a sentence? Science 206:891–902

Turing AM (1950) Computing machinery and intelligence. Mind LIX:236 (Reprinted in Anderson AR 1964)

Towe AL, Amassian VE (1958) Patterns of activity in single cortical units following stimulation of the digits in monkeys. J Neurophysiol 21:292–311

Uttley AM (1955) The probability of neural connexions. Proc R Soc London Ser B 144:229

Uttley AM (1956a) Conditional probability machines and conditioned reflexes (in: Shannon and McCarthy, p 253)

Uttley AM (1956b) Temporal and spatial patterns in a conditional probability machine (in: Shannon and McCarthy, p 277)
Valverde F (1971) Rate and extent of recovery from dark rearing in the visual cortex of the mouse. Brain Res 33:1
Valverde F (1978) The organization of area 18 in the monkey. A Golgi study. Anat Embryol 154:305–334
Vaughan DW, Peters A (1973) A three dimensional study of layer I of the rat parietal cortex. J Comp Neurol 149:355–376
Wall PD, Lettvin JY, McCulloch WS, Pitts WH (1956) Factors limiting the maximum impulse transmission ability of an afferent system of nerve fibres (in: Cherry C)
Ward RR (1971) The living clocks. Knopf Inc, New York
Weir R (1962) Language in the crib. Mouton, The Hague
Weizenbaum J (1966) ELIZA – a computer program for the study of natural language communication between man and machine. Commun ACM 9:36
Wenzel F (1936) Über die Erkennungszeit beim Lesen. Kybernetik 1:32
White EL (1979) Thalamocortical synaptic relations: a review with emphasis on the projections of specific thalamic nuclei to the primary sensory areas of the neocortex. Brain Res 1:275
Wickelgren WA (1968) Sparing of short-term memory in an amnesic patient: implications for strength theory of memory. Neuropsychology 6:235
Wiener N (1948) Cybernetics. Wiley, New York
Willwacher G (1976) Fähigkeiten eines assoziativen Speichersystems in Vergleich zu Gehirnfuktionen. Biol Cybern 24:181
Wilson HR, Cowen JD (1973) A mathematical theory of the functional dynamics of cortical and thalamic nervous tissue. Kybernetik 13:35
Winfield DA, Gatter KL, Powell TPS (1980) An electron microscope study of the types and proportions of neurons in the cortex of the motor and visual areas of the cat and rat. Brain 103:245
Winograd T (1974) Five lectures on artifial intelligence. Stanford AI Memo 246
Winston P (1975) The psychology of computer vision. McGraw-Hill, New York
Winston PH (1977) Artificial intelligence. Addison-Wesly, Reading Mass
Wolff J (1976) Quantitative analysis of topography and development of synapses in the visual cortex. Exp Brain Res Suppl 1:259
Wolff JG (1973) Language, brain and hearing. Methuen, London
Wong R, Harth E (1973) Stationary states and transients in neural populations. J Theor Biol 40:77

Digressions

1 Electrical Signal Transmission in a Single Neuron

Across the membrane of any cell there is a difference in electrical potential of about 60–80 mV, the inside being negative against the outside: the so-called *resting potential*. This potential difference can build up, because the concentrations of various ions inside the cell are different from outside, and the permeability of the membrane is different for different ions.

The activation of synapses causes changes in the permeability of the dendritic membrane leading to changes in the potential, which may cause a "spike" or "action potential" at the "axon hillock", i.e., the place (usually at the cell body) where the axon begins.

A rule of thumb for these changes is that "excitation" corresponds to depolarization (i.e., diminishing) of the resting potential and works in favor of generating a spike, whereas "inhibition" corresponds to hyperpolarization (i.e., enhancing) of the resting potential and works against generation of a spike.

When a spike has been generated, the membrane needs some time to recover, the so-called *refractory period*, during which another spike cannot be generated.

Once a spike has been generated, it moves along the axon, most probably into all its branches without attenuation and at synapses it causes the presynaptic axonal membrane to release some chemicals into the synaptic cleft, which induce the change of the resting potential in the postsynaptic membrane already mentioned.

What about the basic physics (or chemistry) of all this? Imagine a vessel filled with water, which is separated in two halves by an impermeable separating membrane. On one side we put in NaCl, on the other side KCl. Then we have Na^+-, Cl^-- and K^+-ions in the water, which may be distributed as in Fig. 1.

When we take out the separating membrane, K^+-ions will move from right to left and Na^+-ions from left to right, until the concentration of Na^+-, as well as K^+-ions is equal on both sides, i.e., until there is no concentration gradient any more (Fig. 2).

If we have a separating membrane that is permeable for Cl^-- and K^+-ions, but not for Na^+-ions, then at first only the K^+-ions will move from right to left (following their concentration gradient), which causes a volt-

Electrical Signal Transmission in a Single Neuron

	l	r
K^+	0	100
Na^+	100	0
Cl^-	100	100

Fig. 1

	l	r
K^+	50	50
Na^+	50	50
Cl^-	100	100

Fig. 2

	l	r
K^+	40	60
Na^+	100	0
Cl^-	120	80

Fig. 3

age across the membrane, i.e., a difference in the electrical potential of the two sides. This voltage tends to drive positive ions to the right, and negative ions to the left. Therefore not half of the K^+-ions will move to the right, but less, and in addition some Cl^--ions will also move to the right. In the equilibrium for this situation the concentration gradient for the K^+-ions will force them to the left equally as strongly as the voltage (= potential difference) will force them to the right. The same will be true for the Cl^--ions (mutatis mutandis, i.e., exchanging "left" and "right"), and therefore the final equilibrium concentrations might look like Fig. 3.

Thus there will be a permanent voltage across this membrane.

In fact, the membrane of nerve cells is much more permeable for K^+-ions than for Na^+-ions, but it is still possible for Na^+-ions to pass through the membrane into the cell. This "leakage" is compensated for by an active "pumping" mechanism that pumps Na^+-ions back out of the cell, but still there are a lot of Na^+-ions left inside the cell, only their concentration is much lower inside than outside.

Therefore there is a permanent voltage across the membrane of the cell – the inside being negative against the outside. This is called the *resting potential*, and it is about 60–80 mV.

The *action potential* (or *spike*) consists of a transient change in the resting potential, which is basically caused by the fact that the permeability of the membrane for Na^+-ions changes with the potential. If we artificially depolarize the membrane above a certain point, called the *threshold*, it becomes much easier for Na^+-ions to pass into the cell. This tends to cause a further depolarization of the membrane, which in turn further increases the Na^+-permeability of the membrane, etc. . . This mechanism leads within less than a millisecond to a complete breakdown of the potential across the membrane (although actually only a very small percentage of the ions on either side of the membrane passes through it). At this moment the membrane becomes nearly impermeable for Na^+-ions again and the resting potential builds up again.

During some time after the occurrence of such a spike the membrane is quite insensitive to further artifical changes in the potential. This period is called the *refractory period*.

The following figures (4 and 5) illustrate the temporal evolution of the action potential and also its propagation along the axon, which can be explained by the same principle.

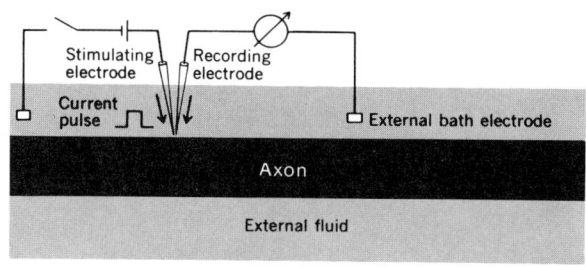
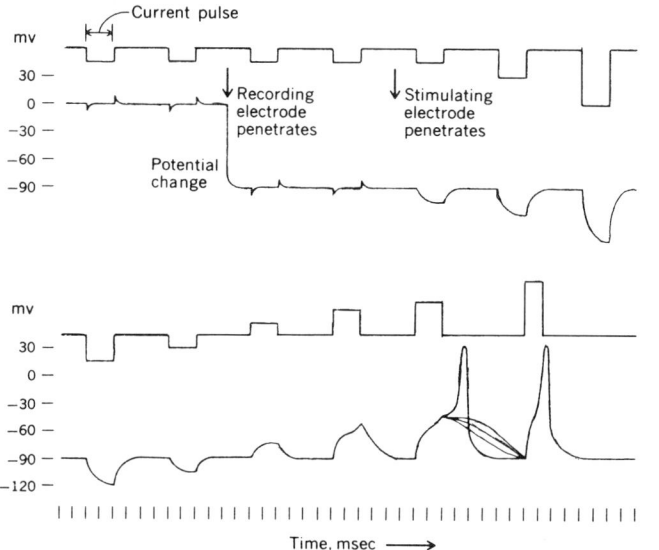
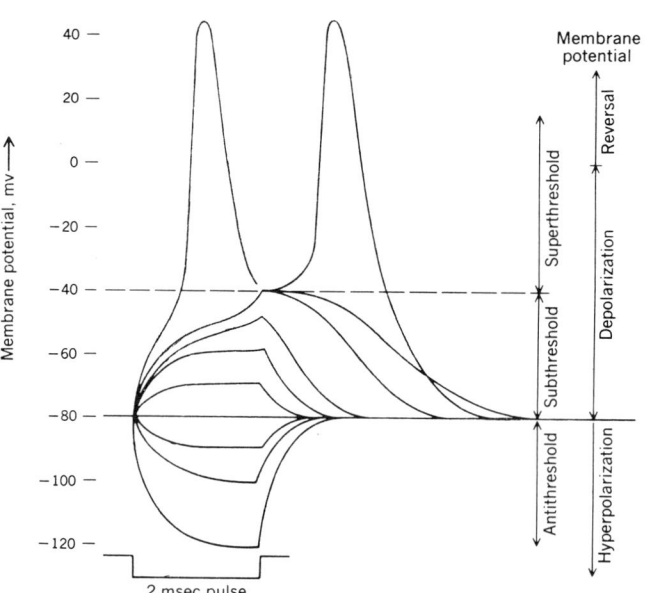

Fig. 4a,b. Variations of the membrane potential caused by stimulating current pulses of variable size and polarity (Katz 1966)

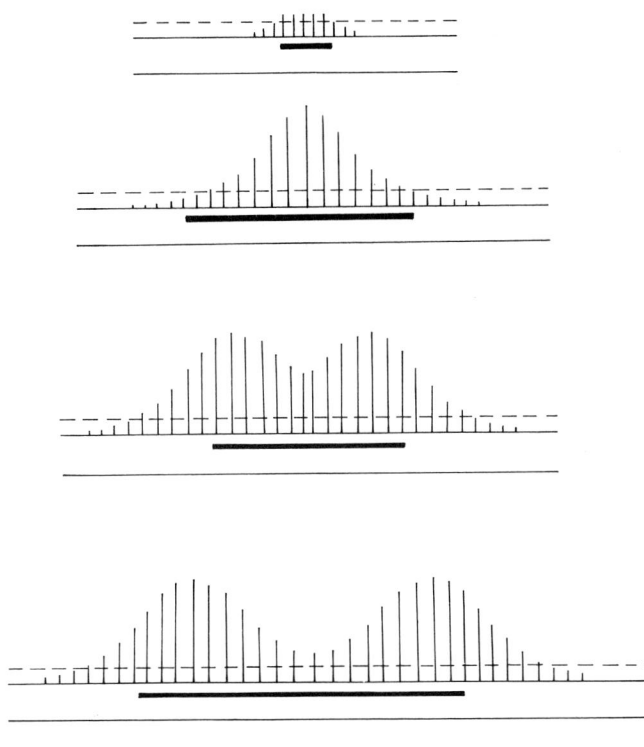

Fig. 5. Evolution in time of membrane potential along a briefly stimulated axon. *Vertical lines* strength of depolarization from the resting potential. *Horizontal bar* zone of the axon that is in the refractory state. *Dotted line* threshold depolarization

Normally the action potential starts at the beginning of the axon, and from this point it runs forward along the axon. When it reaches a synapse, it causes the presynaptic membrane to release some chemicals into the synaptic cleft, i.e., the space between the pre- and the postsynaptic neuron, which in turn changes the permeability of the postsynaptic neuron's membrane for Na^+-ions.

This change causes a depolarization of the membrane, which usually is not strong enough to produce an action potential (it may also be the case that the dendritic membrane does not show this voltage-dependent change in permeability which is characteristic for the generation of action potentials in the axon). But if many synapses are activated in the dendritic tree of a neuron at roughly the same time, the resulting depolarizations of the dendritic membrane will add up and yield an action potential, which

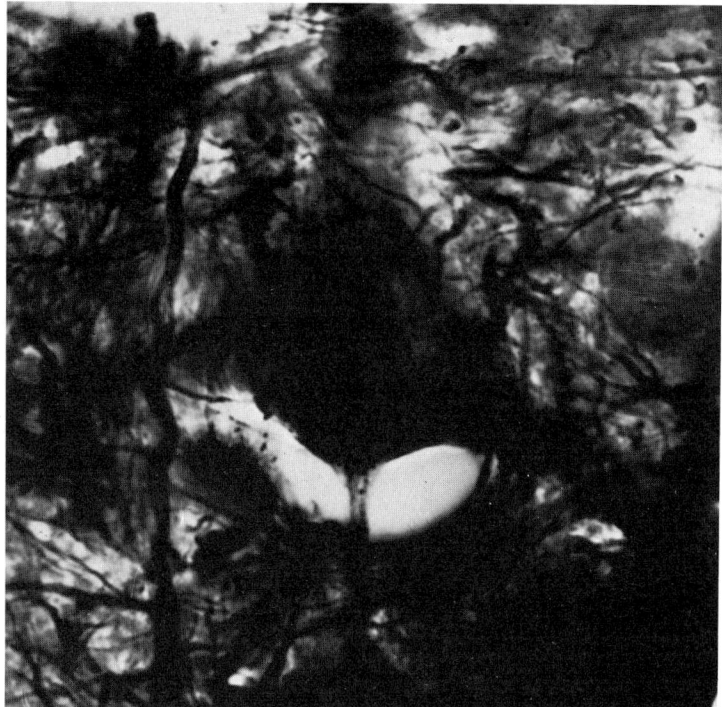

Fig. 6. Axon hillox of a pyramidal cell in a silver-stained preparation (courtesy V. Braitenberg)

usually emerges at a certain point, namely the *axon hillock,* the beginning of the axon. At this point the cell becomes much thinner and much more excitable; starting from this point, the action potential moves along the axon and probably into all its collaterals.

Finally I should mention that a synapse can work not only by changing the permeability of the postsynaptic membrane for Na^+, but that there are (at least) many other ions that can be used, e.g., Ca^{2+}, Na^+, K^+, Cl^-.

For example an increase in the permeability for K^+-ions would lead to a hyperpolarization of the membrane, i.e., the voltage difference of the resting potential would be further increased. A synapse which increases the K^+-permeability of the postsynaptic membrane would therefore act as an inhibitory synapse, whereas a synapse which increases the Na^+-permeability of the postsynaptic membrane would act as an excitatory synapse.

A more detailed discussion of these different mechanisms can be found, for example, in Eccles (1957, 1964), Katz (1966), Rall (1970), Rinzel (1978), Shepherd (1974).

2 Basic Information Theory

1 Roughly, the *amount of information* contained in a message should signify the number of yes/no questions required to guess this message.

We will use this statement as a guideline to define the amount of information. Imagine that the message consists of an answer to a question (e.g., "Claude Shannon is more than 40 years old"). Then, to estimate its information content, we need to know not only the onswer itself, but also the question. For example, the "question" could have been: "Name somebody over 40" or "How old is Claude Shannon?" or "Is Shannon more than 40 years old?"

The information content of the answer also depends on the preknowledge of the person asking the question about the knowledge of the person answering the question. All this preknowledge can be stated formally in the following *scheme:*

$$\begin{pmatrix} a_1, \ldots, & a_n \\ p(a_1), \ldots, p(a_n) \end{pmatrix}$$

containing a list of all (relevantly differing) possible answers $a_1, \ldots, a_n$ to the question and their probabilities, as estimated by the person asking the question.

2 Given this scheme one can work out an optimal *questioning strategy* of yes/no questions that allows to find out the answer (i.e., one of the a_i) to the question.

This strategy should be optimal in the following sense: If it takes n_i yes/no questions to find out the answer, in case it is a_i, the *average* number of questions needed, will be

$$N = \sum_{i=1}^{n} p(a_i) n_i.$$

This number should be minimal.

The actual optimal strategy is called the Huffman Code and it is described for example in Ash (1965). It turns out that it needs approximately

(+) $\quad n_i \approx -\log_2 p(a_i)$

questions to find out a_i.

3 How does the logarithm come in? Obviously, with one yes/no question we can decide between two possibilities, with 2 questions between 4 possibilities, with 3 questions between 8 possibilities, since we can use the first question to divide the 8 possibilities into 2 groups of 4 possibilities each, and decide which group it is, and then use the two remaining questions for the remaining 4 possibilities. In this way, with each additional question the number of possibilities that we can decide between is doubled. This means that with n questions we can decide between 2^n possibilities. If we want to find out the number of questions from the number of possibilities, we have to use the inverse relationship, i.e., for k possibilities we need $\log_2 k$ questions. The logarithm of base 2 will in the following be abbreviated as dual logarithm, $\log_2 x = \text{ld} x$.

For example for 64 possibilities we need ld 64 = 6 questions, since $2^6 = 2 \cdot 2 \cdot 2 \cdot 2 \cdot 2 \cdot 2 = 64$.

If we have 64 equal possibilities, each of them has the probability $\frac{1}{64} = 2^{-6}$, and the information we need to ask for it is $-\text{ld}\frac{1}{64} = \text{ld } 64 = 6$.

But does the formula (+) also work for schemes where not all probabilities are equal, and moreover, what happens if they are not powers of $\frac{1}{2}$ (i.e., of the form $2^{-k} = \left(\frac{1}{2}\right)^k$)?

To see that the formula still works quite well approximatively in these cases, the reader should try to work out the following exercises.

Moreover, it can been rigorously shown that (+) is the best approximation (Ash 1965). One line of argument is given below (Section 4).

Exercise 1. How many yes/no questions do you need to guess a card from a 32-card stack (if the card is drawn completely at random)?

Exercise 2. How many yes/no questions do you need to guess the result of throwing a dice once? (How many questions do you need a) maximally, b) on the average, all exercises 1–4 are meant in this sense.)

Exercise 3. How many yes/no questions do you need to guess the result of throwing a dice once, if you know that the probabilities of the outcomes are *not all equal, but*

$$\begin{pmatrix} 1 & 2 & 3 & 4 & 5 & 6 \\ \frac{1}{32} & \frac{1}{16} & \frac{1}{32} & \frac{1}{8} & \frac{1}{4} & \frac{1}{2} \end{pmatrix}?$$

Basic Information Theory

Exercise 4. How many yes/no questions do you need for the following scheme:

$$\begin{pmatrix} 1 & 2 & 3 & 4 \\ 0.4 & 0.3 & 0.2 & 0.1 \end{pmatrix} \quad ?$$

4 Following our questioning strategy guideline one can formulate the following postulates:

I. The information of the answer a_i depends only on the probability $p(a_i)$ of a_i.
In sympols: $\quad I(q \to a_i) = I(a_i) = I(p(a_i))$.
Indeed, to work out a questioning scheme one needs to know only the probabilities $p(a_i)$ and not the contents of the answers a_i.
Of course, the information of the answer a_i should depend only on the probability $p(a_i)$ of a_i itself in the scheme

$$\begin{pmatrix} a_1 & \cdots & a_n \\ p(a_1) & \cdots & p(a_n) \end{pmatrix}$$

not on the values $p(a_j)$ for $j \neq i$.

II. If an answer has probability $1/2$, its information is one. In symbols:

$$I\left(\tfrac{1}{2}\right) = 1.$$

Indeed, with one yes/no question we could find out the answer for the scheme

$$\begin{pmatrix} a_1 & a_2 \\ \tfrac{1}{2} & \tfrac{1}{2} \end{pmatrix}$$

Intuitively, this scheme contains the most information we can get in one yes/no question, since in a scheme

$$\begin{pmatrix} a_1 & a_2 \\ p & 1-p \end{pmatrix}$$

with $p \neq \tfrac{1}{2}$ we would be "less uncertain" about the answer.

III. If the answer a and a' to the questions q and q' respectively are independent, then the information of both answers is the sum of the information of a and of a'. Independence of the two answers is expressed by the requirement that
$p(q \to a \text{ and } q' \to a') = p(q \to a) \cdot p(q' \to a')$. In symbols this means the following: If $p(q \to a \text{ and } q' \to a') = p(q \to a) p(q' \to a')$ then

$I(q \to a$ and $q' \to a') = I(q \to a) + I(q' \to a')$. Or if we introduce $x := p(q \to a)$ and $y := p(q' \to a')$: $I(x \cdot y) = I(x) + I(y)$.

Requirement (III) shows that $I(x) = c \ln x$, and requirement (II) implies that $1 = I(\frac{1}{2}) = c \cdot \ln \frac{1}{2} = -c \ln 2$, i.e.,

$$c = -\frac{1}{\ln 2}.$$

Thus $I(x) = -\frac{\ln x}{\ln 2} = -\log_2 x = -\mathrm{ld}\, x$.

From requirement (I) we get $I(a_i) = I\, p(a_i) = -\mathrm{ld}\, p(a_i)$.

Therefore the average information obtained by an answer to the question q with scheme $\begin{pmatrix} a_1 & \ldots & a_n \\ p(a_1) & \ldots & p(a_n) \end{pmatrix}$ is

$$I(q) = \Sigma\, p(a_i)\, I(a_i)$$
$$= -\Sigma\, p(a_i)\, \mathrm{ld}\, p(a_i).$$

Clearly, in an actual questioning scheme

$$N = \sum_{i=1}^{n} p(a_i) n_i$$

can only be approximately equal to $I(q)$, since the n_i have to be integers and the values $I(a_i)$ not.

It can be shown that for any questioning scheme $N \geq I(q)$ and that the optimal questioning scheme comes close to $I(q)$ (see Ash 1965). For the scheme

$$\begin{pmatrix} a_1 & a_2 \\ p & (1-p) \end{pmatrix}$$

the information I can be plotted against p:

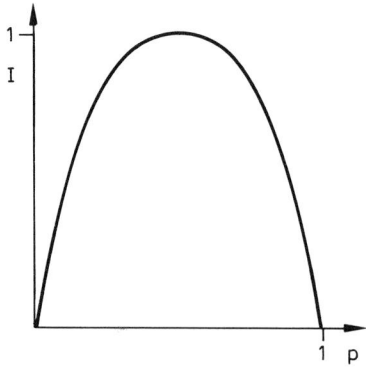

Fig. 1

Basic Information Theory

For the general scheme

$$\begin{pmatrix} a_1 & \cdots & a_n \\ p(a_1) & \cdots & p(a_n) \end{pmatrix}$$

we always have $\Sigma\, p(a_i) = 1$ and the information I attains its minimum, namely 0, at the probabilities $\begin{pmatrix} a_1 & \cdots & a_n \\ 1 & 0 & \cdots & 0 \end{pmatrix}$, $\begin{pmatrix} a_1 & \cdots & a_n \\ 0 & 1 & 0 & \cdots & 0 \end{pmatrix}$, etc. and its maximum, namely ld n, at the probability

$$\begin{pmatrix} a_1 & \cdots & a_n \\ \frac{1}{n} & \cdots & \frac{1}{n} \end{pmatrix}.$$

We have seen that a lot of knowledge about the situation is needed to determine the amount of information contained in a message.

All this is incorporated in the concept of the *information source*. An information source is a device which continually produces messages from a fixed set of possibilities $A_1, \ldots A_n$, about which we know the statistics.

An example is a machine that keeps throwing a dice, here we have

$$\begin{pmatrix} 1, & 2, & 3, & 4, & 5, & 6 \\ \frac{1}{6} & \frac{1}{6} & \frac{1}{6} & \frac{1}{6} & \frac{1}{6} & \frac{1}{6} \end{pmatrix}.$$

Another example may be the notations of the stock-market. Here we have only faint ideas about the underlying statistics. Still another example may be a tele-type giving off letters of English text. Here already a lot is known about the underlying statistics.

In this example another complication comes in:

Let us say the information source produces x messages per second. If we know the possibilities $A_1, \ldots, A_n$ and their probabilities $p_1, \ldots, p_n$, we can calculate the average information of one message as $I_1 = -\Sigma\, p_i\, \text{ld}\, p_i$ but, and from that we could estimate that the source produces $I_1 \cdot x$ bits per second.

It can be, however, that consecutive messages produced by the source are not independent of each other. For example in the English language the letter "q" is with high probability followed by the letter "u". This type of knowledge about the source can be incorporated in the statistics (which we assumed to be known) by considering two consecutive messages as one bigger message (i.e., we get the possibilities

$A_1 A_1, A_1 A_2, \ldots A_1 A_n, A_2 A_1, A_2 A_2, \ldots A_2 A_n, \ldots A_n A_n$ and

$P_{11}, P_{12}, \ldots P_{1n}, P_{21}, P_{22}, \ldots P_{2n}, \ldots P_{nn}.$

This means we get

$$I_2 = -\Sigma P_{ij} \, ld \, p_{ij}$$

bit per message, but we only get $\frac{x}{2}$ of these messages per second, i.e.,

$x \cdot \frac{I_2}{2}$ bit per second.

Clearly one possibility to guess a pair A_iA_j is first to guess A_i and then A_j, but if the choice of A_j is not completely independent of A_i (as in the case "q", "u"), this strategy will not be the best one, so that in general I_2 (the average number of questions needed in the best strategy to guess a pair of messages) is less than $2 \cdot I_1$ (the average number of questions needed in the best strategy to guess a single message). Thus

$$x \cdot \frac{I_2}{2} \leq x \cdot I_1.$$

Of course we could also consider triples or quadruples of messages and get

$\frac{I_4}{4} x \leq \frac{I_2}{2} x \leq I_1 x$ bits per second.

Thus the *information rate* of the source is defined as

$$R = \inf_n \frac{I_n}{n} \cdot x \text{ bits per second.}$$

6 The concept of an information source encounters

1. the *format* of the source, i.e., the set of all different messages $A_1, \ldots, A_n$, that can occur, and the number x of messages that are transmitted per second,
2. the *statistics* of the source, i.e., the probabilities for these messages and also for combinations of consecutive messages.

On the basis of this knowledge the information rate of the source can be calculated in bits per second. If we did not know the statistics of the source, but only the format, we could also guess the messages, but we would need more questions. How many questions would we actually need? Clearly the answer depends only on the number n, and we know it should be ld n.

Therefore the *formatal information rate* F of the source is defined as

$F = x \, ld \, n$.

Clearly we always have $R \leq F$ and the percentage of the formatally possible information rate, that is "wasted" by the special statistical properties of the source, i.e., $\frac{F-R}{F}$ is called the *redundancy* of the source.

Basic Information Theory

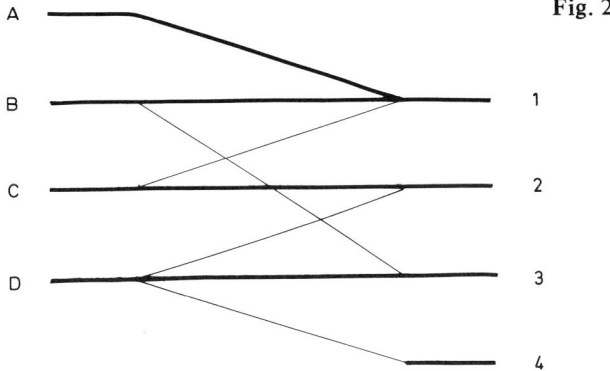

Fig. 2

7   The information or the messages that come out of the information source are then transmitted to a receiver. The transmission of information can be described by the concept of the *channel* (see Fig. 2). A channel is again defined by its format and its statistical characteristics.

The format of the channel consists of the possible input and output messages and the rate at which these messages can pass through the channel.

Of course, if a channel is connected to an information source, the input alphabet should be the same as the alphabet of the source, i.e., the channel should be *formatally adapted* to the source. The statistical characteristics of the channel describe the fact that the transmission of an input signal to the corresponding output signal is sometimes not performed correctly (i.e., as indicated by the solid lines), but may be changed (with a certain probability) (as indicated by the broken lines). Accordingly we have two measures for the information flow through a channel.

I. The *formatal channel capacity* is just the minimum of the formatal information rates as calculated for the output and for the input alphabet. According to (6) in this digression this means: if the input alphabet (set of possible input messages) has n signs and the output alphabet m signs and the channel can transmit x messages per second, then its formatal capacity is

$$C_F = x \text{ ld min}(n,m).$$

II. The (statistical) channel *capacity* is the maximal amount of information that can be transmitted through the channel by an optimally adapted source. This is determined by guessing as before. We connect the channel to a source S with a sufficiently high information rate and try to guess the messages of the source from the output of the channel. The number Q(S) of yes/no questions needed per message in a optimal

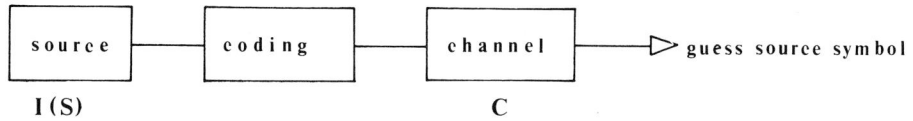

Fig. 3

questioning strategy is the information we need in addition to the channel output, to retain the original information I(S) per message of the source.

Thus the information about the source C, that has been transmitted through the channel is

T(S) = I(S) − Q(S).

The maximal amount of information that can be transmitted through the channel is

T_{max} = max { T(S) : S source for the channel}.

If the channel transmits x messages per second, we get the channel capacity

C = xT_{max} bits per second.

8 In a famous work, Shannon (1948) has shown that the following is possible with arbitrarily small error:

Given a source S with information rate I(S) and a channel with capacity C > I(S), one can code the source output (i.e., connect it via a specially constructed channel to the given channel) such that it is formatally adapted to the channel and the messages of the source can be completely retained from the channel output (with high probability).

In other words: as long as I(S) < C, the source cannot only formatally, but also statistically, be adapted to the channel.

If a channel is connected to a source S (which is not necessarily optimal), the information T(S) = I(S) − Q(S) about the source is transmitted per message and clearly the actual information flow for the source S is

T(S) · x ≦ C ≦ C_F.

Exercise 5. What is the formatal capacity of the five channels below (1 symbol per second is transmitted)? Is it equal to the capacity?

Basic Information Theory

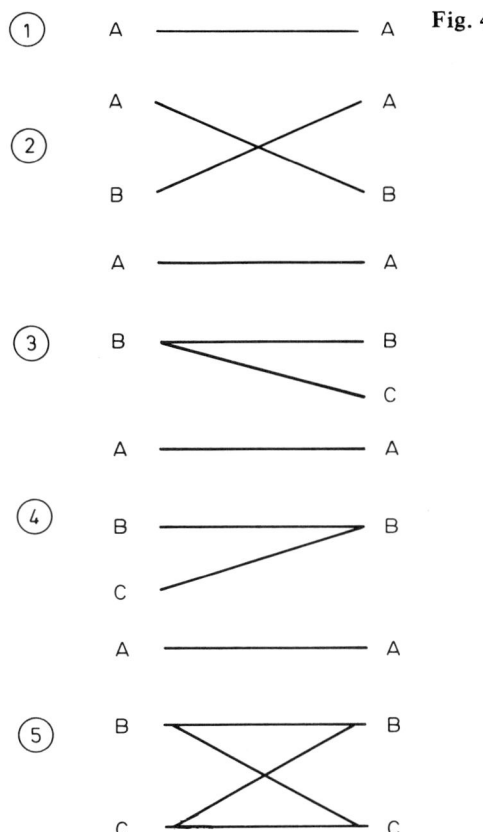

Fig. 4

9 Solutions of the Exerxises

Exercise 1. Five questions.

Exercise 2. A good strategy for guessing the outcome of throwing a dice is the following: Ask "even?" If yes, ask "2?" and perhaps "4?", if no, ask "1?" and perhaps "3?".

This strategy needs two questions to determine the 2 and the 1 and three questions for the other possible outcomes. Throwing a dice is described by the scheme

$$\begin{pmatrix} 1 & 2 & 3 & 4 & 5 & 6 \\ \frac{1}{6} & \frac{1}{6} & \frac{1}{6} & \frac{1}{6} & \frac{1}{6} & \frac{1}{6} \end{pmatrix},$$

the above strategy has $n_1 = n_2 = 2$, $n_3 = n_4 = n_5 = n_6 = 3$ and it is actually optimal.

a) 3 questions.
b) $N = \frac{1}{6}(n_1 + n_2 + n_3 + n_4 + n_5 + n_6) = \frac{16}{6} = 2\frac{2}{3}$ questions.

Exercise 3.
a) Three questions, and one can again use the strategy of Exercise 2.
b) For the average a different strategy is optimal: First question "6?", second question "5?", third question "4?", fourth question "2?" and fifth question "1?".

This strategy has $n_1 = n_3 = 5, n_2 = 4, n_4 = 3, n_5 = 2, n_6 = 1$ yields
$N = \frac{2}{32} \cdot 5 + \frac{1}{16} \cdot 4 + \frac{1}{8} \cdot 3 + \frac{1}{4} \cdot 2 \cdot \frac{1}{2} \cdot 1 = 1\frac{15}{16}$ questions.

Exercise 4
a) Two questions
b) The following strategy is optimal: first question "1?", second question "2?", third question "3?".

This strategy has $n_1 = 1, n_2 = 2, n_3 = n_4 = 3$ and
$N = 0.4 \cdot 1 + 0.3 \cdot 2 + 0.2 \cdot 3 + 0.1 \cdot 3 = 1.9$ questions.

Exercise 5
(1) $C = C_F = 0$
(2) $C = C_F = 1$ bit/s
(3) $C = C_F = 1$ bit/s
(4) $C = C_F = 1$ bit/s
(5) $C < C_F = \text{ld } 3 = 1.585$ bit/s,

if the error probability between B and C is $\frac{1}{2}$, we get $C = 1$ bit/s.

3 Sets and Mappings

This digression will provide the basic concepts of set theory, but I shall try to be as brief as possible. For more details the interested reader should consult a book on naive set theory, for example Halmos (1960).

1 A *set* just consists of several "objects" that are put together to form a new object (which is then called a set). To specify a set, we have to specify the objects belonging to it.

For example {1,2,3} denotes the set containing the numbers 1,2, and 3. 1,2, and 3 are called the *elements* of the set {1,2,3}. If a is an object and A a set we write a ϵ A (read "a in A") to mean that a is an element of the set A, i.e., that a belongs to A. We may write, for example,
7 ϵ {5,6,7,8,9,10}.

In this book we mainly deal with finite sets, this means sets with a finite number of elements (the number of elements of a set is called its *cardinality*).

We will occasionally refer to some infinite sets like

IN = The set of all positive integer numbers
   = {1,2,3, . . .}.
IR = The set of all real numbers.

A finite set can always be specified by listing all its elements, {a,b,c,d,e} for example.

But if it has many elements, it sometimes is more convenient to specify the set by giving a rule characterizing all its elements: For example

A = the set of all integers from 1 to 100
  = {1,2,3, . . .,99,100}.

This can be denoted in the following way:

A = {a | a is an integer between 1 and 100}.

Read:
A is the set of all objects a, such that a is an integer between 1 and 100.

A = {a | a ϵ IN and 1 $\leq$ a $\leq$ 100}.

Two sets A and B are called *equal*, A = B, if they both have the same elements.

We say that A is a subset of B, or that B contains A, A ⊆ B or B ⊇ A, if every object that belongs to A also belongs to B.

By these definitions the following is true:

Theorem. A = B if, and only if, A ⊆ B and B ⊆ A.
Indeed: A and B have the same elements if every element of A also belongs to B and vice versa; and if this is not the case, then there is an element of A not belonging to B or there is an element of B not belonging to A, in either case A and B do not have the same elements.

Theorem. If A ⊆ B and B ⊆ C, then A ⊆ C.

Exercise 1. Explain why this is true.

2 A *mapping* is just any prescription or procedure that works for a certain number of objects and, given one of these objects, produces another object or assigns another object to it.

If the mapping works only for a finite number of objects it can be conveniently specified by writing down a table. For example the mapping $m: a \mapsto 1, b \mapsto 2, c \mapsto 3, d \mapsto 4$ maps a into 1, b into 2, c into 3 and d into 4, and is given by the table

x	m(x)
a	1
b	2
c	3
d	4

The set of all objects on which the mapping works — in this case {a,b,c,d} — is called the *domain* D(m) of the mapping m. The set of objects that are produced by the mapping — in this case {1,2,3,4} — is called the *range* R(m) of the mapping m (cf. Fig. 1).

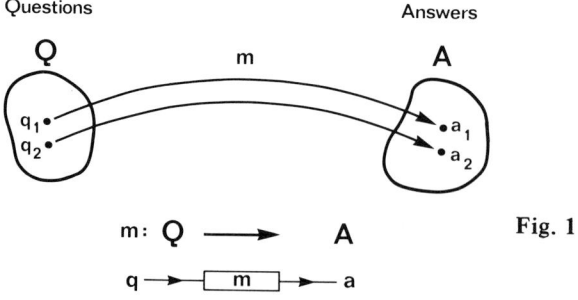

Fig. 1

Sets and Mappings

Given a mapping m and an object x ∈ D(m), the mapping m can work on x and the object that is produced (or assigned to x by m) is called m(x) (read "m of x").

A mapping m is often also called a function or an operator, and an equation like y = m(x) can be interpreted as "x is mapped into y by the mapping m" or "m operates on x yielding the outcome y" or "y is a function of (i.e., dependent on) x, the function (or dependency) being called m".

Often a mapping is more conveniently specified by giving a rule or prescription that defines the assignment.

For example the mapping F: 1 ↦ 2, 2 ↦ 3, 3 ↦ 4, 4 ↦ 5, 5 ↦ 6 maps each of the numbers 1, 2, 3, 4, 5 into the next number, more formally we may write: f: x ↦ x + 1 for every x ∈ {1,2,3,4,5}.

Exercise 2. The mapping h is given by the prescription

$$h : x \mapsto 2^x \text{ for every } x \in \{1, \ldots, 10\}.$$

Give a table for h and find D(h) and R(h).

Exercise 3. The mapping f_1 and f_2 are given by

$f_1 : x \mapsto x^2$ for every $x \in \mathbb{R}$;
$f_2 : x \mapsto \sin x$ for every $x \in \mathbb{R}$.

What is $D(f_1)$, $R(f_1)$, $D(f_2)$, $R(f_2)$? (Hint: Draw a diagram for the functions f_1 and f_2).

A system (Fig. 2) acting on certain inputs x and producing the corresponding outputs y can also be regarded as a mapping S: with D(S) = 𝒥 and R(S) = 𝒪, where 𝒥 is the set of all possible inputs and 𝒪 the set of all possible outputs.

Similar to the action of a mapping m on single objects, we can also consider the action of a mapping m on sets of objects. We write m: x ↦ y to express that m maps x into y; and we write m: A ↦ B to express that m maps the set A into the set B. This means that A is considered as the domain of m [A = D(m)] and that the corresponding range of m is contained in B [R(m) ⊆ B]. If R(m) = B, we say that m maps A *onto* B; in this case the mapping m is called surjective.

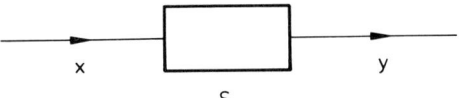

Fig. 2

3 The idea of introducing a *metric* is to provide a notion of "near" and "far", i.e., of distance between two points x and y in a "space" X.

Definition: Let X be a set. A mapping d that assigns to any pair (x,y) of points x, y ϵ X a real number d(x,y) is called a *metric* if it has the following properties:

a) $d(x, y) \geq 0$ for every x, y ϵ X
b) $d(x, y) = d(y, x)$ for every x, y ϵ X
c) $d(x, y) = 0$ if, and only if, $x = y$.
d) $d(x, y) \leq d(x, z) + d(z, y)$ for every x,y,z ϵ X.

Intuitively d(x, y) gives the distance between the points x and y in X.

Clearly, it should have property (a): there are no negative distances. Property (b) means that the distance from x to y is equal to the distance from y to x. Property (c) means that the distance from a point x to itself is zero, and that two different points always have a nonzero distance. Property (d) is called the triangle inequality:

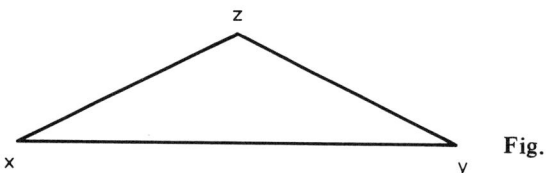

Fig. 3

The way from x to y is shorter than (or equally long as) the way from x to y via z, i.e., the distance from x to y should be less than or equal to the distance from x to z plus the distance from z to y.

4 Solutions of the Exercises

Exercise 1. If every object in A belongs to B, and every object that belongs to B, also belongs to C, then every object in A also belongs to C.

Ecercise 2

x	h(x)
1	2
2	4
3	8
4	16
5	32
6	64
7	128
8	256
9	512
10	1024

$D(h) = \{1,2,3,4,5,6,7,8,9,10\}$

$R(h) = \{2,4,8,16,32,64,128,256,512,1024\}$

Exercise 3

$D(f_1) = \mathrm{IR},\ R(f_1) = \{x : x \epsilon \mathrm{IR} \text{ and } x \geqq 0\}$

$D(f_2) = \mathrm{IR},\ R(f_2) = \{x : x \epsilon \mathrm{IR} \text{ and } -1 \leqq x \leqq 1\}$

4 Local Synaptic Rules

A *local synaptic rule* gives the change in the strength of excitation that a synapse is going to transmit from the presynaptic (axonal) terminal to the postsynaptic (dendritic) receptor, as a function of the momentary local presynaptic and postsynaptic activity.

The presynaptic activity can either be spike or nonspike in the presynaptic axon. The postsynaptic activity is rather a graded electrical potential in the postsynaptic dendrite. If we set up a criterion (e.g., a threshold for the potential), when to call the activity in the dendrite "high" and when to call it "low", a local synaptic rule can be given in the form of a table.

Presynaptic (axonal) activity	Postsynaptic (dendritic) activity	Resulting change in conductivity
High (spike)	High	c_1
High	Low	c_2
Low (nonspike)	High	c_3
Low	Low	c_4

The four numbers c_1, c_2, c_3, c_4 give the change in "conductivity" of the synapse under the four possible qualitatively different conditions on the local activity. Positive conductivity means that the synapse is excitatory, negative conductivity means that it is inhibitory. The changes c_1, c_2, c_3, c_4 are given in some kind of relative units, such that for example the numbers $(2, -1, 1, 0)$ have essentially the same meaning as $(2c, -c, c, 0)$ for any constant c. Let me give some examples how "local synaptic rules" can be expressed by the four numbers (c_1, c_2, c_3, c_4).

I. "All the synapses just grow, independent of the activity" (for example during the first month after birth).
   This is expressed by the rule $(1,1,1,1)$ or (c,c,c,c).
II. "The active neurons develop a lower threshold".
   This is expressed by the rule $(1,0,1,0)$.
III. "The active axons sprout and develop more and/or more efficient synapses".
   This is expressed by the rule $(1,1,0,0)$.

IV. Hebb's rule (cf. Chap. 7.5) is expressed by (1,0,0,0).
V. "Inhibitory synapses become stronger due to activity in the postsynaptic cell".
   This is expressed by the rule (−1,0,−1,0) for inhibitory synapses.
VI. "The inactive neurons develop a higher threshold".
   This is expressed by the rule (0,−1,0,−1).
VII. "The mechanisms of (III) and (VI) both take place independently, but (III) has a stronger effect".
   This is expressed for example by the rule $(1,\frac{1}{2},0,-\frac{1}{2})$.

Rule (VII) is called a *linear superposition* of rules (III) and (VI).

Rules of the type (II), (V), (VI) and more generally all rules (c,d,c,d) with two arbitrary constants c and d, are called *purely postsynaptic rules*.

In these rules the change in conductivity of the synapse depends only on the postsynaptic activity.

Rules of the type (III) and more generally all rules (c,c,d,d) with two arbitrary constants c and d, are called *purely presynaptic rules*.

In these rules the change of conductivity of the synapse depends only on the presynaptic activity.

Let us consider a large network with n neurons and k synapses (where $n \ll k \leq n^2$).

Assume the synapses all work according to a purely presynaptic rule. Then we can add up all the past changes in conductivity for one synapse on the axon of one neuron. This single number is the total change in conductivity of every synapse on this axon, since the changes are caused by a purely presynaptic rule. From this and from the initial conductivity of the synapses we can find out the resulting actual conductivity of every synapse on this axon.

This means that we can determine the conductivity of every synapse in the network from just n numbers (one number per neuron), and we do not need k numbers.

The analogous argument can be made for a purely postsynaptic rule, and even for a linear superposition of a purely presynaptic and a purely postsynaptic rule, where one needs 2n numbers: the total change caused by the purely presynaptic rule for every synapse on the axon and the total change caused by the purely postsynaptic rule for every synapse on the dendrites for each of the n neurons.

In Palm (1980) I have calculated the information-storing capacity of a large network that is arranged as an association matrix and contains k variable storage elements that work according to Hebb's rule (IV). I showed that the storage capacity of such a network increases proportional to k.

The arguments given above imply that for a linear superposition of a purely presynaptic and a purely postsynaptic rule the synaptic storage capacity of the network can only increase proportionally to n, since n numbers are sufficient to reconstruct all the synaptic conductivities.

But n can be small compared to k (in the human brain $n \approx 10^{10}$ and $k \approx 10^{14}$), therefore Hebb's rule works much better than such a superposition (and a fortiori cannot be regarded as such a superposition). In fact, Hebb's rule is based on a true interaction between the presynaptic and the postsynaptic activity. In the following, synaptic rules that can be obtained as a linear superposition of purely presynaptic and purely postsynaptic rules, will be called *noninteractive rules*. All other local synaptic rules will be called *interactive rules*.

How can we decide whether a given synaptic rule is a linear superposition of purely presynaptic and purely postsynaptic rules or not, i.e., whether it is noninteractive or interactive? For example, the rule $(1,0,0,-1)$ is noninteractive (how can it be obtained from purely presynaptic and purely postsynaptic rules?), whereas the rules $(1,0,0,0)$ and $(1,0,0,1)$ are interactive.

In the following I shall work out a systematic way of answering the above question, thus providing a classification of local synaptic rules. It will turn out to be an exercise in linear algebra.

$\mathbb{R}^4$, the set of all quadruples of real numbers, is sometimes called a four-dimensional vector space. This means that the elements (x_1, x_2, x_3, x_4) of $\mathbb{R}^4$ can be written as "linear combinations" of the four so-called canonical "unit vectors" e_1, e_2, e_3 and e_4. Let me explain this a little more:

The *canonical unit vectors* e_1, e_2, e_3 and e_4 in $\mathbb{R}^4$ are defined as follows:

$e_1 = (1,0,0,0)$
$e_2 = (0,1,0,0)$
$e_3 = (0,0,1,0)$
$e_4 = (0,0,0,1)$.

The quadruples $(x_1, x_2, x_3, x_4) \in \mathbb{R}^4$ are now called "vectors" and they are *added* as follows:

$(x_1, x_2, x_3, x_4) + (y_1, y_2, y_3, y_4) = (x_1+y_1, x_2+y_2, x_3+y_3, x_4+y_4)$,

and they are *combined linearly* as follows:
let a and b be real numbers, then

$a \cdot (x_1, x_2, x_3, x_4) + b \cdot (y_1, y_2, y_3, y_4)$
$= (a \cdot x_1 + b \cdot y_1, a \cdot x_2 + b \cdot y_2, a \cdot x_3 + b \cdot y_3, a \cdot x_4 + b \cdot y_4)$

Local Synaptic Rules

is another vector in $\mathbb{R}^4$ which is called a linear combination of the vectors (x_1,x_2,x_3,x_4) and (y_1,y_2,y_3,y_4).

Now any vector (x_1,x_2,x_3,x_4) is a linear combination of the four unit vectors e_1, e_2, e_3, e_4, since

$$x_1 \cdot e_1 + x_2 \cdot e_2 + x_3 \cdot e_3 + x_4 \cdot e_4$$
$$= x_1 \cdot (1,0,0,0) + x_2 \cdot (0,1,0,0) + x_3 \cdot (0,0,1,0) + x_4 \cdot (0,0,0,1)$$
$$= (x_1,x_2,x_3,x_4).$$

It is known that the four unit vectors e_1, e_2, e_3 and e_4 are not the only ones by which every vector can be combined linearly. In fact, the same is true for any four vectors u_1, u_2, u_3, u_4 that are *linearly independent,* i.e.: if a linear combination $a \cdot u_1 + b \cdot u_2 + c \cdot u_3 + d \cdot u_4$ of the four gives the vector $(0,0,0,0)$, then the numbers a, b, c, d must all be 0.

Moreover, it is not possible to combine any vector in $\mathbb{R}^4$ linearly from less than four independent vectors.

Four linearly independent vectors in $\mathbb{R}^4$ are also called a *basis* of $\mathbb{R}^4$.

Now we will classify synaptic rules (c_1,c_2,c_3,c_4) by expressing them as linear combinations of a specific basis u_1, u_2, u_3, u_4 of $\mathbb{R}^4$.

Consider the following synaptic rules:

a) the rule $(1,1,1,1)$ or $(-1,-1,-1,-1)$ or more generally the rule (c,c,c,c) with $c \in \mathbb{R}$ arbitrary,
b) purely presynaptic rules, i.e., the rules $(c,c,d,d,)$ with $c,d \in \mathbb{R}$ arbitrary,
c) purely postsynaptic rules, i.e., the rules (c,d,c,d) with $c,d \in \mathbb{R}$ arbitrary.

We have agreed that the importance of Hebb's rule lies in the fact that it is *not* a linear superposition (i.e., linear combination) of rules of the type (a), (b) or (c).

Let us now determine all linear combinations of these rules:

1. Rules of the type (a) are just multiples of the rule $(1,1,1,1)$, i.e., (c,c,c,c) $= c \cdot (1,1,1,1)$.
2. Rules of the type (b) are just linear combinations of the two rules $(1,1,1,1)$ and $(1,1,0,0)$, i.e., $d \cdot (1,1,1,1) + (c-d) \cdot (1,1,0,0) = (c,c,d,d)$.
3. Rules of the type (c) are just linear combinations of the two rules $(1,1,1,1)$ and $(1,0,1,0)$, i.e., $d \cdot (1,1,1,1) + (c-d) \cdot (1,0,1,0) = (c,d,c,d)$.

Therefore all linear combinations of rules of the type (a), (b) or (c) are just linear combinations of the three rules

$$u_1 = (1,1,1,1), u_2 = (1,1,0,0) \text{ and } u_3 = (1,0,1,0).$$

Therefore not every rule is a linear combination of the types (a), (b) or (c), since not every rule can be combined linearly from u_1, u_2 and u_3, and we need one more vector u_4 to get a basis of $\mathbb{R}^4$. Indeed, the rule

$u_4 = (1,0,0,0)$ is not a linear combination of u_1, u_2 and u_3, so we will choose u_1, u_2, u_3, u_4 as a basis of $\mathbb{R}^4$.

Thus we have to show that u_1, u_2, u_3 and u_4 are linearly independent, which also implies that Hebb's rule u_4 cannot be obtained as a linear combination of u_1, u_2, and u_3.

Finally we will show how an arbitrary vector (c_1, c_2, c_3, c_4) is combined linearly from u_1, u_2, u_3 and u_4.

1. Are u_1, u_2, u_3, u_4 independent?
  Let $a \cdot u_1 + b \cdot u_2 + c \cdot u_3 + d \cdot u_4 = (0,0,0,0)$, i.e., $(a+b+c+d, a+b, a+c, a) = (0,0,0,0)$.
  Therefore $a = 0$, $b = 0$, $c = 0$, and finally $d = 0$.
2. How is a general rule (c_1, c_2, c_3, c_4) combined from u_1, u_2, u_3, u_4?
  Let $(c_1, c_2, c_3, c_4) = d_1 \cdot u_1 + d_2 \cdot u_2 + d_3 \cdot u_3 + d_4 \cdot u_4$, i.e.,
  $(c_1, c_2, c_3, c_4) = (d_1 + d_2 + d_3 + d_4, d_1 + d_2, d_1 + d_3, d_1)$.
  Then $d_1 = c_4$, $d_2 = c_2 - c_4$, $d_3 = c_3 - c_4$, and finally
  $d_1 + d_2 + d_3 + d_4 = c_1$, i.e.,
  $d_4 = c_1 - d_1 - d_2 - d_3$
  $= c_1 - c_4 - (c_2 - c_4) - (c_3 - c_4)$
  $= c_1 + c_4 - c_2 - c_3$.

The new coefficients d_1, d_2, d_3 and d_4 can be used to classify synaptic rules into three classes:

1. *Hebb-like rules* with $d_4 > 0$
2. *Anti-Hebb rules* with $d_4 < 0$
3. *Noninteractive rules* with $d_4 = 0$.

Finally I want to give another basis v_1, v_2, v_3, v_4 of $\mathbb{R}^4$ which has an additional property: it is *orthogonal*, i.e., the inner product $\langle v_i, v_j \rangle$ of any two of the four vectors is zero if they are different ($i \neq j$).

The inner product $\langle c, d \rangle$ of the two vectors $c = (c_1, c_2, c_3, c_4)$ and $d = (d_1, d_2, d_3, d_4)$ is the number

$$c_1 \cdot d_1 + c_2 \cdot d_2 + c_3 \cdot d_3 + c_4 \cdot d_4 =: \langle c, d \rangle.$$

We take

$$v_1 = \frac{1}{2} u_1 = (\frac{1}{2}, \frac{1}{2}, \frac{1}{2}, \frac{1}{2})$$

$$v_2 = u_2 - v_1 = (\frac{1}{2}, \frac{1}{2}, -\frac{1}{2}, -\frac{1}{2}) \quad \text{(which is of type b)}$$

$$v_3 = u_3 - v_1 = (\frac{1}{2}, -\frac{1}{2}, \frac{1}{2}, -\frac{1}{2}) \quad \text{(which is of type c) and}$$

$$v_4 = (\frac{1}{2}, -\frac{1}{2}, -\frac{1}{2}, \frac{1}{2}).$$

Local Synaptic Rules

In this case we can express any vector $c = (c_1, c_2, c_3, c_4)$ as a linear combination $b_1 \cdot v_1 + b_2 \cdot v_2 + b_3 \cdot v_3 + b_4 \cdot v_4$ of v_1, v_2, v_3 and v_4, if we choose

$$b_1 = \langle c, v_1 \rangle = \frac{1}{2}(c_1 + c_2 + c_3 + c_4)$$

$$b_2 = \langle c, v_2 \rangle = \frac{1}{2}(c_1 + c_2 - c_3 - c_4)$$

$$b_3 = \langle c, v_3 \rangle = \frac{1}{2}(c_1 - c_2 + c_3 - c_4)$$

$$b_4 = \langle c, v_4 \rangle = \frac{1}{2}(c_1 - c_2 - c_3 + c_4).$$

Again we call a synaptic rule *Hebb-like*, if $b_4 > 0$, i.e., if

$$(c_1 + c_4 - c_2 - c_3) > 0.$$

5 Flow Diagram for a Survival Algorithm

This digression contains a comparatively simple flow diagram for a survival algorithm, that is built on the ideas developed in Chapter 5 to improve the matchbox algorithm. It works with an associative (feedback) matrix for pattern prediction (as in Chap. 7.2) and with three or four (feedback) matrices for pattern completion (as in Chap. 7.3), but all five matrices could be combined into one big matrix (as explained in Chaps. 11.10, 11.11, 13.2, 13.4).

One of the pattern completion matrices works on the immediate situation $s = (cs,a,v)$ in the sense of Chapter 7.3, the other one works on future situations $s = (cs,a,v)$, where cs is interpreted as a "motive" (for the plan that leads to the prediction of the future situation s). Moreover, in any situation $s = (cs,a,v)$, a is interpreted to contain something like a "plan" (see also Chap. 13.5) and v should also contain a value for the "urgency" of the situation s (see Chaps. 5.5, 5.6).

Apart from the five matrices, the flow diagram contains three short-term memories (for the storage of alternatives) with a comparatively low storage capacity and three simple decision algorithms, which work according to decision criteria that are determined from a few variables.

There are three such algorithms, labeled I, II, III.
I. decides when to stop the running prediction. In this case the three switches controlled by I are briefly opened. This has the effect that the resulting situation at the end of the prediction is transferred to the matrix memory of the next stage (testing of prediction), and that the two matrix memories of the prediction stage are "reset" to the current situation (that is represented in the matrix of the first stage, i.e., the action stage).
II. decides when to stop checking the prediction obtained from the prediction stage; the result is then passed to the next stage (searching for alternatives). The short-term memory corresponding to II can influence the threshold control mechanism of the prediction matrix (P) in order to generate alternative predictions to the most probable prediction which is always produced first. It has to store parameters for the "solidity" of the various alternative predictions obtained, and for the values (and "urgencies") of the corresponding predicted situations.
III. decides when to stop searching for alternative plans or motives. The best plan obtained during the search can be put into action by means of the corresponding switch. The corresponding memory can influence the threshold control mechanisms of the two matrices of the prediction stage in order to generate alternative plans (and to obtain alternative motives). It has to store these plans and motives together with their evaluation (and "solidity")

Flow Diagram for a Survival Algorithm

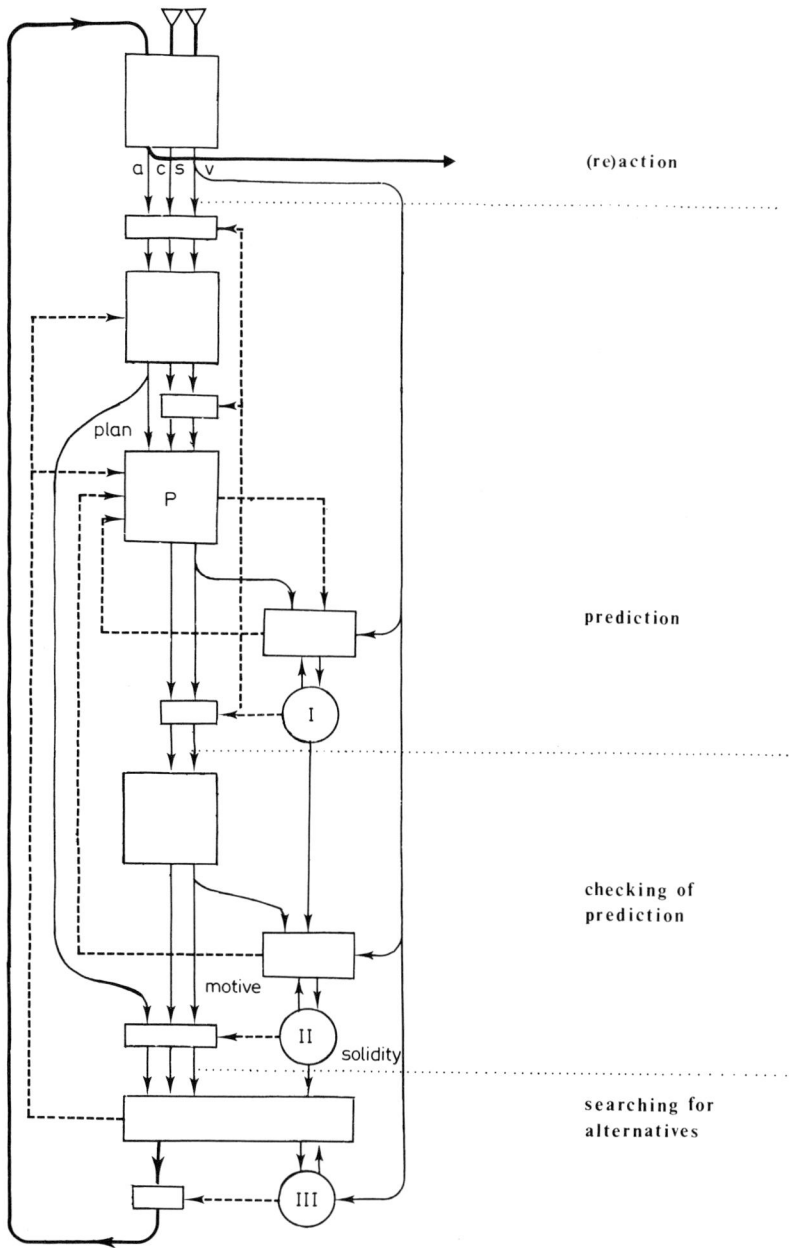

Fig. 1.

⊞ stands for an associative matrix memory with feedback connections as in Fig. 7.2 or 7.8. For reasons of stability it should also contain a threshold control mechanism as in Fig. 12.4. *Broken lines* indicate inputs to and outputs from the matrix relevant for its threshold control mechanism. (Note that the switches could also be realized by a special threshold control)

⊟ indicates a switch for the vertical lines, which is usually switched off, but can be switched on for a short time by the corresponding decision algorithm.

□ indicates a decision algorithm (*circle*) that works together with a short-term memory (*box*)

These decision algorithms are not specified here. In a concrete implementation of such a survival algorithm (for example in a chess-playing machine) it would be no severe problem to specify them, but there would be several reasonable specifications and the choice of a specification (for each of the three decision algorithms) would determine something like the "style" or "character" of the machine (e.g., whether the machine acts quite spontaneously or usually "thinks a lot" before acting).

The following remarks are concerned with a possible realization (or implementation) of this survival algorithm in a mammalian brain:

The five associative matrices, or the one big matrix replacing them could be realized in the neural network of the cerebral cortex. The two short-term memories could be realized in the cortex as well; the contents of such an operational memory could correspond to a pattern of neural activity that "holds", for example in a "higher level P-area" (see Chaps. 7.5, 13.5). Prototypes for the three decision algorithms could be genetically determined (and wired into certain subcortical structures), but see also Chapter 13.8.

6 Suggestions for Further Reading

Anatomy and Physiology

Blinkov and Glezer (1968) The human brain in figures and tables.
Brodal (1969) Neurological anatomy.
Cajal (1911) Histologie du système nerveux de l'homme et des vertèbres.
Eccles (1957) The physiology of nerve cells.
Eccles (1964) The physiology of synapses.
Katz (1966) Nerve, muscle and synapse.
Kuffler and Nichols (1976) From neuron to brain.
Luria (1973) The working brain.
Matzke and Foltz (1972) Synopsis of neuroanatomy.
Mountcastle (1968) Medical physiology.
Schmitt et al. (1967, 1970, 1974, 1979) The neurosciences (I–IV).
Shepherd (1974) The synaptic organization of the brain.
Sholl (1967) The organization of the cerebral cortex.

Psychology

Brown (1970) Psycholinguistics.
Fromkin and Rodman (1974) An introduction to language.
Hebb (1949) The organization of behaviour.
Hebb (1958) Textbook of psychology.
Kohler (1964) The formation and transformation of the perceptual world.
Lefrancois (1972) Psychological theories and human learning: Kongor's report.
Massaro (1975) Experimental psychology and information processing.
Miller (1971) Language and communication.
Miller, Galanter and Pribram (1960) Plans and the structure of behavior.
Milner (1970) Physiological psychology.

Cybernetics and Artificial Intelligence

Braitenberg (1977) On the texture of brains.
Hoffstaedter (1979) Gödel, Escher, Bach.
MacGregor and Lewis (1977) Neural modelling.

McCulloch (1965) Embodiments of minds.
Minsky (1968) Semantic information processing.
Minsky and Papert (1969) Perceptrons.
Neumann von (1958) The computer and the brain.
Polya (1949) How to solve it.
Sampson (1976) Adaptive information processing.
Szentagothai and Arbib (1974) Conceptual models of neural organization.
Wiener (1948) Cybernetics.
Winston (1975) The psychology of computer vision.

Appendices

1 On the Storage Capacity of Associative Memories

This appendix contains a slight modification of a talk given at the University of Salerno in April 1980.

What is memory?
In trying to answer this question you would probably introduce a situation where somebody is asked to remember some fact he has learned before. You might, for example, start your explanation somewhat along this lines:
If somebody knows the answer to a question (e.g., "When was Napoleon born?"), he has acquired that knowledge, i.e., the ability to respond correctly to the question, by "learning". Since the time he has "learned" this answer, he "remembers" it, i.e., he has it in his "memory".
More generally, we usually conceive of our own memory in terms of a flexibility in a stimulus → response mapping: the memory is expressed by a change in our responses to certain "stimuli"; we have learned the correct responses (or at least reasonable responses) in many situations.
On the other hand, the term "information storage" elicits quite a different picture: we typically think of a device like a tape (or a computer memory). In this case the "information" is "stored" by writing it down sequentially on the storage medium (e.g., the tape), and it can be "retrieved" again by reading it out in the same sequence. I shall call a memory that is operated in this way a *listing memory*. Whenever we want to store information externally (not just by remembering it), we use a listing memory. A book is an example for a listing memory. If the task is to remember a sequence of actions (how to assemble a radio) or events (the French revolution) a listing memory like a book can be used in a straightforward way as an external storing device.
If the task is to remember the answers to many different questions, a listing memory cannot be used directly. We need an additional strategy of looking up our question on the list, in order to find the correct answer to it. Indeed, we have invented several good strategies of looking up; the alphabetic ordering that we use in telephone books, for example, is such a strategy.
Would it not be convenient to have an external storing device that is well adapted to the task of storing answers to many questions, i.e., that stores information by adjusting its input → output mapping. Such a memory would work exactly according to the behavioral description of

our own internal memory, given above. From the technical point of view such a memory would have the important advantage that it does not need an additional "looking up" algorithm and therefore works much faster than a conventional computer memory in the question → answer paradigm. Indeed, such memories have been invented: all associative memories (e.g., Gabor 1970, Longuet-Higgins et al. 1970, Kohonen 1977, Rosenblatt 1962, Steinbuch 1961, Uttley 1956a,b) are of this type, which I shall call *mapping memory*. The fact that associative memories are mapping memories is perhaps their most characteristic property.

Unfortunately, this has been widely ignored. For example, in computer sciences it is still a truism that there is a trade-off between the storage capacity of a memory and its access time (because of the looking-up algorithm). This simply is not true for associative memories, which could be built technically and in fact have been built (e.g., Frank 1962).

The main purpose of this appendix is to explain a very simple version of an associative memory (namely Fig. 5.1), which shows the essential features of all associative memories (more refined versions are discussed for example in Kohonen's book 1977) and to present results on the information storage capacity of this memory that have been obtained by Longuet-Higgins et al. (1970) and myself (Palm 1980, 1981a).

Imagine an n by n array of 1 bit storage elements (that can be in two states: 0 and 1). It can be used as a conventional listing memory (Fig. 1).

In this case the message is a string of length 25 which is simply written into the matrix.

It can also be used as a mapping memory (Fig. 2).

In this case the message is a mapping between three pairs of strings of length 5.

The matrix is built up in the following way:

Think of horizontal and vertical wires running through the matrix (as in Fig. 3). Then the first pair of strings is "applied" to the matrix in the following way. The input string is "applied" to the vertical wires, i.e., the first

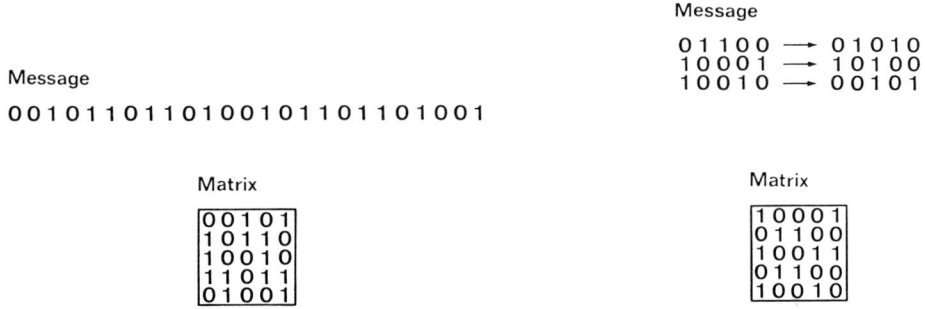

Fig. 1

Fig. 2

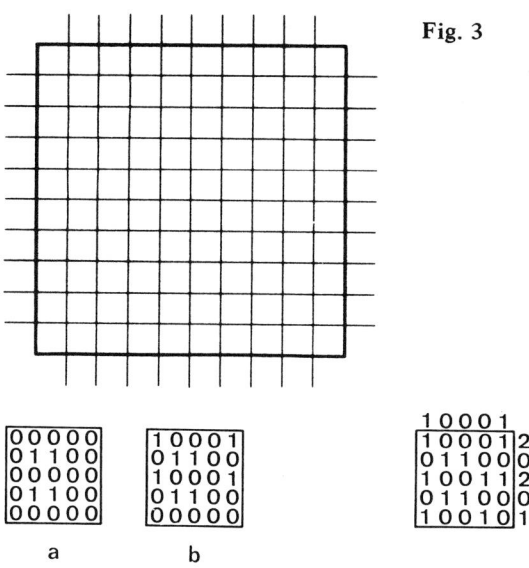

Fig. 3

a

0	0	0	0	0
0	1	1	0	0
0	0	0	0	0
0	1	1	0	0
0	0	0	0	0

b

1	0	0	0	1
0	1	1	0	0
1	0	0	0	1
0	1	1	0	0
0	0	0	0	0

Fig. 4

1	0	0	0	1	
1	0	0	0	1	2
0	1	1	0	0	0
1	0	0	1	1	2
0	1	1	0	0	0
1	0	0	1	0	1

Fig. 5

wire is given activity 0, the second and third ones get activity 1, and the last two wires again get no activity. The output string is "applied" to the horizontal wires in the same way. The storage elements in the matrix have all been set to zero at the beginning. Now each storing element has a vertical and a horizontal wire running through it. If both wires have activity 1, the element is set to one, otherwise it remains at zero. Thus, after "application" of the first pair of strings, the matrix looks as in Fig. 4a; after "application" of the second pair it looks as in Fig. 4b, and finally we get Fig. 2.

The retrieval of the message from the matrix is done simply as follows:

We interpret the state 0 or 1 of each storage element as the connectivity between the two wires running through it. For example, let us apply the second input string to the vertically running wires of the matrix of Fig. 2; on each horizontal wire we add up the activity it gets from the vertical wires through the connections (Fig. 5). We see that we get the maximal value (namely 2) on the first and the third horizontal wires, which corresponds to the output pattern 10100.

In the same way the matrix gives the correct output strings to the other two input strings.

At this point the reader may wonder how many pairs of strings can be stored in the matrix this way. Clearly the matrix will not work correctly any more, if too many pairs of strings have been "applied" to it, because it gets more and more filled with ones.

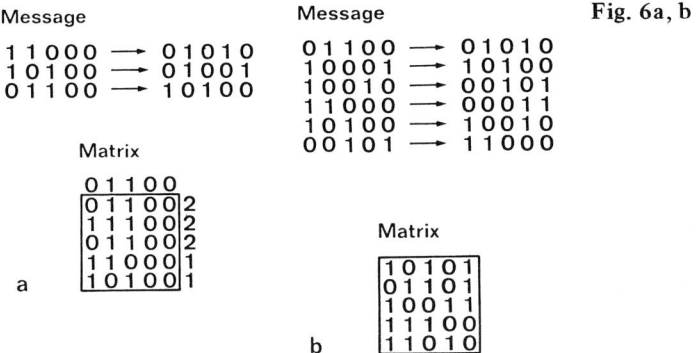

Fig. 6a, b

The problem is that the number of pairs that can be stored (without error) depends on the pairs themselves. For example, in Fig. 6a even three pairs cannot be correctly recalled, whereas in Fig. 6b six pairs can be correctly recalled.

This problem has led to the following approach (cf. Palm 1980): First I specify the format of a set of pairs that is to be stored in the matrix. The format is given by three parameters:

I) the number z of pairs in the set,
II) the number ℓ of ones in every input string,
III) the number k of ones in every output string.

Now I choose at random a set $\mathscr{S}$ of pairs that has this format. Then I can determine the information $\mathcal{I}(\mathscr{S})$ about the list $\mathscr{S}$ that can be retrieved from the matrix. For example, the set $\mathscr{S}_1$ in Fig. 6a has the format $z = 3$, $k = \ell = 2$ and $\mathcal{I}(\mathscr{S}_1) = 8.38$, whereas the set $\mathscr{S}_2$ in Fig. 6b has the format $z = 6$, $k = \ell = 2$ and $\mathcal{I}(\mathscr{S}_2) = 19.93$.

Finally, I try to calculate the average $\overline{\mathcal{I}}$ of $\mathcal{I}(\mathscr{S})$, where $\mathscr{S}$ varies over all sets of pairs with the predescribed format. More accurately, I obtain a number I that satisfies $I \approx \overline{\mathcal{I}}$ and $I \leq \overline{\mathcal{I}}$. This quantity depends on the three parameters z, k, ℓ, and of course on the additional parameter n that determines the dimension of the n x n storing matrix.

Then I can try to find the maximum $I_{max}(n)$ of I, varying the parameter z, k, and ℓ. Finally I can investigate the asymptotic growth of $I_{max}(n)$ with n.

The results of this procedure are the following: For n = 100 I obtain 6508 bits with the parameters $z = 1270, \ell = 3, k = 2$. For n = 1000, I obtain 688,000 bits with the parameters $z = 117,000, \ell = 3, k = 2$.

Another important parameter that illustrates the nature of the difficulty in information retrieval from the matrix is the *overlap,* o. It is defined as the average number of input strings to which an input wire bellongs. It can easily be calculated from the other parameters: $o = \frac{\ell}{n} \cdot z$.

For example, for the above parameters with n = 100 the overlap is o = 38.1 with n = 1000 it is o = 351.

There is still a slight problem in the interpretation of these results: I have optimized just the average value of $\mathcal{J}(\mathcal{S})$, so that I still may get only a small amount of information for every single pair in the set $\mathcal{S}$. Therefore, it seems reasonable to optimize $\mathcal{J}$ under some additional "high fidelity" constraints that guarantee that enough information about every single pair is stored in the matrix. Perhaps the simplest high fidelity constraint is the requirement that on the average 90% of the information of the output string of each pair is stored in the matrix. Under this constraint I get an optimum of 4609 bits for n = 100, z = 417, ℓ = 6, k = 2 (and o = 25), and an optimum of 593,000 bits for n = 1000, z = 34,780, ℓ = 9, k = 2 (and o = 313).

Other high fidelity constraints can be based on the probability p of getting a wrong (additional) maximum in the output of the matrix, when the input string of a pair in the list is applied to the matrix (cf. Fig. 5). For example, one could impose high fidelity constraints on the number p itself, or on the average number $(n-k)p$ of wrong additional output maxima, or on the probability $1 - p^{n-k}$ of getting the correct output pattern without any error, i.e., on the error probability $\delta = p^{n-k}$. All these high fidelity conditions are met in the asymptotic results that are summarized in the following theorem.

Theorem. For any $n \in \mathbb{N}$ and any $\epsilon > 0$, we can find parameters k, ℓ, z such that

$$\frac{I(n,k,\ell,z)}{n^2} \to \frac{\ln 2}{1 + \epsilon} \quad \text{and}$$

$$\frac{\text{Information stored per output string}}{\text{total information of one output string}} \to 1$$

for $n \to \infty$.

The parameters are chosen in such a way that $k = \mathcal{O}(\log n)$,

$$\ell = (1 + \epsilon) \operatorname{ld} n, \quad z \sim \left(\frac{n}{\log n}\right)^2$$

There is a special way of using such an associative memory, namely *auto*-association. It simply means that in every pair of the set $\mathcal{S}$ the input and output strings are identical. In this case the matrix can be used to retrieve the whole string (in the set $\mathcal{S}$) by applying any (sufficiently large) part of it as an input to the matrix. If the matrix is used this way, the same analysis can again be carried out and the results are as follows.

For n = 100, we get 3382 bits with z = 3500 and k = 2 (o = 70); under the constraint that 40% of the information on each string in the bit be extractable from the matrix, we get 3085 bit with z = 294 and k = 5 (o = 14.7).

For n = 1000, we get 346,000 bits with z = 347,000 and k = 2 (o = 694); under the constraint that 40% of the information on each string in the list be extractable from the matrix, we get 335,000 bits with z = 13022 and k = 8 (o = 104.2).

For the asymptotic values we obtain the following theorem.

Theorem. For any $n \in \mathbb{N}$ and any $\epsilon > 0$ we can find parameters k z such that

$$\frac{I(n,k,z)}{n^2} \to \frac{\ln 2}{2} \quad \text{and}$$

$$\frac{\text{information stored per string}}{\text{total information of one string}} \to \frac{1}{2} - \epsilon$$

for $n \to \infty$.

The parameters are chosen such that $k = (1-\epsilon) \text{ld } n$ and $z \sim \left(\frac{n}{k}\right)^2$.

Recently I have finished the asymptotic calculations for another important variation of the associative memory scheme (Palm 1981a). In this case it is no longer assumed that a 1-bit storage element is placed into every entry of the matrix; instead I assume that the storage elements are thrown at random into the matrix. Each entry of the matrix has the probability c of containing a storage element, independent of the other elements. If a storage element is placed at an entry (i,j) of the matrix, it works as usual; if no storage element is placed at an entry (i,j) of the matrix, the connectivity (between horizontal and vertical cable) will remain at its initial value 0.

In this case c gives the density of storage elements in the matrix and $c \cdot n^2$ is the average number of storage elements in the matrix. The asymptotic result for this case is as follows.

Theorem. $\frac{I(n,k,\ell,z)}{n^2 \cdot c} \to \approx 0.05$ and the error probability $\delta \to 0$ for $n \to \infty$.

Here the parameters k, ℓ, z satisfy

$$\ell \approx 9.7 \frac{\ln n}{c}$$

$$k = \mathcal{O}(\log n)$$

$$z \approx \frac{n^2}{\ell k} \cdot 0.35.$$

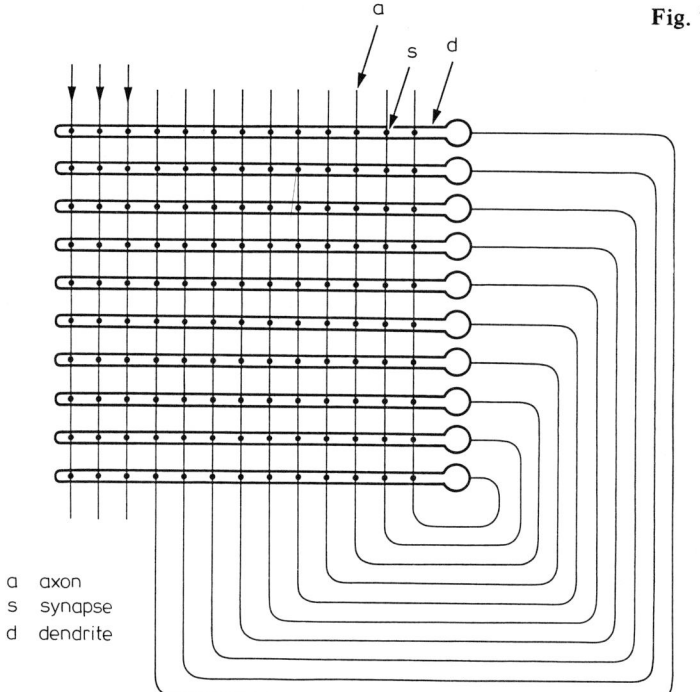

Fig. 7

a axon
s synapse
d dendrite

It has recently been speculated (e.g., Marr 1969, 1970, 1971, Kohonen and Oja 1976, Kohonen 1977, Anderson 1972) that our brain might contain an associative kind of memory. These speculations seem quite natural for two reasons:

I) our own introspection fits more easily with a mapping memory than with a listing memory,
II) the associative matrix memory scheme can be translated quite easily into neurons and synapses (see Fig. 7 and compare Fig. 7.12a).

Figure 7 contains basically only two requirements:

I) In some part of our brain there must be many recurrent connections. This requirement is met by the anatomy of our cortex (see Chap. 8).
II) The synapses in this part of our brain should obey Hebb's law (1949). The strength of a synapse is increased due to the coincidence of pre- and postsynaptic activity. This requirement is very hard to test experimentally, and it is not yet clear whether it is met by (at least some of) the cortical synapses (but see also Chap. 10).

The scheme in Fig 7 can work as an auto-association memory, and if it does so, it will detect and complete certain patterns that have been learned earlier (i.e. strings in the set $\mathcal{S}$).

In this terminology a string corresponds to a pattern of activity in the network and a learned string in the set $\mathcal{S}$ corresponds to a pattern of activity that is self-restoring or self-completing. This is what Hebb (1949) and later Braitenberg (1977) have called a *cell assembly*. Thus one may think of using the results of theorem (3) for a very crude estimation of the size of and overlap between cell assemblies in our cortex.

I do not think that this is a promising approach as yet, mainly for two reasons:

I) The error probability δ chosen in the calculations for theorem (3) is too small (it was chosen to be roughly $e^{-\frac{1}{\ln n}} \approx 0.04$ for $n = 10^{10}$), and we probably do not need such a high fidelity in our brain as opposed to a "commercial" associative matrix memory.

II) The strategy for reconstructing the strings in the learned set $\mathcal{S}$ did not use any information on the actual location of the storage elements in the matrix, which results in a comparatively low estimation of the storage capacity (0.05 bit per storage element). I believe that evolution has led to a more clever location scheme for the storage elements than just random location.

Still I think that theorem (3) can be used to show that the idea of viewing the cortex as an associative memory gives a sufficient storage capacity to make other memory storage mechanisms dispensible. Even if the cortex with its 10^{10} neurons and 10^{14} synapses (both are conservative estimates) is used with the very restricted strategy of theorem (3), it can store about $5 \cdot 10^{12}$ bits.

2 Neural Modeling

The principal motivation for brain modeling is to find a way of representing what goes on in the brain. This can be done by using equations as a kind of language "to fix ideas" — a method that has two disadvantages:

a) This language can be used and understood freely at most by physicists and mathematicians.

b) The equations that are written down usually are too precise and specific, that is, they predict the dynamical behavior of the brain totally or in any case too exactly, and they require too many parameters to be specified, as compared to what the authors often really intend to express by them. This problem gains even more importance by the fact that the equations usually cannot be solved analytically.

Instead of writing down many equations, I shall try to introduce another way of fixing ideas: namely, to use *"blurred matrices"* and *"local synaptic rules"*.

On the other hand, equations for the dynamics of neural networks have the advantage that they can be simulated on a big computer. In Chapter 11 I have presented the results of some of these simulations, since they provide rough intuitive images for what may possibly go on in the brain.

To understand the procedure by which these simulations are obtained, it is important to know at least the basic mathematical (or physical) concept used in investigations on dynamical processes: the concept of state.

By *neural dynamics* we understand rules governing the change of the *state* of the brain in time.

The concept of a state stems from physics and implies that from complete knowledge of the state at some time t_o and the rules governing the change of state, the state of any later time $t > t_o$ can be determined.

In the following I will try to give a very general framework for neuron network theories and to categorize the different theories within that framework (cf. also an der Heiden 1978). To this end it will be convenient to write down a few equations, but I will try to use the mathematical symbols in such an intuitive way that readers not familiar with mathematics can still understand the basic ideas if they skip equations. For their benefit here is a list of symbols with their rough meaning:

Neural Modeling

n	= neuron
a	= activity
c	= connectivity
a_n	= activity of neuron n
$c_{n,n'}$	= synaptic connectivity from neuron n to neuron n'
t	= time
A	= activities of all neurons = activity state
C	= all connectivities between neurons = connectivity state

The *state of activity* of the network can be described by indicating the activity of every neuron in the brain. The activity of one neuron n is usually viewed as a real valued function of time $a_n(t)$. The activity of a neuron at time t can for example be measured as the "instantaneous spike frequency" of that neuron (see, for example, Perkel and Bullock 1968).

Let N denote the set of all neurons in the brain, then the numbers $[a_n(t)]_{n \in N} =: A(t)$ describe the state of activity at time t.

In many models the state of activity alone is not enough to describe the state of the brain, since the connectivity of the synapses also changes. By a synapse we mean a connection between two neurons n, n' ϵ N. Thus we can denote the strength (or connectivity) of this synapse by $c_{n,n'}$.

Then the *state of connectivity* at time t is given by a mapping

$$C(t): \begin{cases} N \times N \to \mathbb{R} \\ (n,n') \mapsto c_{n\,n'}(t) \end{cases}$$

$c_{nn'}(t)$ denotes the connectivity of a (possible) synapse between the neurons n and n' at time t.

If $c_{nn'}(t) = 0$, there is no actual synapse between n and n',
$c_{nn'}(t) > 0$, there is an excitatory synapse between n and n',
$c_{nn'}(t) < 0$, there is an inhibitory synapse between n and n'.

Virtually all neuronal models are based on these concepts, and we can now proceed to classify them.

1 The State of Activity

1.1 The description of the activity of a single neuron n can be either *continuous* or *discrete*.

   a) *Discrete* here means that the neuron n can only be in a finite number of different states of activity. For example a threshold neuron can be either "on" or "off", i.e., its activity a_n can be either 1 or 0.

   b) *Continuous* here means that the activity of a neuron n can be any real number, at least any number in some interval [x,y] (where x < y).

Usually the activity a_n is assumed to be positive, and often the activity cannot exceed some maximal value a_{max}, i.e., $0 \leq a_n \leq a_{max}$, or $a_n \in [0, a_{max}]$.

1.2 The combination of the global state of activity from the states of all single neurons can be either *continuous* or *discrete*.

  a) *Discrete* here means that the set N of all neurons is finite, let us say, it contains k neurons, then we may take $N = \{1, \ldots, k\}$. In this case the state of activity is just a vector $(a_1, \ldots, a_k)$ whose coordinates a_j ($1 \leq j \leq k$) denote the activity of the j-th neuron in N.

  b) *Continuous* here means that the brain is modeled as a three-dimensional mass of neurons or as a two-dimensional sheet of neurons (this continuous view of the brain was already expressed in the model of Beurle 1956, and it leads to "field theories" of the brain, like Griffith 1963, 1965, Wilson and Cowan 1973, Fischer 1973). In this case a neuron n is specified by its coordinates (x_1, x_2) or (x_1, x_2, x_3) in the two- or three-dimensional Euclidean space respectively.

  This means that we can identify N with a subset of $\mathbb{R}^2$ or $\mathbb{R}^3$; in this case $a_{(x_1, x_2)}$ or $a_{(x_1, x_2, x_3)}$ denotes the activity at the point (x_1, x_2) or (x_1, x_2, x_3) in space.

2 The State of Connectivity

2.1 The connectivity between two neurons n and n' is given by a number $c_{n, n'}$. The possible values for the connectivity c can be either *discrete* or *continuous*.

  a) *Discrete* means that c can only have a finite number of possible values, for example 0 for no synapse, 1 for an excitatory synapse, −1 for an inhibitory synapse.

  b) *Continuous* means that c can be any real number — at least any number in some interval [x,y] (where y > x).

2.2 a) If the set N of all neurons is finite, i.e., $N = \{1, \ldots, k\}$ as in 1.2.a, the connectivities $c_{n, n'}$ can be arranged in a matrix C, called the *connectivity matrix*.

$$C = \begin{bmatrix} c_{11} & \cdots & c_{1k} \\ & \vdots & \\ c_{k1} & \cdots & c_{kk} \end{bmatrix}$$

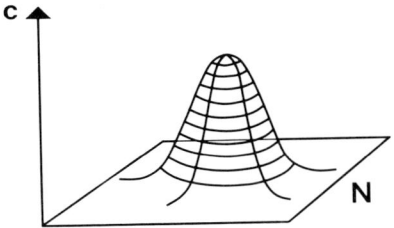

Fig. 1. Typical choice for the function $c_n: N \to \mathbb{R}$ where $N \subseteq \mathbb{R}^2$

Here the element c_{ij} in the j-th column of the i-th row denotes the connectivity from neuron i to neuron j. In this case we can speak of a neuron *network;* an illustration is given in Fig. 11.1.

b) In the case 1.2.b, for example, if $N \subseteq \mathbb{R}^2$, the connectivity from a given neuron (point) $n = (x_1, x_2) \in N$ to other neurons (points) n' is given by a function $c_n: N \to \mathbb{R}$, where $c_n(n') = c_{nn'}$ for example as in Fig. 1; in this case the function c_n is usually required to be continuous.

3 The Initial Conditions

In order to analyze the flow of activity, the initial state of the brain has to be given, from which the development in time starts. Here usually different initial states of activity are used, whereas the initial state of connectivity is not varied in one model, since it corresponds to the genetically predetermined connectivity of the immature brain.

3.1 The initial state of connectivity can either be determined explicitly or statistically.

a) Determined initial connectivity can be given for example as a matrix C in case 2.2.a.
b) Statistic initial connectivity is used more often in brain models. Here only a probability distribution $p_{n, n'}$ for the initial connectivity $c_{n, n'}$ be-

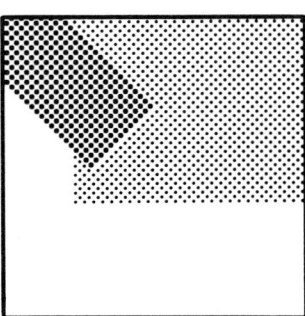

Fig. 2. A blurred connectivity matrix

tween every pair of neurons is given and it is usually assumed that the actual initial connections are formed independently (and according to these probabilities). In this case the probability $p_{n,n'}$ usually does not vary much from neuron to neuron, and we may use the following *blurred connectivity matrix* notation, i.e., we do not give the individual numbers $c_{n,n'}$, but just indicate them by the darkness in the corresponding place of the matrix (see Fig. 2).

Here, in general, we need one matrix to denote the excitatory contacts and another one for the inhibitory contacts.

3.2 The initial connectivity $c_{n,n'}$ — or the corresponding probability $p_{n,n'}$ — may depend only on the actual distance of the cell bodies of n and n'. Formally, distance can be described by a so-called *metric* d: N x N → IR (cf. Digression 3),

a) *metric connectivity* in this context means that there is a metric d: N x N → IR, such that $p_{n,n'}$ (or $c_{n,n'}$) is a function of d (n,n'),
b) *ametric connectivity* means that this is not the case,
c) there may be a mixture of both. For example the rough description of cortical connectivity given in Chapter 8 implies that the short-range connections can be modeled as metric, whereas the long-range connections cannot. For a statistical metric initial connectivity we occasionally use the following "allegorical" blurred matrix notation:
Indeed, if the neurons $n_1, \ldots, n_k$ were really aligned like that, the connectivity in this blurred matrix would only depend on their distance $d(n_i, n_j) = |i-j|$. In reality, however, the configuration of neurons is two- or three-dimensional. Therefore a metric connectivity could not be depicted accurately in a two-dimensional array, like Fig. 3, but a four- or six-dimensional array would be needed, which we cannot draw on paper.

We can now do some exercises in blurred-matrix algebra or "heraldic" — as it may also be called for literally "obvious" reasons:

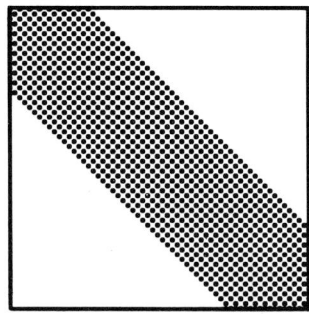

Fig. 3

Neural Modeling

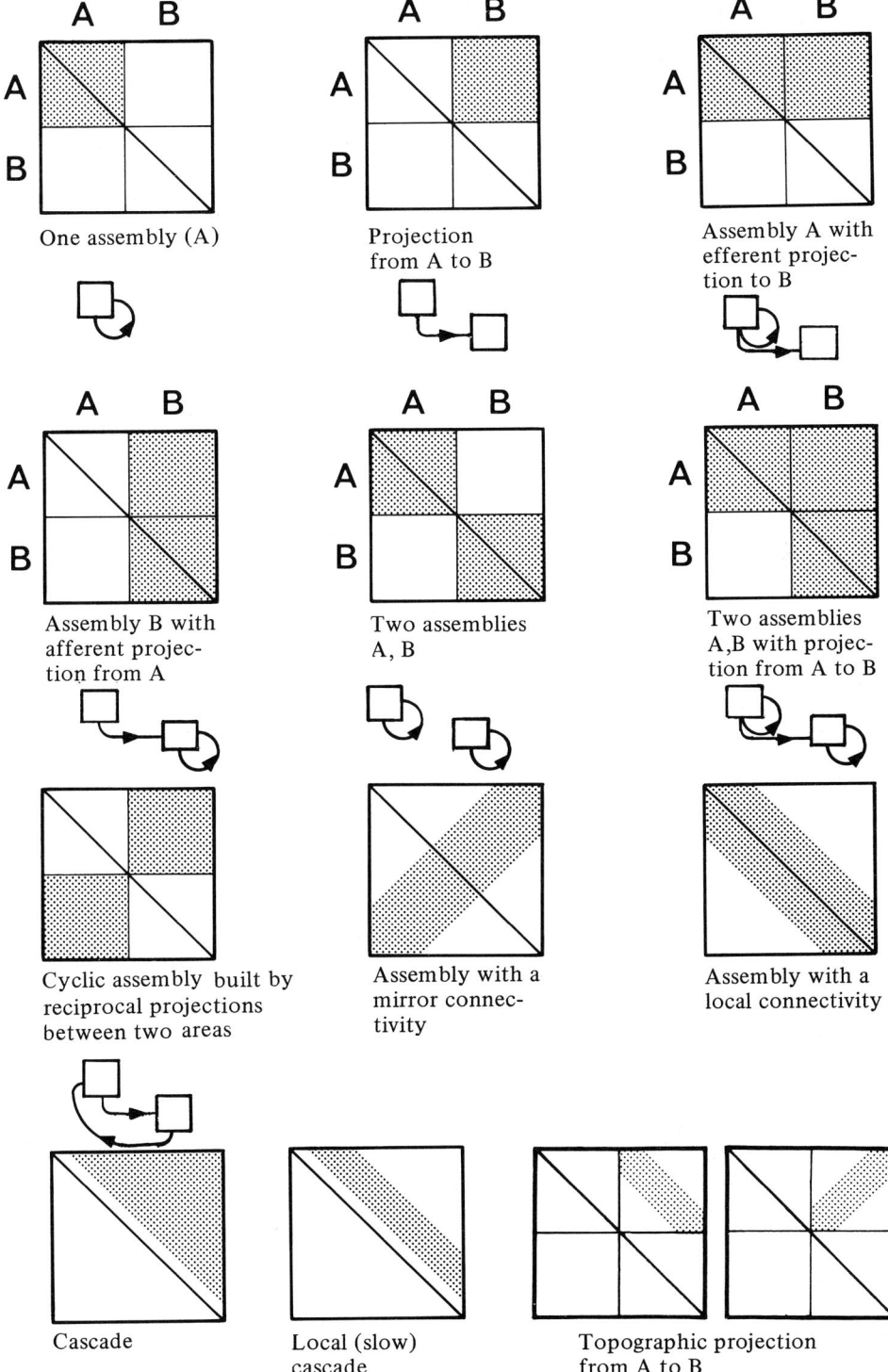

Fig. 4. Heraldic

4 Rules Governing the Change of State

These rules can be divided into rules governing the state of activity A and rules governing the state of connectivity C. Usually the rules are given in a differential way, i.e., the increment of A and C is expressed in terms of A and C:

$$\frac{\Delta A}{\Delta t} = F(A,C)$$

$$\frac{\Delta C}{\Delta t} = G(A,C)$$

These equations have been termed "neuronic equations" and "mnemonic equations" respectively, by Caianiello (1961). The idea behind this distinction between neuronic and mnemonic equations is the following: it is assumed that the dynamics of the activity state is much faster than the dynamics of the connectivity state. Therefore one may first assume fixed connectivities and analyze the dynamics of the activity state for fixed points and limit cycles. Subsequently one may analyze the dynamics of the connectivity state.

4.1 Rules governing the evolution of the state of activity in time.

At a fixed time t we have a certain state of connectivity $C(t)$. From this we want to determine the "next" state of activity — or more exactly the change $\frac{dA(t)}{dt}$ of activity at that moment t.

To do this, we need to know the dynamics of all the single neurons n.

For one neuron n the change in its activity a_n will depend on $a_n(t)$ itself and on the activity of those neurons that are presynaptic to it, i.e., on those $a_{n'}$, where $c_{n',n}(t) \neq 0$. From such a neuron n' our neuron n gets the excitation $a_{n'} \cdot c_{n',n}$ with a certain delay $t_{n',n}$ depending, for example, on the distance between n' and n, i.e., at time t it gets

$$a_{n'}(t - t_{(n',n)}) \cdot c_{(n',n)}(t).$$

In almost every model it is assumed that the excitation from the dendritic synapses of each neuron n is just added; thus the sum

$$z_n(t) = \Sigma_{n'} a_{n'}(t - t_{(n,n')}) c_{(n',n)}(t)$$

is formed.

In continuous models (with respect to 2.2.b) this summation is replaced by integration.

Neural Modeling

In discrete models the definition of the connectivity matrix C in 2.2.a and the assumption of a constant time-distance Δt between the neurons make it possible to write this equation in the following way:

$Z(t) = A(t - \Delta t)C(t)$
where $A(t) = (a_1(t), \ldots, a_k(t))$ as in 1.2.a
and $Z(t) = (z_1(t), \ldots z_k(t))$.

From $z_n(t)$ the increment in the activity $a_n(t)$ of the neuron n is determined by a relationship like

$$\frac{da_n(t)}{dt} = f_n(a_n(t), z_n(t)).$$

Moreover, the equations are usually simplified by assuming that the functions f_n are the same for all neurons n, or only of a few types corresponding to a few types of neurons.

An inspection of simulations of different models gives the general impression that the detailed specification of f_n within reasonable boundaries does not influence the dynamics as much as the choice of the initial connectivity. A particularly simple choice of f_n is provided in the threshold neurons of McCulloch and Pitts (cf. Chap. 3):

$$f_n(a_n(t), z_n(t)) = \begin{cases} 0 \text{ if } z_n(t) < \Theta_n \\ 1 \text{ if } z_n(t) \geqslant \Theta_n \end{cases}.$$

4.2 Rules governing the change of the state of connectivity.

These rules for changes in synaptic connectivity are of special interest for networks that are built to show learning by change of connectivity. They can usually by regarded as variations of Hebb's rule (Hebb 1949). Networks of this type were already described by Uttley (1956a,b), Rosenblatt (1962), and Steinbuch (1961).

Changes in connectivity are often viewed as dependent on the state of activity alone:

$$\frac{dC}{dt} = G(A).$$

Furthermore it can be assumed that the changes in connectivity of a synapses can only depend on the neuronal activity in the immediate neighborhood of that synapse and maybe even only on the (local) pre- and postsynaptic activity.

Here the presynaptic activity is just the activity $a_{n'}$, in the axon of the presynaptic neuron n'.

The postsynaptic activity, however, can in general not be described simply as the "output" activity a_n of the postsynaptic neuron n, since it can be just the activity in the dendrite of neuron n near the synapse s, which for example may be regarded as a weighted sum of activities of other neurons that are presynaptic to n and have their synapses not too far from s.

In any case we may assume that there is a simple qualitative way of classifying the strength of pre- and postsynaptic activity as "high" or "low". For every possible combination of rough descriptions of the pre- and postsynaptic activities as high or low we then note the direction of the postulated change in connectivity of the synapse s.

For example:

Pre	Post	Postulated change
High	High	—
High	Low	+
Low	High	—
Low	Low	+

Such a table I will call a *local synaptic rule*.

The above (quite arbitrary) example of a local synaptic rule would mean that a synapse s becomes more excitatory, whenever the postsynaptic activity is low, and more inhibitory (or less excitatory) whenever the postsynaptic activity is high.

In this scheme, Hebb's rule would be expressed as follows:

Pre	Post	Postulated change
High	High	+
High	Low	0
Low	High	0
Low	Low	0

It can be interpreted in the following way:

The excitation of the synapse s is increased whenever there is *coincidence* of pre- and postsynaptic activity. Here a high postsynaptic activity in neuron n again may mean a coincidence of excitatory axonal activity that is presynaptic to n in the neighborhood of s.

In other words: *By Hebb's rule coincident excitatory presynaptic activity becomes more effective.*

Most models that are designed for studying learning through change of the connectivity use some variation of Hebb's rule (a Hebb-like rule in the sense of Digression 4). This is no wonder, since purely presynaptic and purely postsynaptic rules or linear combinations thereof lead to lower storage capacities (see again Digression 4, where a more elaborated way of classifying synaptic rules is explained).

Of course, in principle every synapse s could have its own synaptic rule, but usually again only one rule is assumed to hold for every synapse — or only a few rules: for example one rule, namely

Pre	Post	Postulated change
High	High	0
High	Low	0
Low	High	0
Low	Low	0

for "unmodifiable" synapses, and perhaps one rule for excitatory modifiable synapses, and one rule for inhibitory modifiable synapses.

Some authors are only interested in the flow of activity in a network with fixed connections, i.e., they only use unmodifiable synapses. One motive for these studies is the stability analysis of large networks (e.g., Amari et al. 1977). In a way, the first analysis of neuronal networks with fixed connectivities has been performed by McCulloch and Pitts (1943), who initiated many formal studies of neuronal networks, when they showed that one can program finite networks of threshold neurons to produce input-output relations of an arbitrary complexity, by fixing all the connectivities in an appropriate way. The simple demonstration I gave in Chapter 3, may give an idea of the flavor of their much more sophisticated result.

In this appendix, however, models that only study the flow of activity in fixed, unmodifiable networks, are regarded as a marginal case. It has turned out that learning is most easily modeled in networks with variable connectivities (Amari 1977, Anderson 1972, Fukushima 1973, 1975, Kohonen 1977, Marr 1970, 1971, Rosenblatt 1962, Steinbuch 1961, Uttley 1956a,b).

5 Technique of Analysis

Given a description of the initial state and a formulation of the rules governing the time evolution of the state of the network (usually in terms of differential equations), the actual evolution has to be described and analyzed.

In most models it is impossible to describe this evolution explicitly — i.e., by solving the equations. The reason is, that there are as many equations for the state of activity as there are neurons (in the set N), and as many equations for the state of connectivity as there are possible synapses.

Only very simplified models, such as that proposed by Kohonen (1977), can be described analytically.

Therefore the behavior of many models is analyzed through computer simulation of the model, with fixed parameters and initial conditions, of course.

Some authors try to give a picture of the behavior of their model in a purely discursive way.

Thus the discussions of brain models can be roughly divided into three groups as to which method of analysis is preferentially used:

a) mathematical
b) computer simulation
c) imaginative − discursive

6 Goal of Modeling

Two main goals are pursued in the brain models discussed here:

a) Understanding of the flow of activity through the brain. Here usually the connectivity between neurons is assumed constant.
Thus only the evolution of the state of activity in time has to be considered.
b) Understanding how organized changes in connectivity can be accomplished through simple local synaptic rules. These changes are then interpreted as the result of learning. Here, I think that the choice of a Hebb-like synaptic rule has turned out to be crucial, whereas the modeling of the dynamics of the single neuron seems to make less difference.

7 Two General Comments

7.1 Using the terminology derived in the preceding classification of models I can now present an overview over several neuron network models simply in form of a table. The various distinctions between continuous and discrete models in (1) and (2) do not seem crucial, with respect to the resulting dynamics (although they may turn out to be crucial for the interpretation, the author has in mind). In computer simulations (which are provided in most cases) a discrete version of the model is analyzed anyway − discrete with respect to time and to spatial coordinates in 1.2.b.

What indeed may be crucial with respect to the dynamics is the distinction between metric and ametric initial connectivity made in Section 3.2 (this Appendix). There is, however, a tendency of continuous models (1.2.b) to assume metric connectivity and in discrete models (1.2.a) to assume ametric (i.e., purely combinatoric) connectivity. A combination of

Neural Modeling

both metric and ametric connectivity can be described most easily in discrete models (cf. Palm and Braitenberg 1979).

7.2 Since most models are stochastic, at least in the sense that they use a statistically discribed initial connectivity, the following should be kept in mind:

Neurons develop their individuality by their small intitial differences from the mean. Therefore, in models that are concerned with learning through synaptic changes, the essence is lost, if just something like the *mean activity* is analyzed, although this may be in many cases mathematically much easier to do.

An analysis of the mean activity in neuron networks is, however, an important tool to investigate questions of stability.

Authors	Dynamics of activity	Dynamics of connectivity	Initial connectivity (shorthand as in Chap. 7)	Technique of analysis
Amari (1977)	Simple, discrete, linear + threshold	a) + 000 b) + 000 and −000 for inhibitory synapses	(1) (2)	Vector analysis
Anderson (1972)	Simple, discrete, linear	+ 000		Vector analysis, S/N calculations
Cooper (Nass and Cooper 1975, Cooper et al. 1979)	Simple, discrete, "nearly" linear	+ 00 −	+ lateral inhibition	Vector analysis, computer simulations
Fukushima (1973, 1975) Fukushima and Miyake (1978)	Simple, discrete	1973 + − − + 1975 } + 000 modified 1978 } postsynaptic activity has to be maximal in a neighborhood	78 73 75	Simulations
Harth (Harth et al. 1970, Anninos et al. 1970)	Simple, discrete	Fixed	+ inhibition	Mathematical (stability, "statistical mechanics"), simulations
Kohonen (1974) Kohonen and Oja (1977)	Simple, discrete, linear	+ 000 − 000 } 74 − + + − } 76		Vector analysis, simulations
von der Malsburg (1973)	Continous 2-dim.	+ − 00 only input synapses are modifyable	+ lateral inhibition	Simulations
Marr (1969, 1970, 1971)	(Qualitative description)	+ 0 − 0 (+ 000)	69 70 71 (+ lateral inhibition)	Qualitative, combinatorical and probalistic calculations
Palm (1980)	Simple, discrete, linear + threshold	+ 000		Mathematical (probalistic calculations, information theory)
Wilson and Cowan (1973)	Continous 1,2-dim.	fixed	+ lateral inhibition	Simulations

Goal of modeling	Emphasis:	New terms	Notes	Quotations mainly
(1) Association (2) Concept formation	Orthogonality, coping of network with additive noise in the input		Approach from matrix memory (matched filters)	Theoretical
Association, matching problem	Linearity of neuron response, strong fast influence vs. weak slow influence		Cortical pyramidal cells are individuals. Models can be simplified as follows:	Experimental
Development of feature detectors	One pattern represented by only one cell		One "column" of visual cortex is modeled	Experimental (visual deprivation)
1973 Temporal sequences 1975 Development of feature detectors 1978 Assoc. memory	Modified synaptic rule (comparison probably realized by glia cells), many layers		Similar results can be achieved with less layers, with "ordinary" synaptic rule by lateral inhibition (see Cooper)	
Evolution of mean activity in randomly connected nets	Finding the right "observables", e.g., average activity in sub-netlets	Netlets, randomness in the small, design in the large	Introduces connectivity matrix notation	Anninos: Theor. Harth: Exper.
Association (+ 000) vs. novelty detection (− 000)	Pseudo-inverse associative memory (matching problem)	Novelty filter	Math. on pseudo-inverse, least squares, assoc. memory, nice pictures and demonstrations of simulations	Theoretical
Self-organization of orientation sensitive cells in striate cortex	Explain organization without genetic prewiring		Retinotopy, movement not considered, inhibition reaches further than excitation	Experimental, Theoretical
69 Cerebellum: matrix memory (storage capacity − cell counts) 70 Neocortex: Classificators, coincidence detectors 71 Archicortex: Auto-association, pattern completion	Stability Associative memory falsifiability of theoretical predictions	Codons, coincidence detectors	Detailed synaptology 69 contains much quantitative Anatomy 70 there are no climbing fibers in Neocortex, no discussion of axon collaterals	Experimental (anatomical)
Calculation of storage capacity of associative memories		Listing vs. mapping	Approach from matrix memory	Theoretical
Spread of activity described and classified	3 Types of dynamics 1. Limit cycles: Thalamus EEG 2. Stationary states: short term memory 3. Transients: sensory cortex		Inhibition reaches further than excitation, Fender-Julesz-Effect	Experimental

3 Cell Assemblies: the Basic Ideas

In this appendix I shall try to put together the main constituents of a theory of cell assemblies, which are scattered throughout this book, and which form the intuitive basis for the more mathematical treatment of Appendix 4.

0 A cell assembly is a set of neurons which often fire together, since every sufficiently large subset of it contributes a significant amount of excitation to the remaining neurons. In other words: the notion of a cell assembly expresses a kind of coherence of a group of neurons in terms of mutual excitation between the members of the group.

Some terms in this definition of a cell assembly are still a bit vague; they will be made precise in Appendix 4. But there are good reasons for keeping them vague here, for example the following problem: A single excitatory synapse between two neurons A and B certainly is not sufficient to produce an electrophysiological effect in the sense that A "fires" B (probably a single excitatory synapse from A to B does not even effect the firing probability of B significantly), and we do not know how many excitatory synapses (nor, how many excitatory neurons) have to work together to yield a significant electrophysiological effect in the postsynaptic neuron.

The idea of talking about the workings of the cortex in terms of cell assemblies and of cell assemblies in terms of the cortical connectivity goes back to the psychologist D.O. Hebb (1949).

The "Tübingen version" of this idea (Braitenberg 1974a,b, 1978a,b, 1981, Legendy 1967, 1968, 1975, Palm 1980, 1981b, Palm and Braitenberg 1979) relies on the following points (of view).

1 The distinction between metric (short-range) and ametric (long-range) intracortical connections (A- and B-system see Chap. 8), and the emphasis on the excitatory ametric connections (between pyramidal cells) as the constituents that bind together large groups of pyramidal cells leads to the idea that a cell assembly usually consists of neurons that are spread all over the cortex, and to the use of networks (graphs) to describe the basic

Cell Assemblies: the Basic Ideas 215

cortical connectivity that is the substrate for cell assemblies ("fibers can override metric", Palm and Braitenberg 1979). This is the reason why I use a discrete and not a continuous model (see Chap. 11 and Appendix 2) of the cortex in Appendix 4.

2 An associative memory (see Appendix 1) can be used for the storage of information, for example as explained in Chapters 5 and 7. In this case (the case of auto-association, cf. Palm 1980) the information is stored in learned patterns of activity and it can be recalled, when part of such a pattern calls forth the rest of it. In other words, information is recalled by completion of stored patterns. Such a stored pattern corresponds to a cell assembly. Therefore cell assemblies (as we conceive them) are formed by learning. A neuronal mechanism for the kind of learning that is performed by associative memories, needs a Hebb-like rule (see Digression 4) for the modification of synaptic connectivity.

3 Positive feedback is the essential prerequisite for holding a cell assembly together. This ingredient was brought into the theory of associative memory by Kohonen (1977); it is essential for the idea that our cortex may work as an associative memory (see Chap. 7), since positive feedback is the outstanding feature of the cortex as pointed out by Braitenberg (1974a,b, 1978a,b), see also Chapter 8.

Negative feedback in neural networks has been widely analyzed by mathematicians and physicists (e.g., Coleman 1971, Coleman and Renninger 1974, Hadeler 1974), whereas the severe problems of stability that occur in a network with strong positive feedback have not been tackled yet.

Appendix 4 can be viewed as a possible starting point for this kind of analysis.

4 The concepts that represent the information upon which we act, should be encoded somehow in our brain. There are three common arguments against the idea that these concepts are represented in the activity of single neurons.

a) Electrophysiologists found neurons that can be said to respond to "features", they also found neurons that respond to complex combinations of various features, but they never found neurons that respond to combinations of features such as one would like to call a "concept".

b) Every day a certain percentage of the cortical neurons die. If a concept was represented in a single neuron, and if that neuron has died, the subject should have lost that concept.

c) The number 10^{10} of neurons in a human brain is large, but in comparison with numbers obtained by counting *possible* configurations, it is not that large. Considering the number of possible input configurations upon which we may have to act someday, or the number of possible concepts that we may need someday, it is certainly important to code in an economic way. Coding in terms of sets of neurons certainly is much more economic than coding in terms of single neurons (for example in 10^{10} neurons there are already about 10^{48} different sets of 5 neurons).

Of course, this large number is partly due to the fact that we have allowed for an arbitrary overlap between different sets of neurons.

On the other hand, the overlap cannot really be arbitrarily large, because two assemblies A and B with too large an overlap could not be distinguished since activity of A would always lead to activity of B (by the above definition 0) and vice versa. The important problem how many assemblies can be placed in a large neuronal network (cf. Legency 1967, 1968) is treated in Appendix 4.

5 An essential device to retrieve the patterns stored in associative memories, is threshold detection (see Chap. 5). In our description of thinking processes in terms of cell assemblies we speak of *threshold control* (Braitenberg 1978a), which works by means of uniform changes of the threshold of almost all neurons in large areas of the cortex (for example through diffusely distributed – excitatory or inhibitory – afferents to the cortex). The basic ideas involved in a description of certain thought processes as different ways of threshold controlling the cortex are listed in Chapter 12 (and 13). For the sake of completeness I will briefly repeat them here.

a) At any moment (cf. also Chap. 1.8) only one assembly is active ("holds").
b) There are two basic reasons for a shift from one assembly to another one:
   I) sensory inputs to the cortex
   II) association governed by a change in threshold like in Figs. 12.3 and 11.6 (which leads to the detection of a new pattern that has a lot in common with the old one).
c) A cell assembly is detected by observing a relatively high activity all over the cortex for a given level of thresholds.
   New assemblies are formed by the intensification of excitatory connections between the participating neurons; the detection, holding, and intensification of a new assembly invoke a pleasant feeling.
d) The "reliability" of an assembly can be tested by finding its "critical threshold", i.e., the maximal threshold at which the assembly still holds

Cell Assemblies: the Basic Ideas

(probably differentially in different areas of the cortex, viz. the reliability of different aspects of an idea in different areas of context (cf. Chap. 12.4).

e) Different states of mind may correspond to different modes of threshold control, which may be performed by comparatively simple inborn algorithms that are initiated in a reflex-like manner. For example:

"Alert": low threshold in sensory areas, high threshold in association areas.

"Absent-minded", "thinking": vice versa.

"All eyes": low threshold in visual areas.

"Acting", "executing a plan": high threshold in (association-)C-areas (see Chaps. 13.2, 13.5), low threshold in (association-)P-areas, sensory areas, and motor areas.

4 Cell Assemblies and Graph Theory

In this Appendix I want to give a mathematical definition for the notion of *"cell assembly"*. This definition should be applicable in the framework of any neuron network model (like those described in Appendix 2).

Furthermore I want to analyze the relations between cell assemblies and to discuss the problem concerning the number of assemblies in large networks (cf. Appendix 3). From Appendix 2, we know that the dynamics in any such model concerns the state of activity and the state of connectivity. For the definition of the cell assemblies contained in a network at any moment we shall rely on the state of connectivity at that moment and on the (much faster) dynamic evolution of the state of activity "around" that moment.

From Appendix 3 we take the intuitive idea of "what a cell assembly should be" and the hint to use a discrete model where the state of connectivity can be described as a finite network or *graph*.

In the following I shall sometimes use a specific neuron model to describe the dynamics of the state of activity in such a network: namely a threshold neuron model (cf. Fig. 3.4), where all the neurons have the same threshold Θ. I shall use this model only because of its utmost simplicity, and because I believe that it is sufficient to show the main features. I do not believe that a more elaborated and more realistic neuron model will add any new phenomena that are pertinent to the definition of and relations between cell assemblies. Of course, this is due to our intuitive notion of a cell assembly as a group of neurons that hold together in a certain sense: this notion is a semistatic one; indeed, the shift from assembly to assembly is conceived to be much slower than the dynamics of the state of activity, probably in the same range as the dynamics of the state of connectivity.

1 Weighted Graphs

To describe the dynamics of the cortical network, it is necessary to know the connectivity of the cortex. One could describe this connectivity by the so-called connectivity (or adjacency) matrix, i.e., by numbering the neurons and denoting by c_{ij} the connectivity from neuron i to neuron j.

Cell Assemblies and Graph Theory

The appearance of this matrix depends to a certain degree on the way the neurons are numbered. The connectivity is given in its purest way as a mapping $c : G \times G \mapsto \mathbb{R}$, where G is the set of all neurons and $c(n,m)$ gives the strength of connectivity from neuron n to neuron m. As usual, positive values of $c(n,m)$ mean an excitatory connection, negative values an inhibitory connection, and the value 0 means no connection at all.

An elegant way to picture such a connectivity mapping c is by means of a graph: the neurons are denoted as points and the connections are indicated by arrows, e.g., $c(n,m) = 3$ is denoted as in Fig. 1a. Arrows with 0 connectivity are, of course, not drawn. For $c(n,m) = 1$ we might also write Fig. 1b instead of Fig. 1c. For $c(n,m) = c(m,n) = 1$ we may even write Fig. 1d or e instead of Fig. 1f. For $n = m$, $c(n,m) = 5$ is denoted as Fig. 1g, and $c(n,m) = 1$ simply as Fig. 1h. Such a connection is called a *self-connection* or *loop*.

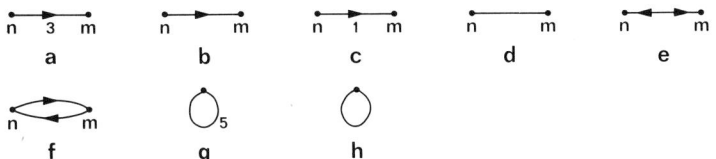

Fig. 1a–h

For example the mapping
$c : G \times G \to \{0,1\}$, $G = \{1, 2, 3, 4, 5\}$, with

$c(1,1) = 0$	$c(2,1) = 0$	$c(3,1) = 0$	$c(4,1) = 0$	$c(5,1) = 1$
$c(1,2) = 1$	$c(2,2) = 0$	$c(3,2) = 0$	$c(4,2) = 0$	$c(5,2) = 0$
$c(1,3) = 0$	$c(2,3) = 1$	$c(3,3) = 0$	$c(4,3) = 0$	$c(5,3) = 0$
$c(1,4) = 0$	$c(2,4) = 0$	$c(3,4) = 1$	$c(4,4) = 0$	$c(5,4) = 0$
$c(1,5) = 0$	$c(2,5) = 0$	$c(3,5) = 0$	$c(4,5) = 1$	$c(5,5) = 0$

can be described by the connectivity matrix

$$C = \begin{bmatrix} 0 & 1 & 0 & 0 & 0 \\ 0 & 0 & 1 & 0 & 0 \\ 0 & 0 & 0 & 1 & 0 \\ 0 & 0 & 0 & 0 & 1 \\ 1 & 0 & 0 & 0 & 0 \end{bmatrix}$$

and can be pictured as in Fig. 2a or b.

Definition: A *weighted graph* is a pair $\langle G, c \rangle$, where G is a set and $c : G \times G \to \mathbb{R}$ a mapping. The elements of G are called *points*. For $x, y \in G$, $c(x,y)$ is called the *strength* or *weight* of the connectivity from x to y.

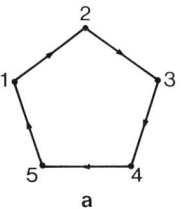 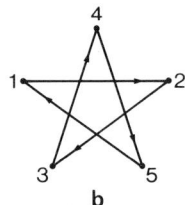

Fig. 2a,b

If $c : G \times G \to \{0,1\}$ and $c(x,x) = 0$ for every $x \in G$, $\langle G,c \rangle$ is called a *directed graph*. If in addition $c(x,y) = c(y,x)$ for every x and y in G, $\langle G,c \rangle$ is called a *graph*.

Thus graphs, as well as directed graphs, do not contain loops.

As an introduction into the theory of graphs and directed graphs I suggest the book of Harari (1969).

2 The Definition of Assemblies

Let us try to define an assembly A as a set of neurons that give enough excitation to each other, to stay active once they are all activated, and such that every (not too small) subset of A significantly contributes excitation the remaining neurons of A.

For the following definition we assume that we are given a finite neuronal network with fixed connectivity and fixed equations that describe the dynamics of the single neurons in the network.

1. Step: A set A is called *persistent*, if — once activated — it stays active. In our model network we may decide to count a neuron n as active (at time t), if its activity $a_n(t)$ exceeds a certain value $\bar{a}$ (Fig. 3).

2. Step: We say that a set A *supports* a set B, if B (alone) is not persistent, but $A \cup B$ is (Fig. 4).

3. Step: We say that a set A *ignites* a set B, if activation of A leads to activation of B. This means the following: if A is activated at some time t then there is another time t' > t such that B (every element of B) is activated at t' (Fig. 5a,b).

4. Step: Every neuron that is eventually activated, once the set A has been activated, belongs to the *hull* of A (Fig. 6).

Cell Assemblies and Graph Theory

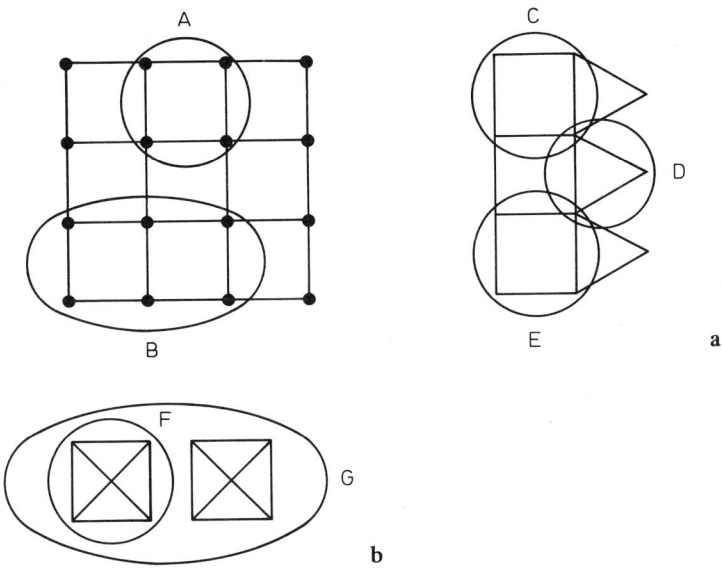

Fig. 3. a A,B,C,D,E are persistent, if every neuron in the network has a 'threshold' of at most 2 (afferent synapses). **b** F and G are persistent at thresholds of at most 3

Fig. 4. A supports B at threshold 2

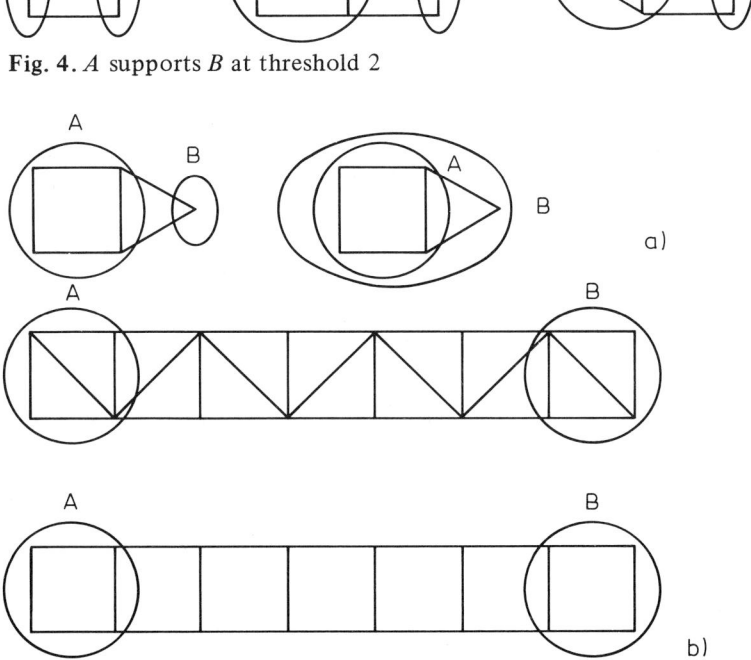

Fig. 5. a A ignites B at threshold 2. **b** A ignites B at threshold 1, but not at threshold 2

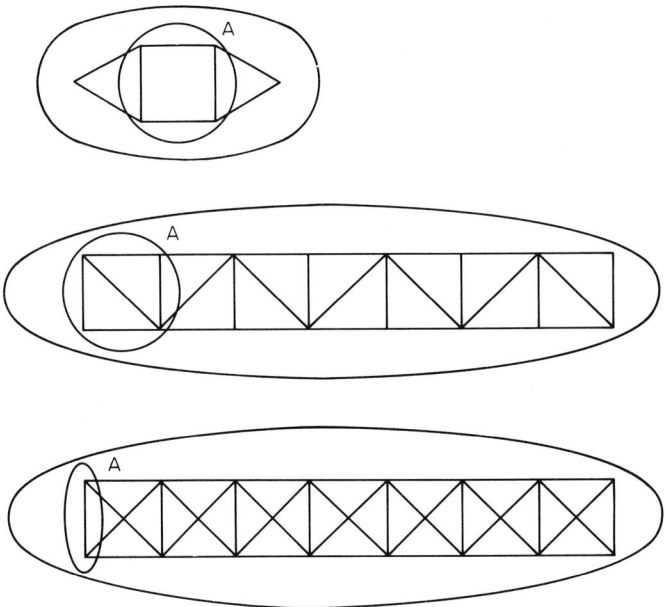

Fig. 6. The hull of *A* at threshold 2

5. Step: A persistent set A is called *tight,* if it holds together in the following sense:

every persistent subset B of A supports or ignites the rest A \ B of A.

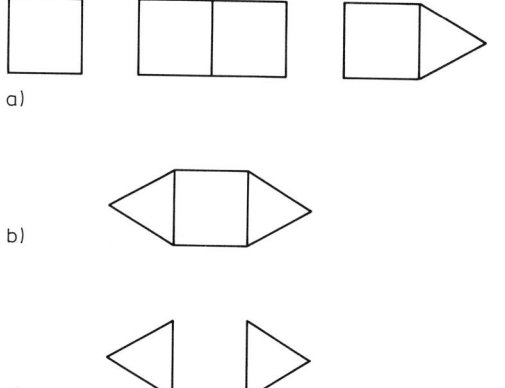

Fig. 7. a Tight at threshold 2; **b** Tight at treshold 1, but not at threshold 2; **c** Not tight at threshold 1

6. Step. The hull of a tight set is called an *assembly* (Fig. 8).

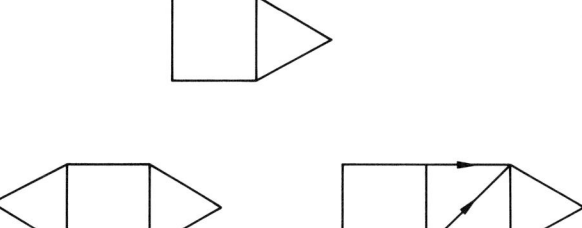

Fig. 8. Assemblies at threshold 2

3 A Simple Model for Neuronal Dynamics

3.1 I want to use such a graph as a simple model for the flow of activity in the brain. This can be done in the following way. The points are identified with the neurons and c(x,y) gives the total strength of the synapses from neuron x to neuron y. Starting from a set M of "on"-neurons, we get the resulting flow of activity through the graph at threshold Θ by interating the mapping

$$f_\Theta : \begin{cases} \mathcal{P}(G) \to \mathcal{P}(G) \\ M \mapsto \{y \in G : \sum_{x \in M} c(x,y) \geq \Theta \} \end{cases}$$

If the set M of neurons is active, this will in turn activate the set $f_\Theta(M)$ at threshold Θ, this in turn will activate $f_\Theta^2(M) = f_\Theta(f_\Theta(M))$ followed by $f_\Theta^3(M) = f_\Theta(f_\Theta(f_\Theta(M)))$, and so on.

This means that I use a very simple dynamical model of the single neuron: the threshold neuron (cf. Fig. 3.4) with threshold Θ, weights determined by the connectivity matrix c, and a fixed time delay of 1 unit.

The overall dynamics is therefore described by a special type of difference equation, namely

$$x(t+1) = h_\Theta(x(t) \cdot C).$$

Here $x(t) = (x_1(t), \ldots, x_n(t))$ denotes the activity vector of the n neurons:

$x_i(t) = 1$ if the neuron is active and $x_i(t) = 0$ otherwise. C is the connectivity matrix, $h_\Theta : z \mapsto \begin{cases} 0 \text{ if } z < \Theta \\ 1 \text{ if } z \geq \Theta \end{cases}$ is a threshold function.

3.2 Threshold Control

The basic idea of threshold control is that the neuronal activity evolves rather fast [it takes at most 5 ms from M to $f_\Theta(M)$; this is a conservative estimate for the conduction time (axonal and synaptic) of a monosynaptic pathway from one cortical neuron to the next] and that it is controlled by comparatively slow variations of the parameter Θ. In other words: in analyzing the flow of activity we may keep Θ fixed at first and let the activity evolve through $M, f_\Theta(M), f_\Theta^2(M), \ldots$ to some final invariant state (or into some cycle). Then we change Θ slightly and look for the new invariant state (that may occasionally be identical to the old one). We can use threshold control to detect cell assemblies: they occur if small variations in Θ do not change the invariant state.

3.3 Cycles

Our graphic model for the dynamics of the brain is too exact in one respect: the activity proceeds from M to $f_\Theta(M)$ and so on, in discrete time steps. In reality, the activity is "smeared out" in time at every synapse with a time constant of a few milliseconds which is in the same range as the time needed by a monosynaptic pathway. Therefore in the long run cycles at fixed threshold Θ are quite improbable in reality, although they will occur in the model.

For example, in the network of Fig. 9, starting with M, the activity will flow around in a cycle forever. In the corresponding real network, the flow of activity will show a cyclic structure at first, but due to the smearing out of activity, the whole net will finally be active.

Thus the real flow of activity in Fig. 9 will be similar to the sequence $M, f_\Theta(M), f_\Theta^2(M), \ldots$ of Fig. 10.

For this reason we will not consider cycles as cell assemblies.

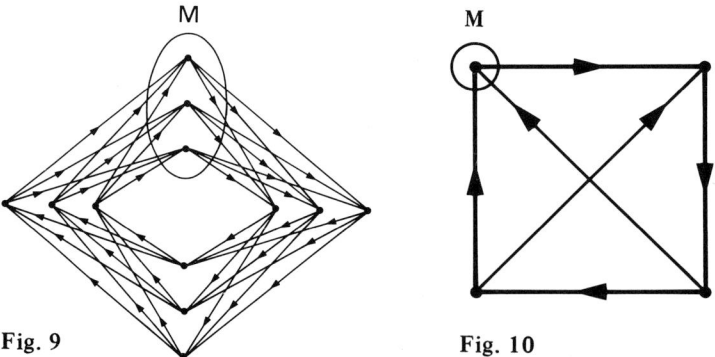

Fig. 9   Fig. 10

3.4 Inhibition

In the next section (4) I shall disregard inhibition in the modeling of cell assemblies, since they are formed basically by the excitatory long range cortico-cortical connections.

Before doing so, it seems important to give a rough qualitative picture of the effects of inhibition that we have to keep at the back of our minds in the next section.

3.4 a Specific Inhibition

This can occur between neighboring cells in the same cortical area, and it implies that a certain part of one assembly selectively inhibits certain other neurons that are part of another assembly (or of several other assemblies). Specific inhibition may, for example, correspond to the phenomenon that we cannot remember some name, because very often another name that is "too" similar in some respect comes to mind first and prevents the desired name from being remembered.

Specific inhibition may be helpful to define concepts from each other that are very similar in some respect. It may be learned through a synaptic mechanism analogous to Hebb's rule: some local inhibitory connections may be enhanced through common pre- and postsynaptic activity (for a theoretical analysis of this mechanism — although in an ametric global model — see Kohonen 1977, Chap. 3.2).

3.4 b Unspecific Local Inhibition

At first glance one might believe that a certain level of diffuse inhibition is equivalent to general permanent increase of the threshold Θ. This is not true, as can be seen in the dynamics of Fig. 11.

Indeed, it turns out that homogeneous diffuse inhibition is equivalent to a "fast" threshold control, whereby Θ is increased proportionally to

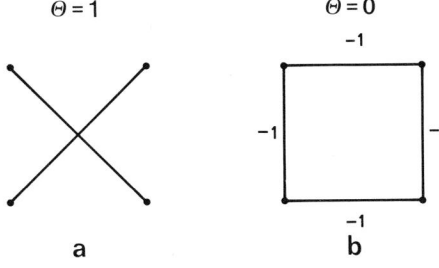

Fig. 11a,b. b is obtained from a by subtracting 1 from the connectivities c (m,n) for m ≠ n

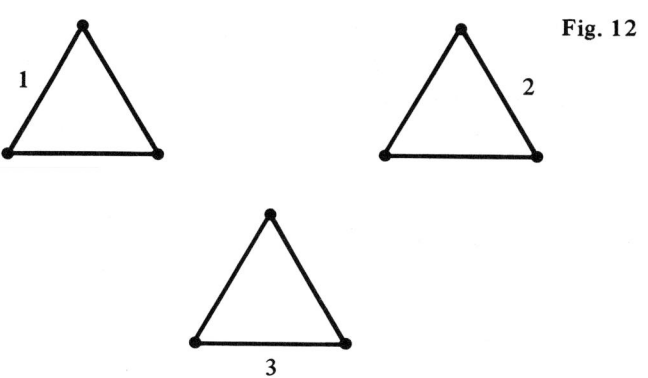

Fig. 12

the number of active neurons (large numbers of active neurons distribute more inhibition than small numbers of active neurons).

This fast threshold control has two implications for the number of cell assemblies:

I. It tends to stabilize the number of active neurons, which is good for cell assemblies, since a constant activity (not zero and not total) implies the existence of a cell assembly.
II. It tends to decrease the number of cell assemblies, as can be seen in the network of Fig. 12. Here we have three obvious assemblies, namely 1, 2, and 3. But also each combination of two of them, i.e., (1,2), (1,3), (2,3) could be regarded as an assembly since it is invariant and stable against small variations of Θ. However, a certain level of diffuse inhibition would forbid a combination — say (1,2) — of two "elementary" assemblies to stay active, simply because it is twice as large and causes twice as much diffuse inhibition. Therefore we would observe a "competition" between 1 and 2 and only one of them could stay active. Thus, a certain level of diffuse inhibition will reduce the number of assemblies in the above network from 6 to 3.

A combination of two assemblies can only be an assembly again if there are some excitatory connections between the two (that help to overcome the increased amount of inhibition).

In the next chapter we shall ignore inhibiton. The last requirement, however, has been incorporated into the definition of a cell assembly.

Let me finally discuss the possible psychological interpretation of the effects (a) and (b).

a) If M denotes a set of neurons (for example an assembly), |M| denotes the number of neurons in the set M. The stabilization of |M| may have the side effect that oscillations of |M| around some mean value do occur. This would mean that some quite large part of an assembly is constantly active, whereas other parts have just an oscillating activity. I think that these oscillations should not alter the concept represented by the assembly. Since we vary the threshold, we must have a large (for low threshold) and a small (for high threshold) set of neurons to represent the same concept, the small set being contained in the large set. Fluctuation in the size of the assembly may be regarded just as fluctuations in the "loudness" of the corresponding concept, as long as they stay within the boundaries of these two sets.

b) The competition between two concepts is a rather common phenomenon in psychology and psychophysics: think for example of ambiguous figures (like Fig. 12.1) and binocular rivalry (Breese 1909).

4 Dynamics at Fixed Threshold

In this section the number Θ is fixed, and we simply write f instead of f_Θ. Moreover, we shall assume that $c(x,y) \in \mathbb{N}_0$ for every $x,y \in G$.

4.1 *Definition:*
a) M *ignites* N (at Θ), if there is a number $n \geq 1$, such that $N \subseteq f_\Theta^n(M)$.
b) M *exhausts* N (at Θ), if $N \subseteq M^* := \bigcup_{n=0}^{\infty} f_\Theta^n(M)$, i.e., if for every element x of N there is a number $n \geq 0$, such that $f_\Theta^n(M) \ni x$.

4.2 *Definition:* A subset M of G is called
invariant, if $f(M) = M$
persistent, if $f(M) \supseteq M$
weak, if there is an $n \in \mathbb{N} : f^n(M) = \emptyset$.

4.3 *Definition:* A sequence $(M_1, \ldots, M_\ell)$ is called a period of length ℓ, if $f(M_i) = M_{i+1}$ for $i = 1, \ldots, \ell-1$ and $f(M_\ell) = M_1$.

4.4 *Proposition:* Let $M \subseteq G$. Exactly one of the following statements is true:
a) M is weak,
b) M ignites an invariant set,
c) M ignites a period.

Proof: This follows from the fact that $\mathcal{P}(G)$ is finite.

If M is persistent, we have $M \subseteq f(M) \subseteq f^2(M) \subseteq \ldots$ and therefore we have case (b). The invariant set generated by M is denoted by cl(M).

The next two propositions are obvious.

4.5 *Proposition:*
a) cl(cl(M)) = cl(M) for M persistent,
b) $A \subseteq B$, A,B persistent, implies $cl(A) \subseteq cl(B)$.

4.6 *Proposition:* If A,B are persistent, then $A \cup B$ is persistent.

Next, we shall define an assembly (at Θ) as a certain subset of G, in terms of the dynamics in G at Θ.

To this end, we shall simply use the definition of Section 2 (this Appendix) in our simple dynamical model.

4.7 *Definition:* A *supports* B, if B is not persistent and $A \cup B$ is persistent.

4.8 *Definition:*
a) A persistent set A is called *tight*, if every persistent subset B of A supports or ignites A\B.
b) An *assembly* is the closure of a tight set.

Figures 7a and 13 show examples of tight sets. The examples of Figs. 6a and 14 show that the closure of a tight set need not be tight again. Figures 7a,b, 8, 13, and 14 show assemblies.

4.9 *Definition:* A subset M of a graph G is called *minimal persistent*, if it is persistent and no proper subset of it is persistent.

4.10 *Proposition:* Every minimal persistent set is tight.

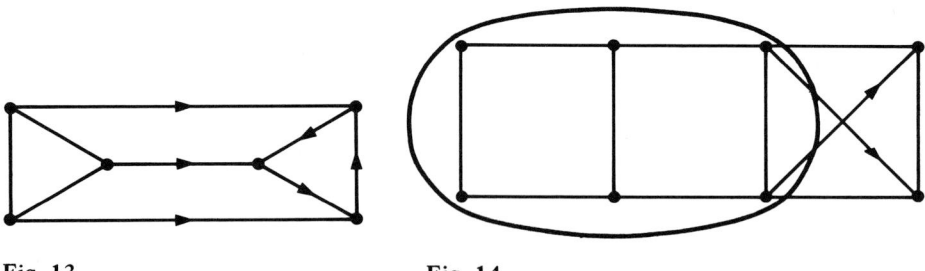

Fig. 13   Fig. 14

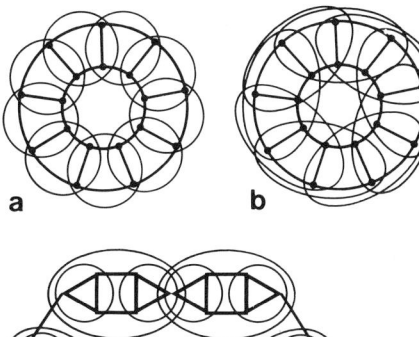

Fig. 15. a shows the 9 minimal persistent sets; **b** shows the 9 additional tight sets (which are assemblies)

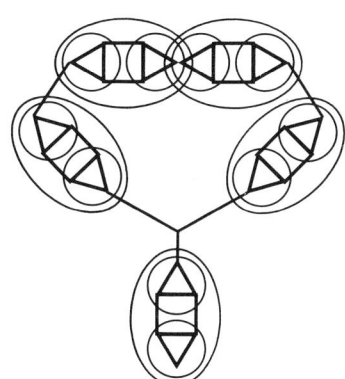

Fig. 16. All assemblies are shown

It is now possible to analyze the structure of weighted graphs (with positive weights) in terms of assemblies, tight sets, and minimal persistent sets.

Let me give some examples (Figs. 15 and 16):
Further examples for assemblies are given in the next section.

5 Inner Structure of and Relations Between Assemblies

In this section I shall define some concepts to describe the inner structure of persistent sets, and especially assemblies. We still assume Θ to be fixed and write f instead of f_Θ. Let A be a persistent set.

We denote by $f_A : \mathcal{P}(A) \to \mathcal{P}(A)$ the mapping $M \mapsto f(M) \cap A$.

5.1 *Definition:* We say that a subset M of A *fills* A, if for every $x \in A$ there is an infinite sequence of numbers n_i such that $x \in f_A^{n_i}(M)$.

For example, in Fig. 17a at $\Theta = 2$, only the square fills, whereas in Fig. 17b, two opposite points of the square fill as well.

5.2 *Definition:*
a) A subset M of a persistent set A is called a *germ* of A, if it fills A and if no proper subset of M fills A.

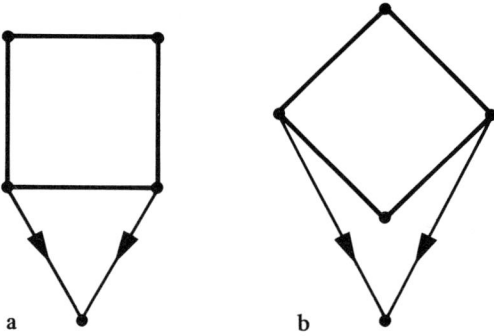

Fig. 17a, b

b) The *kernel* K(A) of a persistent set A is the union of all germs of A.
c) The *halo* H(A) of a persistent set A is cl(A) − K(A).

5.3 *Examples:*

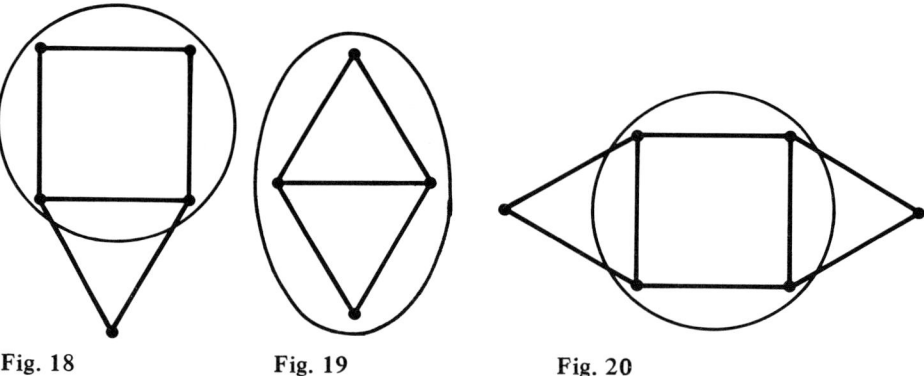

Fig. 18.   **Fig. 19.**   **Fig. 20.**

Fig. 18. This figure shows an invariant set; its kernel is circumscribed. The same conventions are used in **Figs. 19−25**

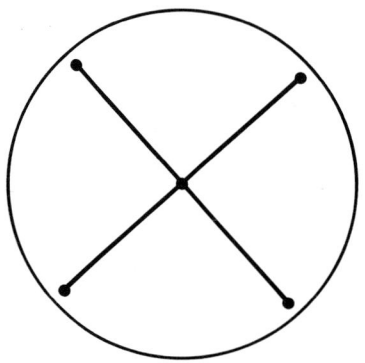

Fig. 21

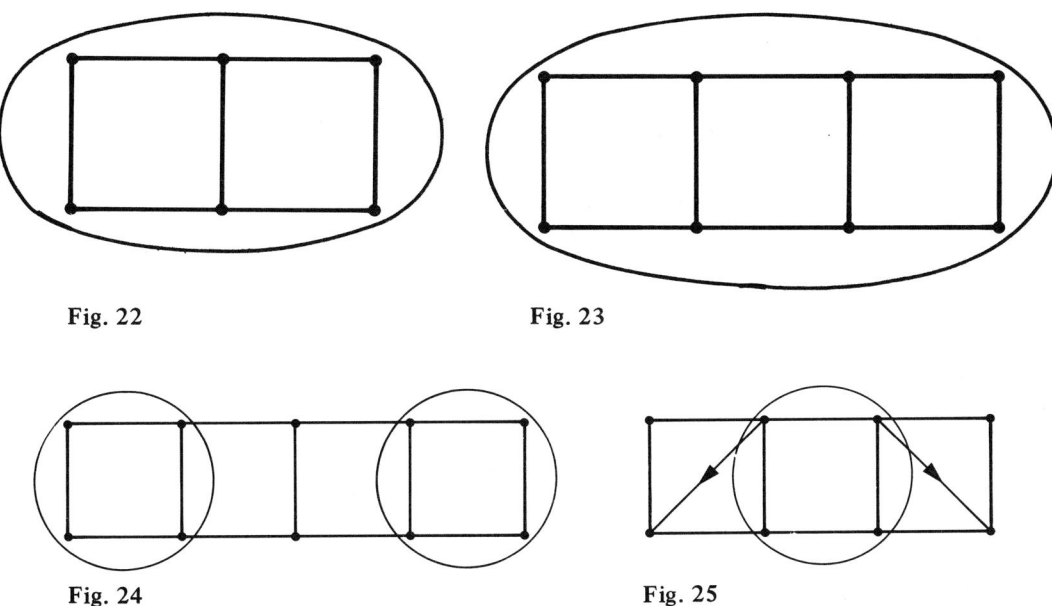

Fig. 22 Fig. 23

Fig. 24 Fig. 25

5.4 Two assemblies may have an excitatory influence on each other in several different ways. In the following I will give examples for the most important cases I can think of.

a) Intersection: Two assemblies A and B have some neurons in common. In Fig. 26a,b the two assemblies form a superassembly.

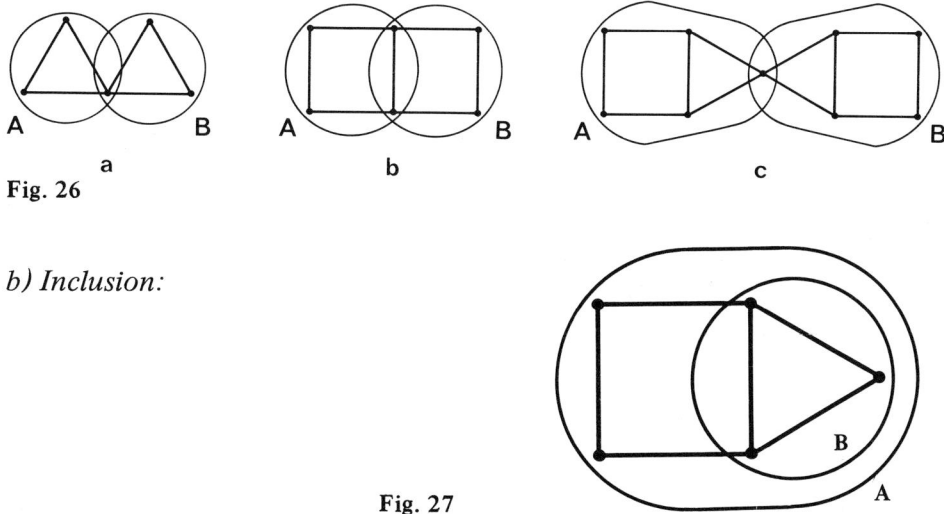

Fig. 26

b) Inclusion:

Fig. 27

c) Projection: **Fig. 28**

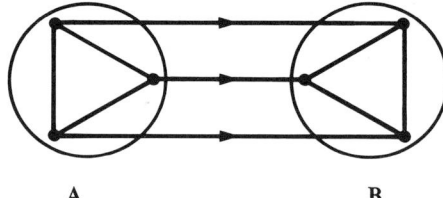

d) Mutual Projection: **Fig. 29**

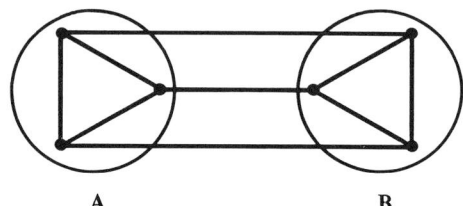

In this case A and B together form a superassembly that holds at higher threshold.

6 Formulation of the Main Problem

Having defined the notion of an "assembly" we can now formulate precisely the main problem of the theory of cell assemblies. Given a weighted graph $\langle G, c \rangle$ with $c(x,y) \in \mathbb{N}_0$ for every x and y in G, we may ask for the number n_Θ of assemblies at threshold Θ and for the total number n of assemblies.

This leads to some very specific graph-theoretical questions that I only want to pose in this section. I have not yet obtained an answer to any of them, but some preliminary results that are hopefully connected to these questions are given in Chapter 8.

In the next section I will introduce some further auxiliary concepts (especially notions of connectivity).

To pose the questions we need one more definition:

6.1 *Definition:* A directed graph $\langle G, c \rangle$ is called *homogeneous,* if for any x, $x' \in G$, $\sum_y s(x,y) = \sum_y s(x',y)$ and $\sum_y s(y,x) = \sum_y (y,x')$.

Remark: This implies that for $e := \dfrac{1}{|G|} \sum_{x,y} s(x,y)$ and any $x \in G$ we have

$\sum_y s(x,y) = e = \sum_y s(y,x)$.

Remember that $|G|$ denotes the number of elements (i.e., points) in G.

6.2 *Question:* Given two numbers k and a, determine a weighted graph $\langle G, c\rangle$ with $|G| = k$ and $e = a$ such that n is maximal.

6.3 *Question:*
a) Is it possible to find a homogeneous weighted graph with this property?
b) Is it possible to find a strongly connected weighted graph with this property?
(Notions of connectivity are defined in the next section.)

6.4 *Question:* What does the function $\Theta \mapsto n_\Theta$ look like, for such a graph?

6.5 *Question:* Given two numbers k and a, consider the set $\mathscr{G}$ of all (homogeneous) (connected) weighted graphs $\langle G, c\rangle$ with $|G| = k$ and $e = a$ and let $\Theta > 0$. What is the average value for n_Θ on the set $\mathscr{G}$? What is the average size of an assembly occurring at Θ in a graph in the set $\mathscr{G}$?

The last question obviously contains several subquestions, which could even be answered in an asymptotic sense for $k, a \to \infty$. In this way one could sharpen the vague conjecture that large randomly connected networks contain many assemblies.

7 Construction of Graphs

In this section I shall introduce some general graphs and some general ways of contructing new graphs from given ones.

7.1 *Definition:*
1. P_n denotes the graph G containing n separate points (Fig. 30a)
2. L_n denotes a single line containing n points (Fig. 30b)
2'. DL_n denotes a directed line containing n points (Fig. 30c)
3. C_n denotes a circle with n points (Fig. 30d)
3'. DC_n denotes a directed circle with n points (Fig. 30e)
4. K_n denotes the complete graph with n points (Fig. 30f)

7.2 *Definition:* The suffix s adds self-connections to the graphs

$$P_n, L_n, K_n, C_n, DL_n, \text{ and } DC_n \text{ (cf. Fig. 31)}.$$

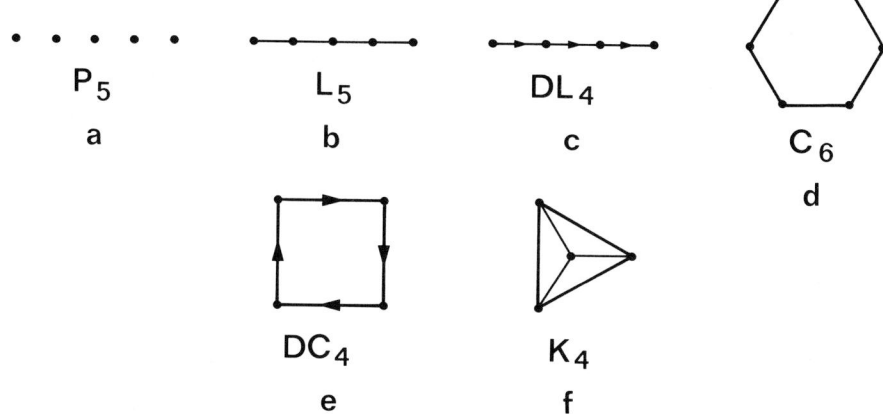

Fig. 30. a shows P_5; b shows L_5; c shows DL_4; d shows C_6; e shows DC_4; f shows K_4

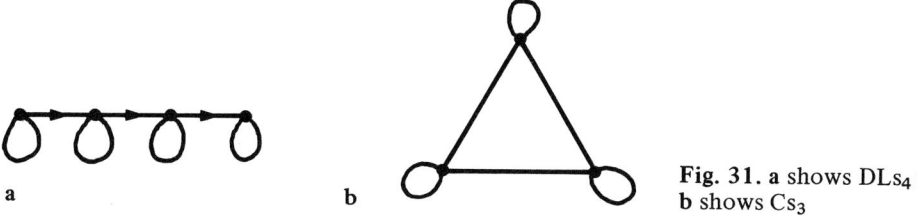

Fig. 31. a shows DL_{S_4}; b shows C_{S_3}

7.3 Given any two directed graphs H and G we may construct the following graphs (compare Fig. 32):

1. $\widetilde{G}$ has connections exactly where G has not, but $\widetilde{G}$ does not have self-connections.
2. G + H means that G and H are placed side by side without any connections.
3. G +$_c$ H, called the connected sum (or join): G and H are placed side by side and every point of G is connected (both ways) with every point of H.
4. G +$_d$ H, called the directed sum: G and H are placed side by side and there is a connection from every point of G to every point of H.
5. G × H: Every point of G is replaced by one version of H and every arrow of G is replaced by |H| arrows connecting the corresponding points of the two versions of H that have replaced the two endpoints of the arrow.

7.4 Some exercises with these notions:
   a) $K_2 = L_2$
   b) $K_3 = C_3$

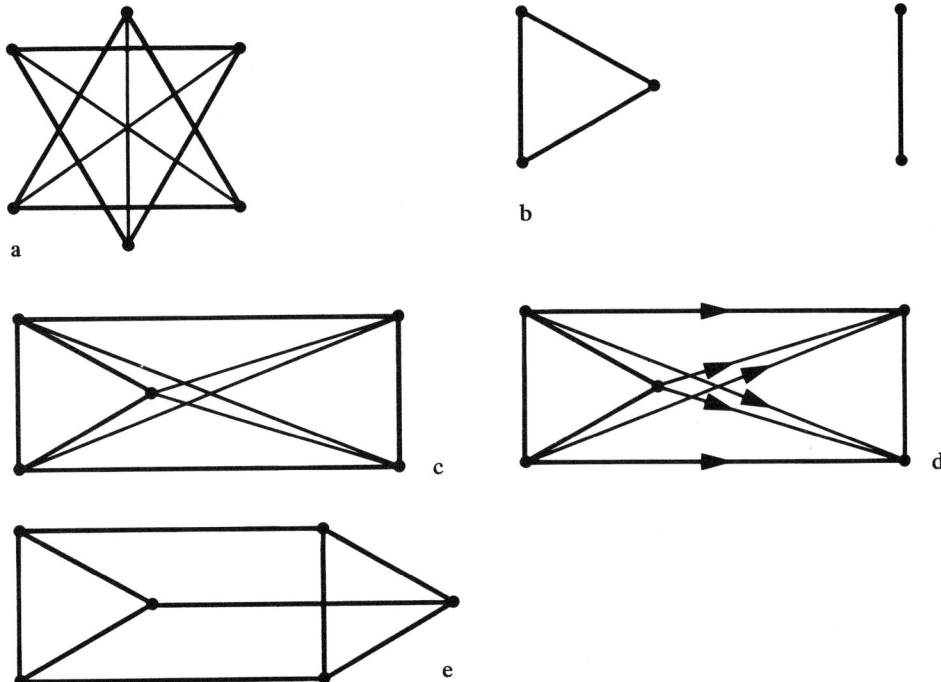

Fig. 32. a shows $\widetilde{C}_6$; **b** shows $K_3 + K_2$; **c** shows $K_3 +_c K_2$; **d** shows $K_3 +_d K_2$; **e** shows $K_3 \times K_2$

c) $\widetilde{C}_4 = L_1 + L_2$
d) $C_4 = K_2 \times K_2$
e) $\widetilde{C}_5 = C_5$
f) $\widetilde{C}_6 = K_3 \times K_2$
g) $Ps_1 \times C_n = Cs_n$
h) $Ps_2 \times C_n = Cs_n + Cs_n$
i) $P_3 \times G = G + G + G$ for any graph G.
j) $P_i + P_j = P_{i+j}$
k) $P_i \times P_j = P_{i \cdot j}$
l) $K_i +_c K_j = K_{i+j}$
m) $G \times H = H \times G$ for any two graphs G and H.
n) $G +_c H = H +_c G$ for any two graphs G and H.
o) $\widetilde{G +_d H} = \widetilde{H} +_d \widetilde{G}$ for any two graphs G and H.
p) $\widetilde{G +_c H} = \widetilde{G} + \widetilde{H}$ for any two graphs G and H.

8 On the Construction of Graphs with Many Assemblies and/or High Connectivity

Let us take $|G| = 6$ and let us try to construct a graph with as many assemblies as possible. Of course, we hope that we should be able to get more than the six assemblies of the rather trivial construction Ps_6 (Fig. 33):

For example we could try Cs_6 (Fig. 34).

This graph is homogeneous and connected and it has 6 assemblies consisting of the six pairs of neighboring points and 6 further assemblies consisting of the six triplets of neighboring points. A set of four neighboring points is no longer an assembly, since it is "combined of" two pairs of neighboring points.

The following weighted graph contains both the assemblies of Ps_6 and those of Cs_6 (Fig. 35):

But using this strong self-excitation we can get a rather trivial solution to the problem, namely the graph G_1 obtained from K_6 by adding self excitation of the strength $c(i,i) = 2$ ($i = 1, \ldots, 6$) (Fig. 36).

In this graph every set of points forms an assembly, since any set of k points is minimal persistent and invariant at $\Theta = k+1$. Thus, $n = 2^6 - 1 = 63$.

In the following it will be more interesting to forbid self-connections or to work only with directed graphs (i.e., to forbid numbers on the arrows). I will now restrict myself to directed graphs without self-connections.

The following general strategy for constructing graphs with many assemblies may have emerged from the previous discussion:

Use the above results with self-connectivity. Replace every point in a "good" graph G with self-connectivity of strength 1 (like Cs_6) by one exemplar of K_2, in other words: try $C_6 \times K_2$.

Replace every point in a "good" graph G with self-connectivity of strength 2 (like G_1 above) by one exemplar of K_3, in other words: try $K_6 \times K_3$.

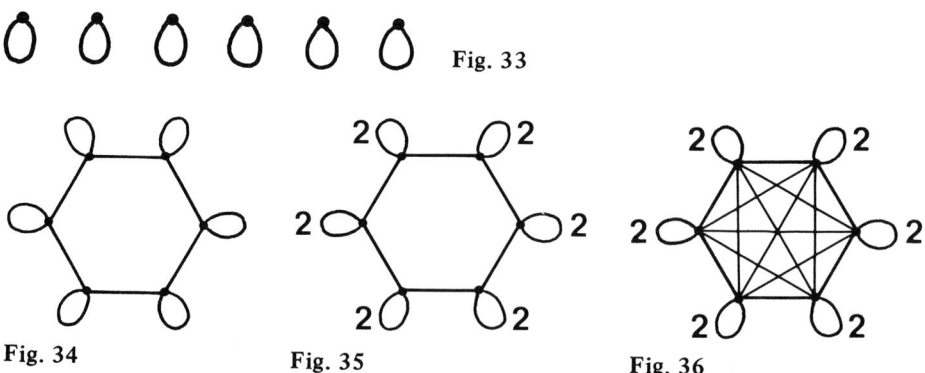

Fig. 33

Fig. 34   Fig. 35   Fig. 36

Cell Assemblies and Graph Theory

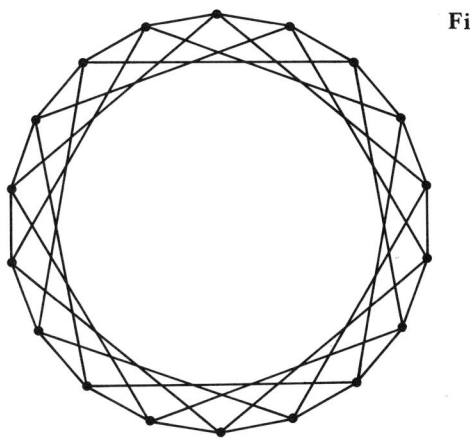

Fig. 37

For $|G| = 6$, this strategy yields $P_3 \times K_2$ with $n = n_1 = 3$ and $K_2 \times K_3$ with $n = 3$.

Up to now I could not find a graph with $|G| = 6$ and $n > 3$. At first sight this may look rather pessimistic but for larger $|G|$ the situation becomes much better:

Let me just show some graphs G with many assemblies for $|G| = 36$. From the first strategy, we may try $K_{12} \times K_3$ with $n \geq 2^{12}$ or for example $G_2 \times K_2$ where G_2 is given in Fig. 37. Here we get $n \geq 2 + 8 \cdot 18 = 146$.

Let me give two more graphs:

$L_6 \times L_6$ with $n = 81$ (all at $\Theta = 2$) and $C_6 \times C_6$ with $n = 99$ (where we get the 18 additional assemblies at $\Theta = 3$).

The champion among all these graphs is $K_{12} \times K_3$, a homogeneous graph with high connectivity.

This graph, however, needs quite a number of connections: the graph $K_n \times K_m$ has $e = n + m - 2$.

Therefore, if we restrict the average number e of connections per point, graphs of the type $K_n \times K_m$ are certainly not the best ones: for example $K_6 \times K_6$ has $e = 10$ and probably $n = 125$ which is not as good as the example $G_2 \times K_2$ with $n \geq 146$ and $e = 5$. But still, the graphs $K_n \times K_m$ do illustrate that it is possible to construct large graphs with a very large number of assemblies:

The graph $K_n \times K_m$ has $n \cdot m$ points, $(n \cdot m) \cdot (n + m - 2)$ connections, i.e., $e = n + m - 2$, and at least $2^n + 2^m - 4$ assemblies.

Let me close these considerations at this still very unsatisfactory state and let me add that I was quite surprised to get n as high as 2^{12} for $|G| = 36$ and that I am very curious to know the maximum value for n in this case.

9 Applications in Other Areas

Clearly, the idea of expressing coherence of a group in terms of mutual excitation (or encouragement, or information flow, . . .) between the members of the group, should have many applications in social contexts. Beyond the "mere" definition of cell assemblies, however, I expect that the proofs and constructions in Sections 4–8 of this Appendix will in most cases not be adequately adapted to the problems occurring in a specific application. Therefore, in this section I only want to hint at possible applications of well-constructed graphs with many assemblies in two other areas of research:

One is the problem of providing connectivity schemes for associative matrix memories.

The other is the problem of designing decentralized communication networks.

9.1 In (Palm 1980) I have described associative matrix memories and especially the case of auto-association.

In the case of auto-association a 0,1-sequence s of length n, $s = (s_1, \ldots, s_n)$ (called a *"pattern"*) is "stored" in a 0,1-matrix by forming $s \otimes s = (s_i \circ s_j)_{i,j}$.

A set $\mathcal{S} = \{s^1, \ldots, s^z\}$ of such patterns is "stored" in the matrix

$$A = A_{\mathcal{S}} = \max_{k=1}^{z} s^k \otimes s^k.$$

If we interpret the matrix A as the connectivity matrix of a graph G_A with n points, we see that each pattern s^k is stored by connecting all the points of G_A that correspond to those places where the 0,1-sequence $s^k = (s^k_1, \ldots, s^k_n)$ contains a *"1"*, to a complete subgraph of G_A.

If these subgraphs do not overlap too much, they will form assemblies and therefore it will be possible to reconstruct the original patterns $s_1, \ldots, s_z$ from G_A by detecting assemblies in G_A.

The matrix A is called the *auto-association matrix* for the set $\mathcal{S}$ of patterns.

9.2 Now the problem is the following:

Does this scheme still work if not every two points in G_A can be connected?

The answer to this question obviously depends on the restrictions that are given to the possibility of connections.

These restrictions are given in a *connectivity scheme* C. C is an n × n 0,1-matrix, where $c_{ij} = 1$ means that i can be connected to j and $c_{ij} = 0$ means that it cannot.

Of course the restriction can as well be described by the directed graph G_c corresponding to C. Given a set $\mathcal{S}$ of patterns, we now form the matrix $C_{\mathcal{S}} := A_{\mathcal{S}} \cdot C$ (where $(X \cdot Y)_{ij} := x_{ij} \cdot y_{ij}$) and the corresponding subgraph $G := G_{c_{\mathcal{S}}}$ of G_c. Then we try to reconstruct the patterns in $\mathcal{S}$ by detecting the assemblies in G. Obviously, if G_c is the complete graph Ks_n, we have no restriction to the connectivity and we are in case 9.1.

But can we design a connectivity scheme C with not too many connections such that the modified procedure still works?

9.3 To this end, we may assume that each pattern in $\mathcal{S}$ contains k "ones". Then we may try to design a matrix C, or a graph G_C, with a small number e of connections, such that any set of k points holds at a high threshold Θ.

This problem can be solved (see Palm 1981) with the following result:

For any homogeneous graph G with $e = n + \Theta - k$ any set of k points holds at Θ.

For any graph G with $e < n + \Theta - k$ some set of k points does not hold at Θ.

This means that we need quite a high number of connections in a graph G_C that is a solution, i.e., we need quite a high number of "ones" in the corresponding matrix G_C.

9.4 The second problem that I announced for this section is the following:

Given n "participants" find a communication network for them with a minimal number of links which connects any two participants via not too many links.

9.5 *Definition:* For M, N ⊆ G we define

$$t_\theta(M,N) := \min \{i : f_\theta^i(M) \cap N \neq \phi\}.$$

Then we define

$$t_\theta(k) := \max \{t_\theta(M,N) : |M| = k, |N| = 1\}.$$

Then $l := t_1(1)$ denotes the number of links through which any two participants can be connected.

The problem can now be exactly formulated:

Given two numbers n and k. Find a (homogeneous) graph G with $|G| = n$ and $l = k$, such that e is minimal. Moreover, find a graph G with the additional property that k does not increase (too much) if any point is removed from G.

The additional property (as well as the homogeneity requirement) is meant to represent the requirement that the network should be decentralized.

I believe that this problem is somehow related to the other problem of this section and also to the problem of cell assemblies, and the following theorem hints in this direction.

9.6 Theorem: Let G be a graph with $|G| = n$ and suppose that $t_\theta(k) = 1$ for two numbers $\theta, k \in \mathbb{N}$ with

$$1 \leq \theta \leq k \leq \frac{n + \theta^2 - \theta}{\theta + 1}.$$

Then $t_\theta(\theta) \leq 2$.

Proof: Assume that $t_\theta(\theta) > 2$.

Then there is $A = \{x_1, \ldots, x_\theta\} \subseteq G$ and $z \in G \setminus A$ such that $t_\theta(A, \{z\}) > 2$.

Obviously $\bigcap_{i=1}^{\theta} f_1(x_i) = f_\theta(A)$ and therefore $z \notin \bigcap_{i=1}^{\theta} f_1(x_i)$ (otherwise $t_\theta(A, \{z\}) = 1$).

1. $|\bigcap_{i=1}^{\theta} f_1(x_i)| < k$, for otherwise $z \in f_\theta(\bigcap_i f_1(x_i)) = f_\theta^2(A)$, and therefore $t_\theta(A, \{z\}) = 2$.

2. Let $M_i = f_1(x_i) \cup \{x_i\}$ for $i = 1, \ldots, \theta$, then $|M_i^c| \leq k - \theta$. Indeed: If $|M_i^c| > k - \theta$, take $A_i \supseteq M_i^c$ such that $x_i \notin A_i$ and $|A_i| = k$ (if even $|M_i^c| \geq k$, simply take $A_i = M_i^c$).

Then $x_i \in f_\theta(A_i)$ (since $t_\theta(k) = 1$), and therefore

$$\sum_{x \in A_i} c(x_i, x) = \sum_{x \in A_i} c(x, x_i) \geq \theta.$$

This means that $\theta \leq |f_1(x_i) \cap A_i| = |M_i \cap A_i| = |A_i \setminus M_i^c|$, but $|A_i \setminus M_i^c| < \theta$.

3. Now $n = |G| = |\bigcap_{i=1}^{\theta} M_i| + |\bigcup_{i=1}^{\theta} M_i^c| \leq |A| + |\bigcap_{i=1}^{\theta} f_1(x_i)| + \sum_{i=1}^{\theta} |M_i^c| < \theta + k + \theta(k - \theta)$, i.e.

$$k > \frac{n + \theta^2 - \theta}{\theta + 1}.$$

Author and Subject Index

acquisition of language   137
action   51, 119, 127f.
− potential   160, 161
afferent   98
algorithm   28, 31, 143
alternating closure   95
ametric   214
amount of information   165
analogy   43
and   21
and-machine   21
anticipation   39
anti-Hebb rule   184
area 17   87
areas (of the cortex)   74
artificial intelligence   18, 49, 143
− squint   95
assembly   116, 119, 120, 144, 199, 214, 218
association   118, 121, 215, 216
associative matrix memory   38, 193, 238
− − with feedback   50, 53, 116, 119
− memory   38, 57, 109, 193, 198, 215
− prediction   50
A-system   84
Attneave   13
auto-association   196, 215, 238
axon   9, 160
− collaterals   9
− hillock   160

babbling phase   137
bar detector   87
basis   183
blood flow analysis   74
blurred matrix   200, 204
brain   8, 60
− model   104, 212, 213
− theory   200f.
Braitenberg   6, 70, 80, 83, 84, 119, 122, 137, 189, 199, 214−216
Brodmann   75
B-system   84
burst   9

Cajal   55, 65, 67, 68, 71, 189
canonical unit vector   182
capacity   10, 171
cardinality   175
C-area   126
candate nucleus   131
cell assembly   116, 119, 144, 199, 214, 218
− types   63
cerebellum   55, 127, 131
cerebral cortex   62
channel   10, 171
− capacity   171
chess computer   18
circumstances   51, 119
climbing fibers   55
coding   19, 49
coincidence   208
− detector   116
collaterals   9
communication network   239
complete   22
completion   112, 119, 215
− area   126
complex cell   87
complexity   28
computer   18, 104, 192, 200
− memory   192
− simulations   104, 108, 110, 112, 210
computing   31
concept   215
conditioning   92
conjunction   21
connectivity   105, 116, 238
− matrix   105, 116, 202, 218
− scheme   238
context   51
continuous   201, 202
cooperative   34
− phenomena   34
cortex   62
cortico-cortical   62
critical threshold   122, 216
Cybernetics   142

cyto-architectonics 74

dark rearing 92
Dawkins 45, 135, 138
dendrites 9
depolarization 160
deprivation 93, 95
— experiment 93, 95
— of information 95
— of intensity 95
— of meaning 95
detector 47
development 93, 138
design 35
diagram 28, 31
diary 131
directed graph 220
discrete 201, 202
disjunction 21
domain 176
dreaming 132, 133

Eccles 164, 189
EEG 47, 133
efferent 10
electrophysiology 47
element 175
evaluation 39, 42
evolution 36, 45, 136, 142
excentricity 88
excitation 10, 80, 160
experience 15

feature 215
feedback 50, 53, 116, 119, 215
— matrix 50, 53, 116, 119
fiber 10
Fichte 17
flow diagram 28, 31
format 170
formatal capacity 10, 171
— channel capacity 171
— information rate 170
freedom of will 145
frontal cortex 129

game playing 18, 39
global connections 84
Gödel 17
Golgi preparation 3
grandmother detector 47
graph 214, 218, 220
— theory 218
grey matter 61

Hebb 1, 56, 92, 104, 116, 119, 140, 189, 198, 199, 207, 214
Hebb-like rule 184, 215
Hebb's rule 56, 94, 116, 181, 198, 207, 208
hemispheres 62
heraldic 204
hierarchical 34
hippocampus 132
holding 53, 112, 117, 120, 216
horizon effect 43
Hubel and Wiesel 8, 87, 95
human behavior 136, 140
— brain 60, 136
Hume 49, 117
hyperpolarization 160

ignition 116
image 128
immediate prediction 120, 125
improved matchbox algorithm 36
information 10, 165
— processing 109
— rate 170
— source 169
— storage 192
— transmitting capacity 10, 171
inhibition 10, 80, 120, 160
initial conditions 203
— state 107
input 20, 62
— coding 49
— region 85
interactionism 146
interactive rule 182
introspection 117, 118
ions 160

Jung 140

Katz 162, 164, 189
Kelvin 45
Kleist 76
Kohonen 110, 112, 113, 193, 209, 215, 225

language 197
Lashley 48
layers 63
learning 92, 192
Lenin 125
lesions 48, 74
Lettvin et al. 47
levels (of investigation) 140
linear algebra 182

Author and Subject Index

linear combination 182
— superposition 181
linearly independent 183
listing 192
— memory 192
local cell 68
— connections 86
— synaptic rule 56, 107, 116, 180, 200, 208
logic 20f.
long-term memory 14
look-ahead algorithm 42, 110
Luria 48, 138, 189

magnification 89
mapping 176
— memory 37, 193
margarine 16
Martinotti cell 68
matchbox algorithm 29
mathematician 6
McCulloch 47, 190
McCulloch and Pitts 24, 207, 209
membrane 160
— potential 160
memory 14, 192
message 193
metaplan 128
metric 176, 204, 214
Miller et al. 128, 129, 189
minimax algorithm 39
Minsky and Papert 26, 190
mnemonic equations 206
moment 13
motor cortex 126
— program 127
movements 127

nand 23
negation 21
negative feedback 215
nerve 10
— cell 9
von Neumann 3, 190
neural dynamics 104, 200, 223
— modeling 200
neuron 9
neuronic equations 206
noninteractive rule 182, 184
nonspecific thalamic afferents 85, 121
nor 24
not 21
not-machine 21
numbers of cells 73, 74, 91
— of fibers 11, 12, 62

occipital cortex 129
ocular dominance 88, 96
one-word sentences 137
or 21
organization 28
orientation 90, 98
or-machine 21
orthogonal 184
output 20, 62
— coding 49
— region 85
overlap 89, 116, 119, 195, 216

parallel organization 32
P-area 125, 126
pattern completion 51, 112, 119, 215
perception 11, 15
perceptron 26
permeability 161
phenomenological model 141, 144
Piaget 138
plan 128
Polya 190
Popper and Eccles 145
positive feedback 215
postsynaptic potential 9
— rule 181
prediction 50, 125
— area 125, 126
preprocessing 49, 125
presynaptic competition 96
— rule 181
programming 31
proprioceptor 126
pruning 40
purpose 142
pyramidal cell 63

questioning strategy 165

range 176
Rauschecker and Singer 98, 100–102
receptive field 87
receptors 10
recurrent organization 32
reductionism 145
redundancy 170
reflex 8
refractory period 160
reliability of ideas 122
resting potential 160
restricted environment 92
reticular formation 132
retina 88
retinal ganglion cell 88

robot 135

Samuel 45
S-area 126
search algorithm 131
− tree 40
self-organization 34
self-reflection 16
sensory area 85, 126
− deprivation 93
sequences of movements 127
serial organization 32
set 175
Shannon 165
short-term memory 13
simple cell 87
simulations 104, 108, 110, 112, 123
situation 51, 119
skeleton cortex 85
sleeping 132
somatosensory cortex 126
source 169
Sperry 48
spike 9, 160
spreading of activity 78f.
stability 108, 215
state 104, 200
− of activity 84, 105, 201
− of connectivity 105, 201
− of mind 121, 217
− transition 107, 206
stellate cell 68
storage (of information) 192
− capacity 193
subassembly 120

surprise 120
survival algorithm 44, 45, 118, 186
synapse 10
synaptic rule 56, 107, 116, 180, 200, 208

teleological arguments 142
temporal succession 112
tendon reflex 8
thalamus 78, 85
theory of games 29
thinking 128
threshold 24, 107, 108, 120, 161, 216
− control 112, 119, 121, 216, 223
− neuron 24, 107, 207
topographical 17, 87, 90
topographic projection 90
TOTE unit 129
Turing 18
Turing test 18
types of neurons 63

unit vector 182
urgentness 42

vector 182
visual cortex 87
− input 87
− pathway 88

weight of connection 25, 219
weighted graph 218
white matter 61
Wiener 142, 190
Willwacher 112, 114, 115

M. Abeles

Local Cortical Circuits

An Electrophysiological Study

1982. 31 figures. VIII, 102 pages
(Studies of Brain Function, Volume 6)
ISBN 3-540-11034-8

The author has developed a unique method for measuring simultaneously the activity of several neighbouring nerve cells, allowing the first experimental observations of spatio-temporal organization of activity in the cortex. The results he obtained over the last 10 years, many of them previously unpublished, are reported here. Several new avenues of research are opened up by such simultaneous measurements of neuronal activity. The strength and abundance of synaptic contacts between neighbouring neurons can be measured. These data may be compared quantitatively with anatomical data. Dynamic changes of connectivity among cortical neurons can also be measured, spatio-temporal codes studied, and the functional parcellation of the cortical nerve-cells into cell assemblies evaluated.

The book shows that the cortical network is not a bundle of simple dedicated chains of neurons, nor a statistical random mass, but a well organized system in which the relevant code is a combination code (i.e. one by which a combination of neurons is fired synchronously). The properties of this novel code are examined in view of the anatomy and physiology of interactions among cortical neurons. The text is developed gradually to allow the non-professional reader to follow the arguments easily.

H. Collewijn

The Oculomotor System of the Rabbit and Its Plasticity

1981. 128 figures. IX, 240 pages
(Studies of Brain Function, Volume 5)
ISBN 3-540-10678-2

The author of this monograph comprehensively describes his studies in the oculomotor system of the rabbit. This is in many respects a simplified model of the more complex system of visually more highly developed mammals, and its study has aided the understanding of eye movements in primates, including man. Main features are the analysis of optokinetics and vestibuloocular reflexes and their interaction, spontaneous oculomotor behavior, the processing and pathways of visual direction-selective signals and their relation to visually elicited eye movements.

Furthermore, the adaptability of the system is described according to physiological and pathological changes in stimulus conditions such as altered visuovestibular relations requiring recalibration of reflexes, dark-rearing, vestibular lesions and albinism. The emphasis is on pricise measurement of eye and head movements in restrained and freely moving animals, for which purpose new techniques were developed.

To illuminate the historical significance of rabbit oculomotor research in our understanding of eye movements, an English translation is included of Ter Braak's classical study of optokinetic nystagmus, first published in 1936, and still a source on inspiration today.

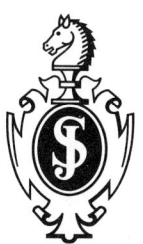

Springer-Verlag
Berlin
Heidelberg
New York

V. Braitenberg
On the Texture of Brains
An Introduction to Neuroanatomy for the Cybernetically Minded

Translated from the German by E. H. Braitenberg and by the author
(Heidelberg Science Library)
1977. 37 figures. IX, 127 pages
ISBN 3-540-08391-X

Contents: Neuroanatomy, Psychology, and Animism. – Physics and Antiphysics. – Information. – What Brains Are Made Of. – How Accurately Are Brains Designed? – Neuroanatomical Invariants: Analysis of the Cerebellar Cortex. – The Automatic Pilot of the Fly. – The Common Sensorium: An Essay on the Cerebral Cortex.

J.-P. Ewert
Neuroethology
An Introduction to the Neurophysiological Fundamentals of Behavior

Translated from the German by Transemantics, Inc. 1980. 171 figures, mostly in color, 9 tables.
VIII, 342 pages
ISBN 3-540-09790-2

The content of the highly successful German original has been up-dated and expanded in this translation with new illustrations and recent experimental findings.

From the reviews of the German edition: "...This book is an introductory work of particular value because it shows the concrete procedures required by experimental analysis without leaving aside the contextual factors implied by every animal act. I am convinced that it will prove extremely useful to biologists and neurophysiologists who need a first technical approach to the problems of behaviour in close relation with underlying mechanisms with which they are already familiar from the anatomical-physiological point of view. It will also help ethologists trained in field observation to grasp the basic problems of comparative physiology linked with overt behaviour phenomena. The book is well illustrated and contains a number of very useful two-colour diagrams. Fundamental problems and findings are well summarized in each chapter in a few clearcut propositions. A basic manual for students in biology, psychology and veterinary medicine taking a first course in ethology."
Behavioural Processes

J. G. Roederer
Introduction to the Physics and Psychophysics of Music
(Heidelberg Science Library)
Corrected reprint of the 2nd edition. 1979.
79 figures, 7 tables. XIV, 202 pages
ISBN 3-540-90116-7

This is the first basic textbook to establish the close relationship of physics, psychophysics, and neuropsychology to music.
The author analyzes the objective physical properties of sound patterns that are associated with the subjective psychological sensations of music. He describes how these sound patterns are actually generated in musical instruments, how they propagate through space, and how they are detected by the ear and interpreted by the brain. The approach throughout is scientific, but complicated mathematics has been avoided.
The main revisions in the second edition reflect recent important developments in the understanding of complex pitch tone perception. Related developments in consonance and dissonance have also been incorporated. Other additions include a section describing the principal information channels in auditory pathways, and a section on the specialization of cerebral hemispheres in regard to speech and music. This reprint incorporates some corrections and slight changes.

Springer-Verlag
Berlin
Heidelberg
New York

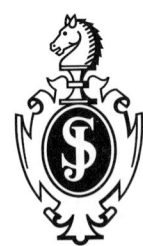